Treating Victims of Weapons of Mass Destruction

Contents

Foreword

Weapons of Mass Destruction? What they are is not well defined. In the following pages, the reader will find precise responses to the major questions on this subject.

"Weapons of mass destruction" have been developed over the last half-century and have undoubtedly left their mark on the last few decades.

They have been, they are, and they will be instruments of coercion, utilized by the powerful against the populace, or more simply against freedom, as well as against displaced minorities, whether they are fleeing from the appropriation of the land where they live or because of political, social, or religious convictions.

They encompass not just one technology, but rather explosives as well as chemical and biological weapons.

Those who would use such weapons have decided that a huge mobilization of mass destruction, as well as justifying a little white lie, to invoke God, the service of "better than worse" or, yet, in the verdict of the rights of man, which is worse? Finally, such persons would like to excuse themselves based on economic blocks, their funeral processions, and their pain, in this manner justifying genocide of a whole population.

Such persons encourage war, the destruction of mankind, and they arm revolutions with which they are identified and promote the annihilation of heritage, blaming the victims as well as destroying their historical works of hundreds of prior years.

In the past, men and women died at the stake rather than renounce their religion. Today, they torture victims by transforming themselves into weapons of mass destruction by the ravages that are created in the areas surrounding their self-sacrifices.

There are diverse weapons of mass destruction, which will have to be considered in future strategic equations in all countries and from insurgent factions. The sole superpower, militarily dominating this world as it has never been dominated before, hasn't it demonstrated its vulnerability to the knives of a dozen terrorists?

The name "weapons of mass destruction" was first used in Hiroshima. The display of weapons of mass destruction has been increased with the Middle East wars, in the Gulf, in Afghanistan, and also with attacks against non-industrialized peoples. Weapons with such power can unexpectedly equalize a conflict, since when utilized by deprived peoples, they shake up the military masters of the planet.

Why Hiroshima – and Nagasaki? Because these two bombs produced the end of a long conflict of extermination which opposed humans by the tens of millions, bombs and cannons by the hundreds of thousands, tanks and airplanes by the hundreds of thousands, and warships by the thousands. They provoked the breakdown of a slow evolution towards a continuous growth of destructive power by a "unity of death." During the gunpowder era, the ravages of weapons covered areas measured in square meters, while new weapons, nuclear in this case, dissipate their energy over areas measured in square kilometers, with persistent radioactivity added to the shock and heat.

In review, the authors of this book, with reference to coercion, emphasize that it is not intermittent in the hierarchy of the means of force. Traditional weapons – called conventional using an "English-ism" used for a long time in France – are commonly allowed by the international community, while those called "weapons of mass destruction" are banned, although the first have been revealed to be as deadly as the second. In reality, it is a matter of a political design with a view to legitimize the possession of instruments of war that accepts a large scientific and above all industrial capacity in eliminating the weapons that threaten this type of monopoly. The "industrialized" nations intend to possess them at the expense of the "non-industrialized" or the "less industrialized" nations.

Campaigns conducted since the beginnings of the atomic era against horizontal proliferation of new weapons are a precedent. The United States has wished – understandably – to possess a weapon exclusively, to gain a strategic and political superiority. It happens that, following an enormous scientific and financial effort, as a modern proof of the "manifest destiny" of this country which has desired to be the only one capable of conceiving this weapon and the only one to benefit at the time from the impunity which it confers and with the power of intimidation, even of compelling others, which are, as it were, substantial.

But here the United States has fallen into its own trap. Their anti-atomic campaigns were much more active when it was a matter of first prohibiting the Soviet Union from upsetting the American monopoly, then, subsequently this was shared out with the USSR to prevent the dissemination of nuclear weapons not susceptible to independent surveillance, even with protest, weakening the system of alliance framework by Washington in order to counter that which Moscow had built. From numerous negotiations a series of treaties were signed with a view towards non-proliferation, notably the prohibition of all experimentation with atomic explosions. Two events finally disrupted the fulfillment of this strategy, one political and the other technical:
- dissolution of the Soviet Union and collapse of the planned economy according to Marxist-Leninist dogma, eliminated the strategic military rivalry;
- the known precision of weapons launched from a distance (ballistic missiles, cruise missiles, guided bombs) has finished the military uselessness of yields in the megaton range and even in the hundred kiloton range: the distance between the launch point and the location of the viewed objective are no longer compensated for by very high yields because they are reckoned now in meters and not kilometers as was the case thirty years ago. The corollary to this form of performance, it is that (relatively) low yields are now militarily sufficient and can be clandestinely experimented with; they are therefore, in the low range, unmanageable. By questioning the treaty prohibiting all experimentation, the United States intends to regain total freedom of action concerning their military panoply. And that in spite of horizontal proliferation, free of constraints, which the international community under the impetus of the United States intends to impose. Another consequence of this revival, the real and psychological gaps between the effects of higher "yield" traditional weapons (for example, a bomb of more than 10 tons) and low-yield atomic weapons tend to become blurred, facilitating the possible passage from one system to the other. Mr. George W. Bush has often made allusion to this new continuity of energies of destruction, going from

a 7.65 millimeter pistol to an atomic projectile in the hundred kiloton range, atomic fission passing from intimidation to use.

Until the United States had begun this dangerous move, nuclear weapons were strongly and fairly condemned. One has not understood, or rather one has not been required to understand, that it has made outlaws of the large disputes with traditional weapons which exerted so much havoc during the last century, the same extent of these ravages has been excluded from all use in creating an exorbitant risk in strategic stakes for all countries which dare to undertake a significant conflict with even a modest nuclear power.

Contemporary history, if its lessons have been correctly interpreted, has owed much to this "weapon of mass destruction" which, paradoxically, has been otherwise a factor for peace, of a means for preventing large-scale wars. Successively, the atomic military has imposed "cold" war between the United States and the USSR, between China and the USSR, between India and China, and between Pakistan and India. During the Kippur War in 1973, because the country of Israel held atomic projectiles, Egypt assigned itself objectives limited to the re-conquest of the Sinai in order not to provoke the use of this weapon of ultimate recourse. It is reasonable, the Chinese Marshall Chen Yi stated to the Reuters Agency in 1958, that: "…the larger the number of nuclear countries, the greater will be the zone of peace which exists on the earth."

In review, besides other factors such as dependence, frustration, misery, xenophobia, and clashes of confessions and of cultures, it must be admitted that political and strategic superiority, results in the invulnerability guaranteed to a group of countries possessing supreme weapons, to contribute to research, then to the generalization of processes capable of weakening, even of neutralizing this overwhelming superiority. From this came the emergence of all other categories of weapons of mass destruction on the international scene which depend neither on a considerable scientific advance nor on a great industrial power as is the case of traditional aerospace weapons and a fortiori for nuclear weapons.

It is poorly understood that these weapons are for circumventing or neutralizing atomic supremacy, and the revelations and details provided by the authors are welcome. At length and furnishing all the scientific, technical, and practical information necessary, they deal with chemical and biological weapons of the present coupled with the panoply of "revolutionaries" as distinguished from "terrorists." Rightly, Doctors Barriot and Bismuth have remarked that, in the offensive cycle of chemical weapons, one finds the same concept of mutual deterrence as that noted in the nuclear cycle.

If the Italians dispersed 700 tons of sulfur mustard onto Ethiopian troops in 1935, it is because the Ethiopians were not able to retaliate with similar weapons. Similarly, when the Japanese dispersed sulfur mustard onto Chinese combatants in 1938 and the following years, they did not have to fear analogous reprisals. The millions of liters of dioxin-containing defoliants sprayed on the Vietnamese jungles could not provoke a similar reaction on the part of the Viet Cong. (Today, the United States is poorly placed to flog Sadam Hussein for using toxic gases against the Iranians and the Kurds who joined with Iran against Iraq, while Tehran also had recourse to chemical warfare against Baghdad; these two belligerents even threatened their own combatants.) In review, in the course of the Second World War and during nearly five years of mutual extermination, the antagonists renounced the use of chemical weapons for fear of reprisals. In their own country, clandestinely, on defenseless men and women, the Germans used a gas in the gas chambers, demonstrating the infamy of their regime.

The authors cite the utilization of toxic chemical products by minorities or terrorist groups alike, as well as by the "secret services" of countries fighting against rebels or terrorists. The processes are relatively simple, with an ease of use such that they are quasi-commonplace. Until now, human losses have been relatively limited but they can, one day, be revealed to be distressing, because as the authors note: "…30 grams of botulinum toxin could kill 60 million persons."

It may be surprising for the majority of readers to find the number of pages dedicated to biotechnologies. It is true that genetic engineering has only been developed in the last thirty years and that the modification of living cells is only familiar to the initiated. Genetic engineering appears, simultaneously, both good genetics and also bad genetics. Good genetics insofar as measured by the fact of numerous processes working towards the preservation of life. But, also, bad genetics since: "…it matters that a biotechnology laboratory could create, voluntarily or involuntarily, a pathogenic agent of unknown power." By the creation of unknown forms of life with their procession of new pathogenic agents, humans learn sorcery in the quest for progress, as in other disciplines, giving birth to new threats to human life in particular, and to all life – already too short – in general. The reader learns of the initial benefits developed for the production of new medications and treatments with a lively interest. Unfortunately, genetic engineering also permits increasing the virulence of infectious agents and rendering the usual treatments based on antibiotics and vaccines ineffective. Life can be threatened in a more underhanded manner: "…biological weapons…can be made up of 'phantom viruses' which could be secretly introduced within a given population and which would remain silent until a signal triggered their pathogenic activity."

And, once again, the sad panoply of means of intimidation, blackmail, and coercion increases. Of course, scientific and also economic power is necessary for such research and the production to which it leads. However, the authors of this fascinating text on the "weapons of mass destruction" do not conceal the dangers of laboratory accidents, human errors by researchers with the best of intentions, involuntary propagation of the results of these works, and harmful exploitation of scientific publications relative to biotechnologies by terrorist organizations.

The 1972 Convention on the prohibition of biological weapons could not prevent the powerful that, having the will and the means, could pursue scientific research for defensive ends – research that a person cannot affirm does not have destructive applications.

In order to learn to defend themselves, it is necessary that mankind know how these evolve, increase, and "perfect" the means of inflicting their will on human communities with more and more virulent antagonists. In these respects, the pages that follow are relevant for readers.

General Pierre-Marie Gallois

Preface

In 1940, while the Battle of Britain killed 100,000 urban civilians under German bombardments, Winston Churchill stated: "Although on my part I am satisfied with existing explosives, I think that we should not stand in the way of progress".

It was the green light given to research on other weapons, biological above all: the British perceived that while the anthrax germ is destroyed by an explosion, the spores are resistant. At the same time, they began studies on sulfur mustard, a chemical weapon which penetrates through the skin, previously utilized during the 1914–1918 war, when it was perceived that gas masks effectively protected against chlorine-based suffocating agents with a purely respiratory toxicity (2% mortality). Finally, the program concerning nuclear weapons in the United States was communicated to their English allies. While the Germans, on their part, between the two world wars, discovered the organophosphate anticholinesterase insecticides and proposed as neurotoxic gases, tabun and sarin, the only chemical weapon utilized during the Second World War was cyanide in closed rooms in concentration camps and not on the battlefield where its volatility reduces its toxicity. At the same time, the utilization of porcelain as a vehicle for cholera by the Japanese Army during the siege of Nan King was a long shot: the germs did not seem to disseminate the infection in this population, where it was already endemic.

In this self-limitation of use by the belligerents, the difficulty of militarization of these different weapons called "unconventional" came into play, as well as the discovery of antibiotics in the years 1940–1944 to counteract possible epidemics caused by the development of powerful nuclear weapons, as well as the conclusions of weapons designers: everything being equal, the attrition due to firearms is seven times greater than that due to unconventional weapons, with the exception of nuclear weapons, which alone merit the name of "weapons of mass destruction".

At the time, the Allies preferred to use explosives – the bombardments of German cities killed 600,000 persons from 1942 to 1945 – and the atomic weapons were released against Hiroshima and Nagasaki.

Since then, chemical weapons have been mainly utilized during the Iran-Iraq war with an overall mortality of 4% and moreover on several occasions by a Japanese sect. Mailing germs through the Postal system in the United States has not up to now been proven to have a terrorist origin.

During the terrible genocides or attacks in recent years, the machete and the knife, the explosives or the crashes of vehicles (airplanes and cars), packed with flammable materials, have perfectly played their role as death machines to kill and demoralize targeted populations.

With the attack in Moscow at the end of 2002, some new chemical weapons were tested, but this time in a counter-terrorist setting: some medications which were justified because they are active in medical treatment are also dangerous, and which, if they can neutralize hostage takers who were later slaughtered, also killed one hostage out of seven during their use.

And what about the anxiety provoked in the civilian populace, which due to their numbers and the diffuse nature of the threats, and who cannot benefit from the same level of protection as exposed military personnel? Those in charge of safety and physicians responsible for treatment are not entirely without resources. Vaccines, antibiotics, decontamination measures, maintenance of vital function (supportive care), administration of antidotes when they exist, limiting the capacities of terrorists to cause harm and the fact of only twelve deaths in Tokyo in 1995 in a population trapped in public transportation with several millions of potential victims emphasize this point.

The major chemical accidents of the 20th Century were of industrial origin, such as Bhopal in India in 1984 where 2500 persons died in one hour during a release of methyl isocyanate, or as a combination of suicide and murder, as in the Moon sect in Guyana with some 900 deaths from cyanide during the 1970s.

At the beginning of the 21st Century, it nevertheless appears that the dangers of explosives and blades, responsible for more than 95% of violent deaths from warfare or terrorism, do not loom large in the collective consciousness despite the fear of harm during tribal conflicts, clashes between ideologies, or during wars declared between countries.

In August 2002, the World Health Organization published data on non-accidental violent deaths from the preceding year: 1,600,000, of which 815,000 were suicides, 52,000 were domestic crimes, sordid or street brawls, and approximately 225000 were from war or terrorism.

The citizens, the structures for safety and health and the media inform us more and more about the means of countering the utilization of unconventional weapons. This book attempts to respond to their concerns.

Chantal Bismuth

About the Translator

Alan H. Hall, M.D. is a Board-Certified Medical Toxicologist, President and Chief Medical Toxicologist of Toxicology Consulting and Medical Translating Services, Inc. Wyoming, USA, and Clinical Assistant Professor of Preventive Medicine and Bio metrics at the University of Colorado Health Sciences Center, Denver. He is a member of the Advisory Board for the Forensic Sciences program at Weatherford College, Weatherford, Texas, USA. Dr. Hall has served as a Flight Surgeon in the United States Air Forces Reserves and is also a U.S. Army (Vietnam era) veteran. He holds two Distinguished Alumnus awards from Indiana University South Bend. He has been translating medical/scientific information from several international languages into English for over 20 years. Dr. Hall travels extensively worldwide as a consulting Medical Toxicologist.

List of Contributors

David J. Baker
Fellow of the Royal College of Anaesthetists London, UK, Department of Anesthesia-Intensive Care, Hôpital Necker, Paris, France.

Patrick Barriot
Anesthesiologist-Intensivist, former chief physician of the Unités d'Intervention de la Sécurité Civile [Intervention Units for Civil Security], former Medical Advisor for the Directeur de la Sécurité Civile [Director of Civil Security], Director of the "Biological Risk" Department of Point Org Safety, 26 quai Carnot, 92212 Saint-Cloud Cedex, France.

Frédéric Baud
Professor of Medical Intensive Care, University of Paris VII, Director of the Medical and Toxicological Intensive Care Service, Hôpital Laribosière, Paris, France.

Chantal Bismuth
Professor of Medicine, University of Paris VII, former Advisor for Defense, International Consultant in Toxicology, Hôpital Fernand-Widal, Paris, France.

Stephen W. Borron
George Washington University, Washington, DC, United States; Physician Researcher at INSERM U26, Hôpital Fernand-Widal, Paris, France.

Pierre Carli
Professor of Medicine, University of Paris V, Director of the SAMU Service, Hôpital Necker, Paris, France.

Arnaud Delahaye
Attaché, Medical and Toxicological Intensive Care, Hôpital Lariboisière, Paris, France.

Pierre-Marie Gallois
General, Designer of French Nuclear Entente, author of numerous works on Global Strategy, among them publications for the Epoch of Man.

Timothy C. Marrs
Fellow of the Royal College of Pathologists, Food Standards Agency, London, UK.

Robert L. Maynard
Fellow of the Royal College of Physicians, Department of Health, Skipton House, London, UK.

Bruno Mégarbane
Director of the Paris VIII Faculty Clinic, Hospital Practitioner, Medical and Toxicological Intensive Care, Hôpital Lariboisière, Paris, France.

Andreas Schaper
Surgeon and Intensivist, North German Poison Center, University of Göttingen, Germany.

Caroline Telion
Hospital Practitioner, Paris SAMU, Hôpital Necker, Paris, France.

Vladimir Volkoff
Author of numerous works regarding disinformation, 1989 International Peace Prize.

1

Ambiguous concepts and porous borders

Patrick Barriot and Chantal Bismuth

Efforts employed to eradicate non-conventional weapons of the enemy – nuclear, chemical, biological, radiological, and nuclear (CBRN) weapons, or special weapons – opportunely grouped together as 'weapons of mass destruction', have some suspicious things about them. The ambiguity of the concepts, the permeability of the classifications, and the plasticity of the doctrines seem to have no other goal than to frustrate international conventions and manipulate public opinion. The prohibition publicized for certain weapons allows the development, with little noise, of still more terrible weapons that no one wants to name, and the risk of their legalization and the justification of worse extortions is high [1–3]. All physicians are susceptible to being engaged at the initial level in case of conflict. It is therefore necessary to question the conception and utilization of high-technology weapons that do not make a great effect on civilian populations.

Conventional Weapons and CBRN Weapons

The first question one must ask is: 'What is the distinction between conventional weapons and special weapons?' Is the criterion a power to kill extensively or a barbaric lethal mechanism of action? In other terms, is it qualitative or quantitative? In theory, 1 kg of a neurotoxicant could kill a million persons, and 30 kg of botulinum toxin could kill 60 million persons. An epidemic of variola (smallpox) could kill millions of humans. In practice, chemical or biological weapons have not to this day responded to the expectations of their promoters and have not caused mass destruction, unlike classic bombs. The only weapon of mass destruction is unquestionably the megaton thermonuclear bomb, which is not, at this time, in the hands of countries qualified as 'rogue'. For the physician, all mechanistic classification that relies on describing the effects or mechanisms of action of weapon systems is not only odious with regard

Treating Victims of Mass Destsuction Edited by Patrick Barriot and Chantal Bismuth
© 2008 John Wiley & Sons, Ltd

to human suffering, but also unfounded. The power of conventional firearms is also totally more deadly than the effects of weapons called 'special'. The carpet bombs released more than 50 years ago by vast campaigns of high-altitude aerial bombardment, that made up a part of the official doctrines of civilized countries, rival the destructive power of the CBRN weapons utilized at present, yet carrying the most atrocious conventional weapons rouses only little official reprobation.

The 'thermobaric' bombs, such as fuel air explosive (FAE), BLU or massive ordinance air blast (MOAB) bombs, had a powerful blast effect and caused the rapid disappearance of oxygen by burning a flammable aerosol product. The FAE was utilized in Vietnam and the BLU-82 bomb was utilized in Afghanistan and Iraq. The bomb BLU-82, also named the 'Daisy Cutter', weighed nearly 7 tons. It was the most powerful classic bomb in the American arsenal. In March 2003, the Pentagon tested in Florida the MOAB (also called the 'Mother Of All Bombs'), which is now the largest non-nuclear bomb in existence. This munition has a massive blast effect and weighs nearly 10 tons, and is launched from a Hercules C-130 aircraft and then guided on its course by means of a global positioning system (GPS) satellite system. It spreads a cloud of flammable product over the objective, of which the fire uses the oxygen in the air as a fuel and results in an extraordinarily powerful explosion. This bomb, which possesses a destructive power equivalent to a small nuclear device, is even qualified as ' subatomic'. Furthermore, today, the treaties and declarations of intent remain impotent to eradicate, among others, antipersonnel mines or fragmentation munitions. The cluster bomb is a fragmentation bomb that disperses, on impact or above the ground, submunitions that explode and project hundreds of fragments. This bomb has been released on civilian populations in Iraq, Kosovo, and Afghanistan. Approximately 10% of these bombs do not explode on impact and become veritable antipersonnel mines that injure farmers and children who venture into the fields. Some thousands of civilians have been killed in this way in Iraq, Kuwait, Afghanistan, and Kosovo.

On their part, terrorists, as pragmatic as inhumane, have willingly had recourse to conventional means whose efficacy no longer needs to be demonstrated – home-made bombs, vehicles packed with explosives, rocket launchers. A kamikazi who explodes himself in a public place kills more human beings than the 39 Scuds fired by Iraq into Israel during the first Gulf War. A SAM-7 missile fired by a single man can knock down an airplane on take-off and cause hundreds of deaths, while an aircraft hijacked by a small group of kamikazis can knock down a high-rise building and cause thousands of deaths. By way of comparison, the sarin gas attack in the Tokyo subway by the Aum sect caused the deaths of 12 persons on March 20, 2005, and anthrax-containing letters caused the deaths of five persons in the USA in the autumn of 2001, while attacks with explosives in Bali and Grozny caused 192 and more than 80 deaths, respectively. Timothy McVeigh did not require a 'dirty bomb' to launch the terror attack in Oklahoma City, causing 186 deaths in April 1995; a single rudimentary charge was sufficient to kill French citizens at the Port-Royal metro station; and some knives permitted the commando suicide of September 11, 2001, to accomplish a true carnage in New York City with more than 3000 victims. When there exists a very large technological disparity between existing forces, the battlefield can be displaced to the cities and the strategies of the weak against the strong are based on terrorism. The imbalance of forces gives rise to the equilibrium of terror.

In fact, the only valid classification would be one that takes into account the suffering inflicted on human beings. But how about a thermal burn from a conventional weapon or a burn by microwave weapons? Could it be less disturbing than a chemical burn from a chemical vesicant agent? How about a bomb that depletes oxygen, such as the FAE, the BLU-82, or the MOAB, creating a veritable gas chamber in the open field? Is it more tolerable than a cyanide bomb that blocks the utilization of oxygen? How about a retinal burn from a combat laser? Is it more 'conventional' than a corneal burn from sulfur mustard? If a burn or toxicology specialist can establish pathophysiological distinctions, it is less probable that the victim can make the same distinction, and for the physician it is not a conventional matter to destroy a human being. Furthermore, the mechanisms of action of the last-generation weapons, coming from the laboratories of countries, are classed as 'secret-defense' (in reality 'secret-aggression') weapons. These non-classified weapons need only time to benefit from passing for conventional weapons, preserving the secrets of their fabrication and increasing their power of terror and deterrence. The strong have bet on the fact that unconventional weapons of tomorrow will not be weapons banned by the conventions, but weapons compatible with being 'outside of convention' by virtue of their secret and indescribable technology.

The radioactive and nuclear (RN) weapons of the last generation are not even mentioned in treaties, which is also the situation for miniaturized nuclear weapons with selective effects, high-power microwave weapons, or particle beam weapons [4–6]. In playing on the miniaturization of nuclear weapons and modulating their effects, it is possible to maintain them in a twilight classification favorable to the violation of all the conventions. The new generation of miniaturized nuclear weapons, such as the Robust Nuclear Earth Penetrator, or 'mini-nuke', can deliver an energy of less than 1 kiloton (in the range of hundreds of tons). Let us recall that the power of the bomb at Hiroshima was 15 kilotons. The designers of the B 61-11 nuclear bomb put forward a light version (0.3 kiloton TNT equivalent), but remain discreet about the higher-yield version, equivalent to several times the power of the bomb at Hiroshima. This plutonium-based device, supposed to explode 30 meters underground, was developed in total infringement of the Nuclear Non-proliferation Treaty. What can be said about the situation where the threshold for legal proscription is situated beyond that at which an anti-forces weapon becomes an anti-cities weapon, or where a tactical weapon becomes a pre-strategic and then a strategic weapon? It is thus possible to pass imperceptibly from a 'subatomic' weapon to a subkiloton atomic weapon (or hundred kiloton weapon), and then to a megaton weapon.

Concerning biological weapons, the progress of genetic engineering permits from now on the sequencing and manipulation of the genomes of biological agents pathogenic for humans [7,8]. Faced with an emerging virus, such as influenza or an atypical pneumonia, it would be difficult to distinguish between a natural epidemic and the spreading of a militarized pathogenic agent. An infectious agent can be transported in several hours from all over the planet by a traveler: West Nile fever was installed in the USA and new strains of Dengue fever imported from Asia colonized South America. Crimea-Congo hemorrhagic fever and Ebola fever represent a permanent danger in Africa. So-called 'fourth-generation weapons' could be developed in countries' laboratories, possessing some effects which initially would be difficult to detect, indescribable or unclassifiable. Biological weapons would probably not disseminate plague or smallpox. They could have effects more and more selective on certain functions, particularly cerebral, some effects more and more subtle and, we are tempted to say, more and more 'natural'. They could strike targeted ethnic groups, inactivate very precise genes, and set in motion physiological cell death (apoptosis). Which treaty decries these effects? What convention prohibits them?

Chemical weapons benefit equally from the porosity of the classifications and technological progress. The militarization of medications which followed the militarization of biological agents constitutes a new awkwardness forced on the physician. An emerging concept is that of 'assault medications' placed in service for counter-terrorism to be a halfway-house between an anesthetic gas and a combat gas. Chemical weapons of the future may perhaps already be hidden in the Vidal® Dictionary of Medications. These weapons, presented as non-lethal, in reality possess a lethal power in two ways: it is a matter of paralyzing the enemy before executing him. During the taking of hostages in Moscow, which caused at least 117 deaths (hostages not included), the essential problem was to understand whether the product utilized was, yes or no, proscribed by the International Convention on Chemical Weapons. If it involved a halogen or opioid product, its use would be legal and the drama of the theater on Doubrovka street could be classified as a therapeutic hazard, the prescribers having made an error in dosing. These series of 'pass–pass' technologies and semantics allow the threshold critique of proscription to be erased, passing on to a binary system of armament systems (authorized weapons/proscribed weapons). We emphasize here the hypocrisy of 'non-lethal' weapons. The use of irritant or incapacitating agents, qualified as 'non-lethal' weapons, is proscribed by the International Convention on Chemical Weapons. Riot control agents cannot, therefore, be employed as weapons of war. We come to see that the 'non-lethal' character of these weapons is subject to caution. During the Vietnam war, irritant agents were dispersed before aerial bombardments in order to dislodge the Vietnamese infantrymen from their shelters. It was therefore not a matter of limiting human losses but, on the contrary, of increasing the fatal efficacy of the air raids by depriving the enemy of his protection. The American Secretary of Defense, Donald Rumsfeld, justified recourse to such weapons in his speech on February 5, 2003, to the House of Representatives Armed Forces Committee. Rumsfeld declared:

> 'We are in a very difficult situation. Our forces are authorized to shoot at people and to kill them, but not authorized to utilize a non-lethal agent for combat control. It is an embarrassing situation. There are some moments where the usage of non-lethal agents is perfectly appropriate, when it is necessary to transport prisoners in a confined space, in an aircraft for example, or for example when enemy troops are in a cave in Afghanistan and you know they have their women and children with them.'

It was at one time more a matter of paralyzing the enemy, of blinding or disorienting them before striking them. In the same fashion, combat lasers which blind the enemy by causing retinal burns are declared 'non-lethal' by the Pentagon. They only prevent the adversary from utilizing his weapon. A person can only ignore what happens to a combatant blinded when facing his enemy. A thousand leagues from all forms of compassion or humanity, it is a matter of substituting some technological processes for the human suffering and some words for facts. Must it be necessary to hunt for the category of conventional weapons, the homemade bomb packed with nails or small shot and accept in the same category 'non-lethal combat control agents', combat lasers, microwave weapons, and particle beams?

To add to the confusion, recall that conventional weapons are likely to be used to release non-conventional agents. Bombardment of an industrial site by means of conventional bombs can set in motion a contamination (chemical, radiological, or biological) of the environment, with catastrophic public health consequences. The administration of Bill Clinton envisioned, in the 1990s, bombarding the North Korean nuclear reactor at Yongbyon. During the first Gulf war, allied aviation bombarded many Iraqi NBC armament sites: the nuclear armament site in Tuwaitha, the biological armament site in Taji, and the chemical armament site in Falluja. In the course of the war against Serbia, NATO did not hesitate to bomb the petrochemical complex of Pancevo, liberating products as toxic as certain combat gases. This confusion of effects can be put to profitable use for concealing the use of non-conventional weapons in the cadre of 'preventive strikes'. In effect, who can say whether the contamination observed following a bombardment is due to the bomb dropped or to the bombarded site? Above all, if one takes precautions, before the strike, to convince international opinion that the target country has available in its territory numerous sites with non-conventional weapons! Not to be outdone, terrorist groups have available at low cost a sort of binary weapon, because a classical explosive charge can liberate CBRN agents from a nuclear center, from a protected biotechnology laboratory (a P4 laboratory), or an industrial chemical site.

In the end, one can ask how setting a classification of weapons serves to elaborate conventions that are systematically distorted or violated. In making a range of miniaturized nuclear and launching devices the focus of a recent program of anti-ballistic missile defense, the USA also distorted the Nuclear Non-proliferation Treaty as well as the 1972 Anti-Ballistic Missile (ABM) Treaty. In opposing all procedures for verification in its territory in the context of the 1972 Convention for the prohibition of biological weapons, it rendered this convention inapplicable. Some other countries who were signatories to this Convention pursue programs of offensive research on materials of biological weapons under cover of 'defensive research'.

'Surgical strikes' and weapons of mass destruction

A second question should not be eluded. Modern high-technology weapons – are they instruments of precision, contrary to weapons of mass destruction, which seem to be held exclusively by the enemy? The war rhetoric, which repeatedly has recourse to the medical vocabulary, does not clarify the debate. According to this rhetoric, intelligent weapons allow the operation of 'surgical strikes', of striking the objectives while limiting the adverse effects. This can be compared to an electric scalpel, whose intensity is regulated in such a way as to excise pathological tissues without damaging the adjacent healthy tissue. If 'pathological tissues' represent a blow to the enemy forces, the 'healthy tissues' in general represent the hand that holds the scalpel; NATO says otherwise, as does the civilian population of the bombarded country. In recent wars, we have learned that the border between anti-forces strikes and anti-cities strikes is poorly drawn and tortuous. Not only are civilian populations not spared, but they can be the admitted targets. In the course of wars in the second part of the twentieth century, the percentage of civilian victims rose from 10% to 90%. The 'conventional' bombardment of Dresden and the 'non-conventional' bombardment of Hiroshima were comparable in horror. The Mitchell doctrine, in force since the 1930s, makes massive aerial strikes preliminary to all American military attacks. The strategic aerial bombardments above all destroy civilian and industrial installations, leaving intact a great part of the military potential. NATO rules of engagement impose the practice of high-altitude bombardments (higher than 5000 meters) to protect the pilots against aerial defenses. At this altitude, it is illusory to visually make a distinction between civilians and military personnel. It is therefore at the price of 'collateral damage' that NATO forces have not sustained any losses during the latest aerial campaigns. The concept of 'zero military personnel mortality' is associated with the 'effect' of 90% civilian victims. During the war against Serbia, the Alliance openly demanded research of the 'Dresden effect', that is to say the exhaustion of the morale of a people which goes with the bombing of their apartment buildings, their bridges, their hospitals, their electricity centers, their factories, their petroleum refineries, their telephone centers, and their television relays. The distinction between anti-forces strikes and anti-cities strikes is eclipsed to the benefit of 'legitimate military objectives'. On the night of April 22–23, 1990, NATO aviation took for its target the studios of the Serbian National Television (RTS), located in the heart of Belgrade, killing 16 journalists at their workstations; for NATO, the media entered into the definition of a legitimate military objective. During the 1991 Gulf war, the supplies of potable water for Iraq were deliberately targeted. Destruction, by means of 'conventional' bombs, of a network for potable drinking water of a country is probably the most effective method for propagating natural infectious agents by the basic route of dirty water. This form of biological warfare does not strike soldiers, but rather children who die in epidemics of infectious gastroenteritis.

Economic embargos, such as those for water, take an entire people hostage and organize their deficiencies by depriving them most often of products of primary necessity, such as foodstuffs and medications. The embargo against Iraq caused more human beings to perish than the bomb of Hiroshima, taking into account the respective medical sequelae. For all these reasons, physicians consider with much skepticism the notions of surgical strikes and reduced collateral effects. From all the evidence, the ambiguous concept of 'reduction of collateral damage' is attached more to the preservation of the economic potential of a country than to the losses amongst its civilian population.

Again, it is more a matter of semantic distortion and Orwellian manipulation of the language than the cruel reality of the facts. Of course, terrorists do the same and do not hesitate to blindly strike innocent victims.

The only means of justly evaluating the human damage is to look at the victims and not to read the technical instructions for the weapons employed. High-technology weapons are presented as inoffensive for civilian populations on the grounds that they are equipped with selective anti-forces effects – inhibition of the enemy's communication systems with graphite bombs or electromagnetic bombs, better penetration of bunkers with miniaturized nuclear weapons, better penetration of steel armor plate with depleted uranium munitions. However, the high-technology weapons are a long way from proving their innocuousness. The graphite bomb, a veritable 'finger on the switch' of a country, could cut the electricity to hospitals and maternity wards, indirectly threatening the lives of hospitalized patients, as was observed in 1999. An article in a major French daily paper described the graphite bomb in this manner:

'The American weapon available is the future of weapons, temporarily switching off the electrical systems of a country. It is a matter of graphite bombs (BLU 114), utilized for the first time in 1999 in Serbia. These weapons spread carbon filaments on transformers, causing a short circuit. On several occasions, the current was switched off in Belgrade. The damages are minor, and it suffices to clean up the electrical facilities for them to resume operation.'

This journalist has probably never found himself in a hospital suddenly deprived of electricity, in particular in an operating room, an intensive care service, or a neonatal intensive care service. It appears that the damages are not 'minor' and that it does not suffice to clean up so that all operations can be resumed. And what can be said about the health consequences of inhaling graphite particles or exposure to radioactivity released from mini-bombs or depleted uranium munitions? Will there be few people who care about the health consequences, in particular the risk of oncogenic effects, for the civilian populations of sprayed regions? Must it be recalled that, during the Vietnam war, the American authorities affirmed the innocuousness of the aerial spraying of defoliants vis-à-vis the civilian populations? Furthermore, the distinction between the anti-matériel effect and the anti-personnel effect is sufficiently fuzzy for this type of weapon. By way of example, a microwave weapon can be utilized to neutralize electronic systems but it can also serve to cook human beings by adjusting the intensity.

From non-proliferation to counter-proliferation

The third question concerns the future of the Western techno-industrial society that combines aggressive strategies and technological supremacy [9,10]. We assist the passage from a defensive doctrine founded on deterrence to an offensive doctrine by multiplying innovative concepts: revisions of treaties and conventions, preventive war, counter-proliferation interference. This process was begun well before the attacks of

September 11, 2001. It is too often justified in the name of moral or humanitarian concepts. Once again, physicians have participated, voluntarily or involuntarily, in the war effort. The notion of a right of humanitarian interference together with the simultaneous dropping of bombs and a lively maintenance of confusion serves some tactical interests. In the same fashion, the USA has attacked, attacked, still attacks, and will still attack Iraq without caring about the advice of the Security Council and of the Iraqi people. It is a matter of maintaining confusion and dramatizing the threat to justify fatal preventive strikes.

Scientific progress has permitted the development of high-technology weapons. Shortly after the discovery of nuclear fission, Frederic Joliot, Lew Kowarski, and Hans Heinrich von Halban filed a patent with the title, 'Improvement of explosive charges'. In fact, firearms have been modernized with striking regularity since the Battle of Crécy, and the canons of the Black Prince were the precursors of the artillery of the Napoleonic campaigns, the Civil War and modern slaughter. In his Directive of August 30, 1941, to the Committee of the Heads of Major Countries, Churchill took a position in favor of developing a uranium bomb in the name of progress:

'Although I am for my part satisfied with existing explosives, I think that we must not make obstacles to progess.'

The physicist, Edward Teller, architect of the A bomb and designer of the H bomb, affirmed that, for him, the technology was a measure to save the free world. Today, specialists in genetic engineering rival physicists for improving CBRN weapon systems and inventing new forms of apocalypse. One could think, like Edward Teller, that the free world would be saved by technology, but one could also think, like Theodore Kaczinsky, that the techno-industrial society has involuntarily created the instruments of its own destruction [11]. A technology developed is a technology for immanent application. By its technological supremacy, the Western techno-industrial society has set in motion an imbalance of world forces that would inevitably give birth to the terrorist threat. In effect, no force, working or open, can oppose it on the classical front with comparable systems of armaments, and accordingly the concept of counter-proliferation has a view to destroy, in the enemies' countries, all potential for the production of sophisticated weapons. The imbalanced conflicts therefore go on to proliferate and no national sanctuary will be safe. Neither a vaccine against smallpox nor the ballistic anti-missile shield will prevent armed kamikazis from using means, more or less conventional, to sow terror in our society.

Faced with such threats and with such stakes, physicians must resist all manipulation. Their vocation is to denounce confusion of types and refuse to place at the disposition of the war makers their vocabulary, their medications, their designs, or their staffs. They must refuse to participate in offensive research under cover of defensive programs, and oppose themselves to the instrumentalism of humanitarian interference with the aim of transforming this latter into an agent for military interference. Nevertheless, on the occasion of recent conflicts, few physicians expressed themselves on the ethical and moral problems posed by the warmakers' strategies and the weapons systems [12]. They too often remain confined in the role of technical advisers to which they are assigned by the authorities, even if this role is essential. Treatment of war victims or attackers, whether they are civilians or military personnel, makes in effect an appeal to medical competencies in very diverse fields and specialties. These competencies will be crucial in cases of technological or industrial accidents, accidents that constitute a permanent threat for the future of our societies. We must not forget the disastrous cost of the catastrophe in Chernobyl, and also not forget that the gas leak in Bhopal caused more deaths than the September 11, 2001, attacks in the USA.

References

1. Amnesty International. Armes nouvelles au service des tortionnaires. *Le Monde Diplomatique*, April, 1997; 3.
2. Najman M. Les Américians préparent les armes du xx1^e siècie. *Le Monde Diplomatique*, February, 1998; 4–5.
3. Wright S. Hypocrisie des armes non létales. *Le Monde Diplomatique*, December, 1999; 24.
4. Abdelkrim-Delanne C. Ces armes si peu conventionnelles. *Le Monde Diplomatique*, June, 1999; 11.
5. Poupée K. Un test pour les armes électromagnétiques. *Le Monde Diplomatique*, April, 2003; 15.
6. Vidal G. Ces armes si peu conventionnelles (réponse à l'article de Christine Abdelkrim-Delanne). *Le Monde Diplomatique*, August, 1999; 2.
7. Rifkin J. Bioterrorisme high-tech et révolution génétique. *Le Monde*, October 6, 2001; 16.
8. Rifkin J. *The Biotech Century: Harnessing the Gene and Remaking the World*. New York: Jeremy P. Tarcher/G. P. Putnam's Sons, 1998.
9. Conférence des Laureates du Prix Nobel. *Promesses et Menaces à l'Aube du xx1^e Siècle*. Paris: Éditions Odile Jacob, 1988.
10. Pisiani F. Penser la cybergurerre. *Le Monde Diplomatique*, August, 1999; 4–5.
11. Kaczynski T. *La Société Industrielle et Son Avenir*. Paris: Éditions de l'Encyclopédie des Nuisances, 1988.
12. Bismuth C, Barriot P. De destruction massive ou conventionnelles, les armes tuent les civis. *Le Monde Diplomatique*, May, 2003; 16–17.

2

Introduction to chemical weapons

Patrick Barriot and Chantal Bismuth

On April 29, 1977, the international convention was entered into effect that interdicted the development, production, stocking, and use of chemical weapons [1–3]. This convention also prohibits dispersion devices as well as the use of herbicides or riot control agents in the arsenal for wartime operations. It is accompanied by a mechanism for international verification.

Chemical agents and dissemination devices

The chemical agents likely to be used for military, police, or terrorist purposes come from several large families (Table 2.1). Gases utilized by the armed forces or law enforcement agencies are generally volatile liquids that are dispersed in the form of aerosols. They penetrate into the body by the respiratory route. It is classic to distinguish the lethal agents from the non-lethal agents or incapacitating agents. The lethal potential of a chemical agent is evaluated by its LD_{50}, otherwise called the dose that causes death amongst 50% of exposed subjects. When one envisages respiratory or percutaneous absorption, the LD_{50} is expressed in mg/min/m^3 or in mg/kg (Table 2.2). For those who hold that chemical weapons are 'weapons of mass destruction', 1 kg of a neurotoxic agent can kill 1 million people and 30 g of botulinum toxin can kill 60 million. In reality, it is very difficult to establish a correlation between the quantity of the product utilized and the number of victims. Numerous factors, such as the physico-chemical characteristics of the product, the dispersion devices utilized, or the meteorological conditions, can frustrate predictions or disappoint criminal attacks. Moreover, the distinction between lethal and 'non-lethal' weapons is not always so clear-cut. We emphasize this point. Defoliants or ecocidal weapons are utilized to destroy the trees in the rain forest and result in persistent contamination of soils that causes nutritional difficulties for the enemy. The majority of chemical agents can be utilized by terrorist groups with a view towards contamination by inhalation or ingestion. The synthesis and militarization of these agents does not constitute a major technological obstacle.

Treating Victims of Mass Destsuction   Edited by Patrick Barriot and Chantal Bismuth
© 2008 John Wiley & Sons, Ltd

Table 2.1   Classification of chemical agents

Physical incapacitating agents
    Orthochlorobenzylidine malononitrile (CS)
    Diphenyl-amino-chloroarsine (Adamsite) (DA)
    Fumigants

Psychiatric incapacitating agents
    Quinuclidinol benzylate (BZ)
    Lysergamide (LSD)

Assault medications
    Halogen or opiate agents
    'Calmative' agents

Combat gases
    Choking agents: phosgene, chlorine
    Vesicants: sulfur mustard, Lewisite
    Neurotoxic organophosphates: G agents (tabun, sarin, soman)
    or V agents (VX)
    Cellular poisons: hydrocyanic acid, cyanogen chloride, arsine

Toxins
    Botulinum toxin
    Ricin
    Trichothecenes
    Staphylococcal enterotoxins

Poisons and heavy metals
    Arsenic
    Cyanide
    Mercury
    Uranium
    Plutonium
    Thallium

Herbicides and ecocidal agents
    Cacodylic acid
    2,4,5-Trichlorophenoxyacetic acid
    Tetrachlorodibenzodioxin (TCDD)

It must only be noted that industrial installations producing fertilizers, pesticides, or pharmaceutical products can be converted from these civilian objectives and secretly engage in an offensive process. For this reason, the production techniques are called 'dual'.

The toxic substances of warfare can be dispersed by artillery shells, bombs, or low-altitude aerial spraying by means of numerous dispersion devices. The pressurized cylinders of World War I, which liberated clouds of chlorine derivatives, were rapidly replaced by toxic substances projectors, in particular the British 'Livens Projector',

Table 2.2 Lethal doses (LD50)

Choking agents
  Chlorine: 19 000 mg/min/m^3
  Phosgene: 3200 mg/min/m^3

Vesicants
  Sulfur mustard: 1500 mg/min/m^3 (100 mg/kg)

Cyanide derivatives
  Hydrocyanic acid: 2500–5000 mg/min/m^3
  Cyanogen chloride: 11 000 mg/min/m^3

Neurotoxic organophosphates
  Tabun: 300 mg/min/m^3 (14 mg/kg)
  Sarin: 200 mg/min/m^3 (24 mg/kg)
  Soman: 60 mg/min/m^3 (0.7 mg/kg)
  VX: 20 mg/min/m^3 (0.15 mg/kg)

Toxins
  Botulinum toxin: 0.2 mg/min/m^3

then by artillery shells, rockets, bombs, and missiles. The major problem of explosive munitions resides in the mechanical and thermal constraints exerted on the chemical product at the time of detonation. This latter is charged with rupturing the envelope of the tube that contains the chemical agent in order to disperse it, but it usually destroys a part. Certain munitions, called 'binaries', are made up of two distinct compartments, each containing a non-toxic product. During the detonation, the two products are mixed and produce the lethal agent. Numerous munitions have been adapted to chemical weapons, including large aerial bombs such as the Iraqi R-400 bomb or ballistic missiles. In countries called 'proliferators', the majority of the missiles are derived from the Soviet Scud. Iraq possessed Al-Hussein missiles, with an 850 km range, equipped with chemical warheads. The ground-to-ground Al-Samoud missile, with a range of 150 km, existed in two versions: one with liquid propellant and the other with solid propellant (Ababil-100). Numerous countries have developed missiles capable of being adapted to chemical warheads: for example, North Korea (Nodong, Taepodong), Iran, (Scud B, Shahab), Syria (Scud D), Israel (Jericho rocket). Low-altitude aerial spraying can be carried out by modified fighter aircraft, such as the Soviet Sukoi, the American F-16, or the French Mirage F1, equipped with tanks of 1000 or 2200 liters. Czech L-29 airplanes and Polish M-18 crop-dusting airplanes can also be utilized for this purpose. Finally, aircraft without pilots (unmanned aerial vehicles or UAVs) or drones, in particular the Hunter drone, are capable of being equipped with large reservoirs filled with chemical products.

A terrorist group could envision the dispersion of toxic products by means of the light aircraft mostly utilized for crop dusting. The destruction of chemical installations by means of conventional explosives is equally likely to release and disperse extremely dangerous chemical agents into the environment. The most likely scenario, however, is the dispersion of an aerosol in an enclosed or confined space (underground transportation system, hotel, office building, congress center) by means of more or less rudimentary devices. An aerosol generator connected to a system of air conditioning, ventilation, or humidification could result in a large number of victims. Another possibility is the contamination of products destined for consumption, in particular foods and beverages.

Warfare utilization of chemical agents

At the beginning of the twentieth century, the combined efforts of German entomologists and chemists opened the way for the industrial production of lethal chemical agents. Under the influence of Professor Karl Escherich (1871–1951), entomologists conducted the initial experiments with gases based on cyanide, in the arsenal for controlling insects that threatened the old forests of Germany. Professor Fritz Jacob Haber (1868–1934), Nobel Prize winner in Chemistry in 1918 and dubbed the 'father of chemical warfare', suggested that technologies derived from the battle against insect control could be applied on the World War I battlefield. The first chemical artillery shells of the Great War were 105 mm lacrimator shells, fired by German artillery at Neuve-Chapelle on October 27, 1914. But the Great Chemical War, as it was first named by Olivier Lepick, actually began on April 22, 1915, at Langemarck (Ypres). On that day, more than 5000 pressurized cylinders, placed in the trenches, released 150 tons of chlorine in the form of 'derived gaseous clouds', causing the deaths of about 1000 soldiers and the poisoning of 3000 soldiers. Choking agents were used from 1917. Hydrocyanic acid, available at the beginning of the war, was not utilized. The second date marking this chemical warfare was July 12, 1917, which saw the appearance on the Ypres battlefield of sulfur ethyl-dichloride, or mustard gas. Nearly 50 000 'Yperite' (sulfur mustard) artillery shells were fired by the German artillery, causing 14 200 victims, of whom 489 died. Chemical injuries represented 3.4% of the total number of the victims of this war.

At the end of World War I, the German zoologist Albrecht Hase (1882–1962) united his efforts with those of Fritz Haber to develop a program of research on chemical weapons. Under cover of studies on insecticides, these two scientists performed, among others, experiments on gases based on cyanide, Zyklon, which was utilized in the gas chambers in World War II. The aircraft manufacturer, Junkers, placed at their disposal an engine specially conceived for dispersing chemical agents such as arsenic over large areas. Some confidential notes have revealed that the 'battle against insect pests' achieved public opinion acceptance for a program of research on offensive chemical weapons. Sarah Jannsen, historian for sciences at the Max-Planck-Institut in Berlin, has placed in evidence the transfer of technology between entomologists and chemists that allowed the development of war gases. On his part, during the 1930s, a chemist from the firm I. G. Farben, Dr Gerhard Schrader, discovered the neurotoxic organophosphates in conducting some research on insecticides. Tabun was discovered in 1936 and militarized in 1939. Sarin was discovered in 1939. Simultaneously, as well as work on new agents, the product tested for the first time at Ypres (sulfur mustard) was utilized several times in the period between the two World Wars. In 1935, Italian forces carried out aerial spraying with 700 tons of sulfur mustard on Ethiopian troops in Abyssinia, causing some 15 000 victims. The Japanese Imperial Army also used sulfur mustard and Lewisite against the Chinese, beginning in 1938.

During World War II, no chemical weapons were employed by the belligerents on the battlefield. However, the Wehrmacht stored more than 10 000 tons of chemical agents and the Allies also accumulated large quantities of chemical weapons. Methyl cyanoformate or Zyklon-B was utilized in the gas chambers.

During the Vietnam War (1961–1973), the American forces mainly had recourse to herbicides and incapacitating agents. Spraying of herbicides had the purpose of destruction of the Vietnamese rain forest that served as natural camouflage for the adversary. Nearly 20 000 aerial operations dispersed 83 million liters of defoliants on Vietnam, principally in the south of the country, between 1961 and 1971. The numerous toxic agents utilized (Agent Orange, Agent Purple, Agent Pink, etc.) were manufactured in the USA in the 1960s, in particular by the Monsanto firm. They were heavily contaminated with tetrachlorodibenzodioxin (TCDD), a powerful dioxin. This latter, very persistent, accumulated in the environment and in the food chain. Few epidemiological and ecological studies have been carried out on the long-term consequences of the widespread use of defoliants in Vietnam. About 4.8 million persons were directly affected by the spraying and, according to the Vietnamese Red Cross, more than 1 million persons still suffer today from the ill-effects of the dioxins. Lymphomas and sarcomas are the two cancers most often suspected of being due to defoliant exposure. The American forces also employed incapacitating agents during military operations. In particular, irritating agents were dispersed before bombardments to dislodge Vietnamese snipers from their trees. It was a matter of increasing the lethality of air raids by depriving the enemy of this protection.

During the war between Iran and Iraq (1980–1988), which caused hundreds of thousands of deaths, the two protagonists had massive recourse to chemical weapons. The Iraqi military–industrial complex produced large quantities of sulfur mustard, nerve agents, and toxins under the direction of Rihab Tuha (dubbed 'Doctor Germ'), spouse of General Amer Rachid, also implicated in the development of chemical weapons. These latter had also been utilized by the regime of Saddam Hussein against the Kurdish populations to punish them for having supported Iran. Ali Hassan al-Majid, called 'Chemical Ali', leader of the Baas Party in Kurdistan, was able to subdue the Kurdish rebellion in this fashion. It has always seemed that the chemical bombardment of the town of Halabja, in March 1988, was not part of an operation of anti-Kurdish repression. The town was in fact the site of confrontation between the Iranian army and the Iraqi army, both of which had recourse to war gases. The number of civilian victims killed by chemical weapons during the Battle of Halabja seems to have been overestimated.

Iraq seems to have ceased manufacturing chemical weapons after the first Gulf War in 1991, during which no war gases were utilized. In January, 1991, some days before the beginning of air raids against Iraq, the American Secretary of State, James Baker, declared that Washington could deploy overwhelming force, implying nuclear, if Baghdad used chemical or biological weapons. Of the 39 Scuds launched by Iraq against Israel in 1991, none had chemical warheads. Under pressure from the USA, who accused Iraq of having preserved its stock of weapons of mass destruction, the Security Council of the United Nations voted on November 8, 2002, for Resolution 1441, imposing a program of 'intrusive' inspections and the complete disarmament of Iraq. The Hans Blix inspectors only discovered residuals of prohibited weapons that were subsequently destroyed. Steve Allison, British chemical engineer, UNO expert within the group of inspectors, qualified the intelligence furnished by London and Washington on the claimed sensitive sites as 'absolute nonsense'. In March 2003, an American–British coalition claimed to have obtained proof that Saddam Hussein still possessed weapons of mass destruction susceptible to threaten the Security of the USA and its allies. This theme was invoked by George Bush to launch the 'Iraqi Freedom' campaign, a conflict during the course of which no chemical weapons were employed by the Iraqi troops. No weapons of mass destruction were discovered after the invasion of Iraq by the American–British coalition. On several occasions, American television announced the discovery of 'suspect products', which were revealed to be pesticides. In April 2003, the USA announced the dispatch of 1000 experts equipped with mobile laboratories and charged with adding to the research of hundreds of American military personnel already in place. Overall, about 5000 military personnel carried out research for weapons of mass destruction retained by Iraq. The chief of the inspectors in the disarmament of Iraq, Hans Blix, proposed the services of his group to lend an international legitimacy to any eventual discovery of chemical weapons, but the USA rejected his offer. The Iraqi general Amer Hammondi Al-Saadi, scientific counselor to Saddam Hassein, declared during his surrender to the American Forces:

'I tell you for History: we have nothing'.

General Tommy Franks, chief of the coalition armed forces, declared himself disappointed because 'we haven't found anything yet' in matters of weapons of mass destruction. In his last report to the Security Council, submitted June 2, 2003, the chief of the UNO disarmament inspectors, Hans Blix, once again emphasized:

'The inspections have not allowed discovery of proof of the continuation or resumption by Bagdad of programs for weapons of mass destruction.'

It is important to recall the process of disinformation that allowed justification of the preventive attack on Iraq [1,4–6,7–29].

On February 5, 2003, the American Secretary of State, Colin Powell, in a 90-minute exposé before the Security Council, presented satellite photos and recordings to support a long enumeration of weapons of mass destruction retained by Iraq. According to him, the Iraqi menace was imminent and the quantity of chemical agents was evaluated to be 100–500 tons. A week later, the photographs presented by Colin Powell were publicly contested by Hans Blix, the inspector responsible for the disarmament of Iraq.

Hans Blix declared later that at the approach of the war, Washington 'had pressured' the UNO inspectors so that the terms of their report would become unfavorable to Iraq. The Office for Special Plans (OSP) of the Intelligence Agency at the Pentagon, created after the attacks of September 11, 2001, by Paul Wolfowitz, second of the Department of Defense, was also charged with dramatizing the menace of Iraqi weapons of mass destruction in order to justify a pre-emptive attack. A classified document from the CIA emphasized, during September 2002:

'Reliable information does not exist on the production or stocking of chemical weapons by Iraq.'

Some CIA agents, uneasy about the diversion for 'political ends' of their reports on Iraq, made internal complaints. After the war, Donald Rumsfeld declared:

'It is possible that Saddam Hussein had decided to destroy (the weapons) before the beginning of the conflict.'

However, this hypothesis was qualified by Tony Blair as 'manifestly absurd' during a debate at the European Community, at the onset of hostilities. On Tuesday May 27, 2003, during a conference in New York, Donald Rumsfeld, Secretary of Defense, responding to a questioner who asked him why Iraq had not utilized biochemical weapons against the American–British forces, said:

'We don't know that that is what happened.'

In an interview given by Paul Wolfowitz to the monthly magazine *Vanity Fair*, the Number Two of the Pentagon declared:

'For the motives which have often been seen with the American Government bureaucracy, we have fallen into accord on the question which seems to be gathering everyone, to know that weapons of mass destruction should be the principal reason for the war.'

On Thursday May 29, a 'memorandum' addressed to President Bush by a group of senior experts from the CIA and the State Department emphasized that 6 weeks of unfruitful research for weapons of mass destruction proved that:

'... either these weapons were simply not there, or that they were not in sufficient quantity to justify the repeated affirmations according to which Iraq posed a great threat to the security of our country.'

The group emphasized, in passing, that some intelligence had:

'... already been falsified for political reasons but never in so systematic a fashion for deceiving our elected representatives in order to authorize a war.'

The Republican Senator from Virginia and President of the Armed Forces Committee, John Warner, declared:

'We are in a situation where the credibility of the administration and the congress is directly threatened.'

Two dossiers established that the British government, with a view towards justifying the war, were made the object of comparable manipulations. The first dossier, published in September 2002, was designed to convince the country of the severity of the Iraqi threat. It claimed, based on a report from the British intelligence services, that Saddam Hussein could make use of his chemical and biological weapons 'in 45 minutes'. The BBC revealed that the British intelligence services were constrained by Tony Blair to rewrite their dossier on weapons of mass destructions in order to render them more alarmist. Tony Blair's Director of Communications, Alastair Campbell, rewrote the dossier established by the Joint Intelligence Committee in order to render it more disturbing. A high-level official of the intelligence services confided to the BBC:

'The news according to which the weapons of mass destruction could be activated in 45 minutes was a typical example. It did not figure in the original example. It was added against our will because it was not reliable.'

The Secretary of State for Defense, Adam Ingram, confirmed that this key element, which contributed to defeat the hesitation of Parliament, had not been 'corroborated'. The British Minister of Foreign Affairs, Jack Straw, did not hesitate to emphasize that:

'... the discovery of weapons of extermination was not of crucial importance.'

Robin Cook, Labour Minister for Parliamentary Relations, who resigned in March 2003, demanded of a committee of Parliamentary enquiry:

'We have said that Saddam Hussein had weapons ready to be utilizable in 45 minutes. It has now been 45 days since the war was concluded and we have not discovered any .... It is becoming clear that Saddam never had any which would have allowed him to attack us first.'

The second report involved was developed by the Downing Street information service and made public in February 2003. It denounced the practices of the Iraqi regime for misleading the UNO disarmament inspectors. The British Parliamentary Commission in charge of secret services and interior security confirmed in its annual report the stupefying thoughtlessness of this report. Of the 19 pages of the dossier, 13 were reproduced word for word from a university thesis by an Iraqi–American student, written 10 years previously and available on the internet. The rest was 'borrowed' from *Jane's Defense* magazine, without the least reference to the plagiarized documents.

The document was presented as a synthesis by the intelligence services and constituted a new dossier slanted against the Iraqi regime.

Mr Tony Benn, former Labour minister, emphasized the severity of the disinformation:

> 'I believe that the Prime Minister has lied to us, more and more, and that this sets in motion long-term damage to democracy. If one cannot believe what the ministers say, it is the entire democratic process which is in peril.'

Malcolm Savidge, elected Labour minister, affirmed:

> 'I don't know of an accusation more serious than that of having led a people and a Parliament into a war under a false pretext. It is, according to me, much more serious than Watergate.'

According to a public opinion poll published on Saturday June 14, 2003, by *The Times*, 58% of Britons considered that Tony Blair and George W. Bush had 'knowingly' exaggerated the threat of weapons of mass destruction to justify the intervention of Anglo-American troops in Iraq. Also, 34% of Britons asserted that they were not disposed to have confidence in the head of the government on any subject, taking into account the manner in which he had manipulated the Iraqi dossiers. An editorial in the daily paper, *Le Monde*, on May 30, 2003 concluded:

> 'It is thus, without doubt, the greatest lie of State in recent years. A campaign of manipulation undertaken probably in all knowledge of things, in all cases despite all the contrary indications, to foster belief in world public opinion that Iraq retained and fabricated weapons of mass destruction.'

Terrorism and counter-terrorism

The utilization of chemical agents by terrorists is far from being unusual, and the evaluation of threats should take into account measures to frustrate them or cause these efforts to fail [30]. Some cultures of *Clostridium botulinum* were discovered in October 1980 in a cache of the 'Red Army Faction', and more recently ricin was discovered in London.

Analysis of recent events imposes the attentive contemplation of the threat of contamination of food or beverages by means of chemical agents. In a wartime scenario, the objective is more or less to starve the population by destroying their food resources. For terrorist groups, the intended effect is not to kill a large number of persons but rather to produce a panic reaction or to ruin an economic network. In 1977, mercury contamination of citrus fruits in a province of Israel that were destined for European markets was reported. Only a dozen persons were poisoned, but the export of Israeli citrus fruits was markedly decreased. In March 1989, Chilean grapes imported to the USA were contaminated with cyanide. No human poisonings were observed, but many countries suspended the importation of fruits grown in Chile. There is thus a discrepancy between the severity of the poisoning and its economic repercussions. The contamination of water by various chemical agents (botulinum toxin, thallium, cyanide, etc.) represents a permanent risk in crisis situations. The dispersion of botulinum toxin into a potable drinking water reservoir does not summarize the terrorist risk and chlorination of water does not eliminate all danger. In the 1980s, Iraqi dissidents were contaminated with drinks and food containing thallium. In March 1992, lethal concentrations of potassium cyanide were discovered in the water reservoirs of a Turkish army camp in Istanbul. This chemical attack was claimed by the Kurdistan Workers Party (PKK). In January 1995, a dozen Russian military personnel died in Tadjikistan after having drunk champagne contaminated with cyanide. Contamination with a chemical agent is not limited to food and beverages. Cosmetic and pharmaceutical products offer, to diverse agents, a favorable route for penetration into the body, particularly the muco-cutaneous route (i.e. eye lotions, creams, lipsticks, aerosols, inhalers, etc.). A bottle of Chanel No. 5 perfume has, for example, been filled with the neurotoxicant, sarin.

On two occasions, the Japanese Aum Shinrikyo ('Supreme Truth') provoked attacks with Sarin gas [31,32]. The first was in Matsumoto in June, 1994. On that day, the sect attempted to assassinate a judge by disseminating sarin in proximity to his residence. There were seven deaths and 144 poisoned persons. The second attempt, on March 20, 1995, was an extensive chemical attack against the civilian population. Some packages containing sarin were placed in five cars on three subway lines in Tokyo during the rush hour, causing 12 deaths and more than 5000 poisoned persons. The Aum sect also attempted to disseminate botulinum toxin by spraying.

Chemical agents are utilized by secret services or 'security services' of different countries to eliminate opponents, rebels, or terrorists. In September 1978, the Bulgarian secret service assassinated Georgi Markov in London by means of an umbrella whose point was filled with ricin. We have already mentioned thallium poisoning, in the 1980s, of Iraqi dissidents by means of contaminated foods and beverages. The KGB and later the Russian FSB, the American CIA, and the Israeli Mossad have, amongst others, also had recourse to this type of 'targeted action for neutralization'. The utilization of an anesthetic gas by the Russian security forces during a hostage-taking in the Doubrovka theater posed another significant problem. It seemed in effect that these units had utilized a militarized medication before making the assault, which cost the lives not only of the Chechnyan commandos, who were executed in their sleep, but also of 117 hostages who were submitted to the uncontrolled effect of a general anesthetic. The gas utilized, a true 'assault medication' placed into service for counter-terrorism, was vaguely presented as a 'non-lethal' agent. It was proven to be mortal in two ways. The terrorists were paralyzed before being executed. Regarding the hostages, no measures were taken at the site to palliate the effects, which were revealed to be lethal. The employment of a halogen or opiate medication during police or military operations could fall outside the scope of the international convention on chemical weapons and become legitimate, in favor of a medical definition of the product. Moreover, it is known that many national laboratories have developed medications suitable for diffusion in the form of aerosols and capable of inducing disturbances of vigilance or of behavior. Numerous small molecules (endogenous peptides, neuromediators, bioregulators) can provoke submissive behavior and in this manner act as true 'chemical straightjackets'.

It is important to emphasize that, on the battlefield, the classical chemical weapons are only efficacious when they are used against unprotected combatants: soldiers in World War I surprised by clouds of chlorine, Ethiopian soldiers sprayed with sulfur mustard in Abyssinia, Vietnamese combatants exposed to incapacitating agents and defoliants, Iranian military personnel bombarded with sulfur mustard. When the combatants are well-prepared and supplied with respiratory and skin protection, the loss of human life is limited. Recourse to chemical weapons, which are tactical weapons, supposes that the enemy cannot reply with strategic nuclear weapons. The civilian population is always vulnerable and very poorly protected [33]. New molecules, issuing from research on cerebral biochemistry and placed into service for counter-terrorism, probably reserve some strongly adverse surprises for those who inhale them [34].

References

1. Affaire Kelly: mauvaise onde à la BBC. *Libération*, July 22, 2003; 7–8.
2. Lepick O. *Les Armes Chimiques*. Paris: Presses Universitaires de France, 'Que sais-je?', 1999.
3. Meyer C. *L'Arme Chimique*. Paris: Ellipses, 2003; 447 pp.
4. Armes irakiennes: George bush tente de désamorcer la crise. *Le Monde*, July 15, 2003; 2.
5. Armes irakiennes, mensonges et manipulations. *Le Monde*, July 17, 2003; 1–3.
6. Arsenal de Saddam Hussein: Blair sur la sellette. *Le Figaro*, June 4, 2003; 5.
7. Bush et Blair: ont-ils menti sur les armes irakiennes? *Le Monde*, May 30, 2003; 1–2.
8. Bush et Blair sous le feu de la polémique. *Le Figaro*, July 15, 2003; 2.
9. Des armes de destruction massive introuvables. *Le Figaro*, June 16, 2003; 3.
10. Guerre d'lrak, affaire Kelly: Tony Blair et la BBC accuses. *Le Monde*, July 22, 2003; 1–2.
11. Irak: ces mensonges d'État qui déstabilisent Bush et Blair. *Le Monde*, July 19, 2003; 1–2.
12. Irak: la grande manip de Bush et Blair. *Libération*, May 30, 2003; 10.
13. Irak: lemont de trop pour Tony Blair. *Le Monde*, July 20 and 21, 2003; 1–2.
14. L'absence d'armes de destruction massive destabilise Blair. *Le Figaro*, July 11, 2003; 3.
15. L'aveu américain. *Le Monde*, May 30, 2003; 10.
16. La BBC au coeur du scandale Kelly. *Le Figaro*, July 22, 2003; 1–3.
17. La disparition de David Kelly menace le gouvernement Blair. *Le Figaro*, July 19 and 20, 2003; 3.
18. La menace irakienne gonflée par Bush et Blair. *Libération*, June 4, 2003; 14.
19. Lacran A. L'arsenal oublié des Américains. *Le Figaro*, July 5 and 6, 2003; 13.
20. Le cadaver qui menace Blair. *Libération*, July 19 and 20, 2003; 1–3.
21. Le mort et le mensonge (editorial). *Le Monde*, July 22, 2003; 8.
22. Les declarations américaines sur les armes en Irak sont mises en doute. *Le Monde*, June 5, 2003; 4.
23. Les désarmants aveux de Donald Rumsfeld. *Le Figaro*, May 29, 2003; 3.
24. Polémique aux États-Unis sur la presence d'armes de destruction massive en Irak. *Le Monde*, June 3, 2003; 6.
25. Ramonet I. Mensonges d'État. *Le Monde Diplomatique*, July, 2003; **592**: 1, 7.
26. Selon Paul Wolfowitz, la presence d'armes mortelles en Irak n'était qu'un prétexte 'bureaucratique'. *Le Monde*, May 31, 2003; 4.
27. Tony Blair contre-attaque après la mort de David Kelly. *Le Figaro*, July 21, 2003; 1–3.

28. Tony Blair épinglé par les parlementaires britanniques. *Le Figaro*, June 12, 2003; 3.
29. Un rapport parlementaire sur les ADM critique le Premier minister (Tony Blair) mais blanchit son 'spin doctor'. *Le Monde*, July 9, 2003; 2.
30. Lepick O, Daguizan JF. *Le Terrorisme Non-conventionnel*. Paris: Presses Universitaires de France, 2003.
31. Nozaki H, Aikawa N, Fujisima S *et al.* A case of VX poisoning and the difference from sarin. *Lancet*, 1995; **346**: 698–699.
32. Suzuki T, Morita H, Ono K *et al.* Sarin poisoning in Tokyo subway. *Lancet*, 1995; **345**: 980–981.
33. Tucker JB. National health and medical services response to incidents of chemical and biological terrorism. *J Am Med Assoc*, 1997; **278**: 362–368.
34. Blanchet JM, Noto R, Pailler FM *et al. Les Aggressions Chimiques*, Collection dirigée par Fusilier R. Aubervilliers, Éditions France-Sélection, 1997.

3

Chemical weapons

Chantal Bismuth

History and doctrines

Chemical weapons, like biological weapons, are the modern incarnations of combat processes that have produced ill-effects on civilian populations reported since antiquity. From the rhizomes of Hellebore thrown into the Pleistos on the order of the sage Solon (600 BC), to the irritating ashes of the Athenians (reported by Thucydides in 429 BC), to the suffocating and sulfurous fumes of the Roman Legions, to the Greek fire of the Byzantines, to the arsenical bombs recommended to the German horse soldiers for extermination of the Turks, there exists a thick chronicle of diabolical ingenuity. This was combined with an empirical knowledge of natural toxicants, the art of isolating them, and the conditions for neutralizing or destroying soldiers and civilian populations.

Modern chemical weapons (Table 3.1) result from the capacity for production on an industrial scale and under varied conditions for the synthesis of toxic products. In this form, they have a history and a topicality. The first spraying of chlorine against armed forces was launched in April, 1915. The repeated use of suffocating and vesicant gases in the European theater during World War I installed in the collective conscious of developed countries the feeling of the persistent plausibility of chemical threats. The idea persists that it is necessary to make dispositions to respond to aggression of this nature. Today it is also generally admitted, even by the most rigorous theoreticians of nuclear deterrence, that the threat of the use of chemical weapons is a necessary element in the development of a crisis between nuclear powers. Not utilized during World War II– at least as a combat method – chemical weapons were employed, although indirectly, during the Vietnam War (in the form of defoliants). Although not commonplace, they were used in the Iran–Iraq War and since then appear to be a permanent threat in acts of terrorism. In the future, the civilian population appears at once the initial target and the first victim of the utilization of chemical agents because of their concentration, the very great difficulty of systematic protection, and the ravaging effect on the collective mentality of these threats, alleged or real.

Treating Victims of Mass Destsuction   Edited by Patrick Barriot and Chantal Bismuth
© 2008 John Wiley & Sons, Ltd

Table 3.1 Some 'inventors' of war gases*

Common name	Formula	Discovered by	Date
Chlorine	Cl_2	G. Scheele	1774
Cyanogen chloride	CNCl	Cl. Berthollet	1790
		G. S. Serullas	1827
Phosgene	$COCl_2$	J. Davy	1812
Chloropicrin	O_2N-CCl_3	J. Stenhouse	1848
Diphosgene	$CCl_3-OCOCl$	W. Hentschel	1887
Mustard gas (sulfur mustard)	$S(CH_2CH_2Cl)_2$	F. Guthrie	1860
		A. Niemann	1860
		V. Meyer	1886
'Organophosphates'		W. Lang and G. von Krueger	1932
Nitrogen mustard	$N(CH_2CH_2Cl)_3$	K. Ward	1934
Tabun	$Me_2N-P(O)(OEt)CN$	G. Schrader	1937
Sarin	$(Me)_2-CHO-P(O)(Me)F$	G. Schrader	1937
Soman	$(t-BU)(Me)CHO-P(O)(Me)F$	'Heereswaffenamt'	1944
Perfluoro-isobutene	$(F_3C)_2C=CH_2$	T. J. Brice et al.	1952

*Personal communication, J. Jacques, Laboratory of Molecular Interactions, College of France, Paris.

An effective threat

There thus exists an effective chemical threat [1]. It is revealed by the existence of large stockpiles of munitions or of toxic products for military usage in the former USSR, the USA and certain terrorist countries, and above all by the active pursuit of research tending to develop new toxicants or dispersal methods with an efficacy superior to that of existing munitions.

A correct analysis of the chemical threat should, in effect, clearly distinguish between the *weapon* and the *munition*. The weapon includes an extensive range of products with variable effects (see Table 3.1). The different munitions are outlined at the end of this chapter.

Limits of use and effects

Chemical weapons are difficult to use. They are formulated in unstable physical states (gaseous or liquid) that limit the possible methods of contamination and only guarantee a limited military efficacy. The chemical weapon utilizable in some conditions allows ballistic firing and its concentration up to saturation for a given reliable objective and a reduced yield. As volatiles, vaporized or sprayed, semi-persistent (neurotoxicants) or persistent (thickened soman, sulfur mstard), the chemical toxicants have a reliable direct capacity for physical harm in classic combat. It is admitted that, to be efficacious, they must be administered at the rate of a ton per square kilometer, concentrations that can be obtained neither by spraying nor by artillery fire, nor even by bombardment. Conversely, their toxic effects, psychological or physical, have a multiplied impact in the case of bioterrorism. Some of their physical properties are listed in Table 3.2.

Table 3.2 Some properties of various agents that could be utilized for chemical warfare

#	Tabun* Sarin* Soman*	VX*	Hsydrocyanic acid	Cyanogen chloride	Phosgene	Mustard gas	Botulinum toxin	BZ	CN	CS	DM
1	Tabun* Sarin* Soman*	VX*	Hsydrocyanic acid	Cyanogen chloride	Phosgene	Mustard gas	Botulinum toxin	BZ	CN	CS	DM
2	Lethal agent (neurotoxic gas)	Lethal agent (neurotoxic gas)	Lethal agent (hemotoxic gas)	Lethal agent (hemotoxic gas)	Lethal agent (pulmonary irritant)	Lethal and incapacitating agent (vesicant)	Lethal agent	Incapacitating agent (psychotropic)	*All 3*: neutralizing agent		
3	Vapors, aerosols or sprays	Aerosol or spray	Vapors	Vapors	Vapors	Spray	Aerosol or dry powder	Aerosol or dry powder	*All 3*: aerosol or dry powder		
4	All types of chemical weapons	Large bombs	Large bombs	Large bombs	Motor shells, large bombs	All types of chemical weapons	Small bombs, tanks, sprayers	Small bombs, tanks, sprayers	*All 3*: all types of chemical weapons		
5	1000 kg	1000 kg	1000 kg	1000 kg	1500 kg	1500 kg	400 kg	500 kg	*All 3*: 750 kg		
6	100%	1–5%	100%	6–7%	Hydrolyzed	0.05%	Soluble	?	Slightly soluble	Insoluble	Insoluble
7	12 100 mg/m³	3–18 mg/m³	873 000 mg/m³	3 300 000 mg/m³	6 370 000 mg/m³	630 mg/m³	Negligible	Negligible	105 mg/m³	Negligible	0.02 mg/m³
8 (a)	Liquid	Liquid	Liquid	Solid	Liquid	Solid	Solid	Solid	*All 3*: solid		
(b)	Liquid	Liquid	Liquid	Vapors	Vapors	Liquid	Solid	Solid	*All 3*: solid		

Table 3.2 *Continued*

9 (a) 15 min–1 hour	1–12 hours	Several minutes	Several minutes	12–48 hours	—	—	—	—	—	—
(b) 15 min–1 hour	3–21 days	Several minutes	Several minutes	2–7 days	—	—	—	2 weeks for CS1 Longer for CS2	—	—
(c) 1–2 days	1–16 weeks	¼–4 hours	¼–1 hour	2–8 weeks	—	—	—	—	—	—
10 >5 mg/min/m^3	>0.5 mg/min/m^3	>2000 mg/min/m^3	>7000 mg/min/m^3	>1600 mg/min/m^3	>100 mg/min/m^3	0.001 mg (oral route)	100 mg/min/m^3	5–15 mg/m^3 (concentrate)	1–5 mg/m^3 (concentrate)	2–5 mg/m^3 (concentrate)
11 100 mg/min/m^3	10 mg/min/m^3	5000 mg/min/m^3	11 000 mg/min/m^3	3200 mg/min/m^3	1500 mg/min/m^3	0.02 mg/min/m^3	—	10 000 mg/min/m^3	25 000–150 000 mg/min/m^3	15 000 mg/min/m^3
12 1500 mg/person	6 mg/person	—	—	4500 mg/person	—	—	—	—	—	—

*Organophosphates.

1. Common name; 2, military classification; 3, most probable form for dissemination of the agent; 4, type of device proposed for dissemination of the agent; 5, approximate maximum weight of the agent effectively deliverable by a single light bomber (bomb load, 4 tons); 6, approximate solubility in water at 20°C; 7, volatility at 20°C; 8, physical state, (a) at –10°C, (b) at +20°C; 9, approximate duration of risk (by contact or in the air after evaporation) to be anticipated at ground level, (a) 10°C, modified by rain, moderate wind, (b) 15°C in sunny weather, light breeze, (c) –10°C in sunny weather, without wind, snow showers; 10, efficacious doses (lesions or incapacitation of military value); 11, Ct_{50} in humans by the respiratory route (in cases of reliable activity, ventilation approximately 15 liters/minute); 12, estimated lethal doses in humans by the percutaneous route.

After Bismuth C et al. Toxicologie Clinique. Paris: Flammarion Médecine-Sciences, 2000.

Currently proven facts

Chemical weapons thus remain a restless threat in all conflicts, armed or not. Terrorists utilize this fear to alarm civilian populations, sometimes into states of mass panic, which they create to serve their purposes, since the desired end is obtained before use.

The utilization of chemical weapons was massive during the 1914–1918 war: initially, suffocating gas (1915), dispersed by trucks into the enemy trenches (chlorine–phosgene); then, from 1917, mustard gas or Ypérite (from the name of the Belgian city, Ypres). The mortality due to chemical weapons represented 1% of the total mortality of this war, after having involved 2% of the soldiers under fire [2].

During World War II and despite the production and synthesis, essentially in Germany, of numerous organophosphates, similar to widely utilized insecticides but toxic at much smaller doses and more persistent, their employment for warfare purposes (suppression of combat action or civilian victimization) was not carried out, except for the tragic massacres, in enclosed sites, of Jewish and gypsy populations in concentration camps with Zyclon-B, a derivative of hydrocyanic acid. Since then, the use of chemical weapons in different conflicts worldwide has been constantly feared and anticipated. The defoliants utilized during the Vietnam War in the 1970s could be considered chemical weapons.

We review that:

- The Italian fascists interrogated their suspects after having made them swallow ricin oil, which induced diarrhea and reduced their means of resistance.

- The injection of ricin (alkaloid from the seed) into the Bulgarian agent, Georgi Markov, in London in 1978 caused his rapid death. The toxicity is thus, in effect, systemic and can be lethal.

- It seems that throughout the Cold War, the Soviets conducted their interrogations of suspects or dissidents using neuroleptics. These antipsychotic medications are strong modifiers of behavior and overcome all psychological resistance.

- During the 1980–1988 Iran–Iraq war, sulfur mustard-containing aerial bombs or rockets were frequently used, contaminating military personnel as well as civilians. The military hospitals were at that time overwhelmed with those wounded by firearms (this murderous war caused many hundreds of thousands of deaths by one party or the other). Amongst those injured by chemical weapons, only the severe cases were hospitalized; of these hospitalized cases, representing about one-third of the victims, the military physicians deplored a mortality of 4.8%.

- Finally, there were reports by the Iranian authorities on 12 000 chemical injuries, including 50 combatants [3] and 130 'martyrs' (who died) out of 4500 hospitalized victims [4].

Organophosphates (probably tabun) were denounced in the attack on a water treatment facility in Koramshar (rockets launched from helicopters), causing 15 deaths amongst

100 victims [5]. Some Iraqi solders were themselves injured by sulfur mustard-containing munitions without being able to certify that these were Iranian weapons and not their own weapons fired in error. Finally, the Iraqis utilized chemical weapons in 1988 against the Kurdish village of Halabja, which was occupied by the Iranians during the conflict between the two countries. The attack was done by bombardment. The Iranians organized a visit to the site by 'Medecins sans Frontiers' ('Doctors without Borders') that took place 5 days later. Two toxic substances had been utilized: sulfur mustard (the injured were immediately transported to Iranian hospitals) and a neurotoxic gas, tabun and/or sarin. Cyanides were excluded. The inspectors counted 100 dead lying in the streets, 80 bodies in a common grave, and 50 children killed in their school. Moreover, 406 injured were treated in the hospital in Bakhtran. Many of the victims had already left the treatment centers on the fifth day to return to their homes [6]. During the First Gulf War, the utilization of chemical weapons was an obsession. It was known that Iraq possessed large stockpiles of sulfur mustard and organophosphates.

During the bombardment of Israel (a non-belligerent country) by Scud missiles, in fact containing conventional charges, the observers bizarrely seemed nearly relieved ('it was not chemical', as though conventional charges were innocent), suggesting that their early protests had dissuaded Iraq. Another possible explanation is that Iraq had not gone to the expense of equipping its missiles to carry toxic chemicals for more than 600 kilometers.

After the destruction of Iraqi industrial chemical sites during the armistice, without immediate symptoms, certain military personnel have incorporated into the 'Gulf War syndrome' a certain number of chronic complaints that they attribute to these chemical emissions. However, toxicologists accept that reports of chronic lesions developing from a single exposure do not exist in the medical literature if the exposure has not caused acute manifestations. We have reviewed this (see Chapter 7).

In the 1990s, the Japanese Aum sect attacked an apartment complex with sarin, an organophosphate, causing 300 injuries and seven deaths. This sect reproduced the same act of terrorism in the Tokyo subway, with larger amounts of sarin that were dispersed in several locations from perforated sacks: 550 000 passengers complained of varied effects; 1500 victims were treated, and 12 deaths occurred. This situation demonstrated controlled evidence of the possible efficacy of good medical action management in case of chemical attack. Catastrophe is not inescapable.

Finally, in the most recent manifestation in 2002, in order to free the hostages from a Moscow theater, the Russians utilized a gas whose composition remains conjectural (opiate or volatile anesthetic?), which certainly neutralized the terrorists but also caused the deaths of 117 hostages, apparently from respiratory distress. The gas utilized was not prohibited by the Geneva Convention, the authorities said, which leaves one to suppose that it involved a medication, the more so since the antidote carried by the rescuers was naloxone, a powerful opioid antidote. Thus, a new page for toxic chemicals was opened to our communities, a phenomenon physicians know well – an efficacious medication always has a certain danger and necessitates prudence in its application and medical knowledge for its control. We will see later in this book that 'counter-terrorism' operations have a future and their own risks (see Chapter 10).

Analysis of the different chemical agents utilized or currently available

For some years, an international consensus authorized the utilization by countries of two types of chemical weapons:

- *Defoliants*, in operations against guerillas. Their massive utilization by the aerial route in Vietnam, Cambodia, and Laos, carried out during 1962–1970, was a true 'ecocide'.

- *Lacrimator gases*, in street disturbances and in all anti-riot police operations.

Neutralizing agents

Neutralizing agents were supposed to interrupt ongoing aggressive action. The lacrimators (Table 3.3) above all are tolerated and have become commonplace

Table 3.3   Lacrimator grenades (in France)

Mobile gendarmes: composition
  Chloroacetophenone (CN), 25%
  Diphenylaminochlorarsine (DW), 5%
  Kieselguhr excipients, 70%

Police
  Type 0
    Ethylbromacetate, 86.6%
    Mixture 6.3%, ethyl acetate
    Bromine products, 7.1% monobromoacetic acid
    (strong acid)
  Type 1
    Chloroacetophenone, 32%
    'Cosiba' silica flower, 10%
  Type 2
    ortho-Chlorobenzalmalononitrile (CS), 1.5%
    Ammonium chloride, 8.3%
    Ammonium perchlorate, 37.6%
    Lacotose, 35.4%
    Talc, 7.2%
    Zinc oxide, 4%
    'Araldite' mixture, 6%

Toxicity
  Ethylbromoacetate and chloroacetophenone: very weak
  ortho-Chlorobenzalmalononitrile: moderate or high
  (Some organophosphates acting at the level of the motor
  end-plates have been introduced into certain lacrimator
  grenades)

'riot-control' agents and are also currently proposed in self-defense sprays. They are basically essentially either omega-chloroacetophenone (CN), or *ortho*-chlorobenzalma-lonitrile (CS), or Adamsite (10-chloro-5,10-dihydro-phenarsazine; DM). They are lacri-mators, sternutators, and irritants.

These neutralizing agents ('short-term incapacitants', according to military terminology) rarely bring about hospitalization, either because some mucosal and ocular lesions are more mechanical than chemical, due to the propulsion of the gas, or because of bronchospasm. With regard to the latter, the possibility of development of reactive airways dysfunction syndrome (RADS, as described by Brooks: Brooks SM occupational asthma. Toxicol Lett 1995; 82–83 39–45.) following a single exposure has recently been suggested. One can consider individual variation for certain effects of neutralizing agents.

omega-Chloroacetophenone (CN)

This is a lachrimator generally disseminated in the form of aerosols at high concentra-tions. It produces an intense irritation of the nasal passages and upper airways, followed by itching and a burning sensation. Some allergic reactions have been observed.

ortho-Chlorobenzalmalononitrile (CS)

Personal defense aerosols sold commercially in France usually contain ortho-chlorobenzalmalontrile, in solution in methylene chloride, methylethylketone, and/or 1,1,1–trichloroethane. The propellants for these bombs are freons.

Symptomatology *ortho*-Chlorobenzalmolononitrile is highly irritating. Projection at a distance (greater than 1 meter) outdoors produces conjunctival hyperemia, production of tears, a burning sensation of the eyes and respiratory passages, and erythema of un-covered areas. However, prolonged exposure to high concentrations or direct splashing with the liquid (aggression from less than 1 meter) on the skin or the mucous mem-branes is responsible for caustic lesions (cutaneous burns, corneal and conjunctival ulcerations), bronchospasm, and acute pulmonary edema. *ortho*-Chlorobenzalmalono-nitrile is also a sensitizer (producing contact eczema).

Treatment Immediate cutaneous or ocular decontamination with prolonged water lavage. Initially, water exacerbates the burning sensation because it facilitates the dissociation of *ortho*-chlorobenzalmalononitrile. This effect is transient, and continu-ation of the lavage is indispensable. Decontamination for 10–15 minutes is necessary for the prevention of caustic effects. Secondarily, the treatment of cutaneous and ocular lesions is symptomatic.

The persistence of signs of respiratory irritation 1 hour after exposure requires hospitalization of the victim. Medical monitoring should be continued for at least 24 hours because of the risk of delayed acute pulmonary edema.

DM (Adamsite: 10-chloro-5,10-dihydrophenarsazine)

In aerosols at low doses, this agent provokes irritation of the upper airways, the sensitive nerve endings, and the eyes; it also irritates the skin, but to a lesser degree. At higher doses, it attacks the lower airways. This irritation is accompanied by a painful oppressive feeling and, rapidly, by vomiting, dizziness, extreme debility and generalized trembling. DM begins to act in 2–3 minutes; recovery is generally complete in 1–2 hours.

Capsaicin (pepper spray or pepper gas)

Capsaicin, from now on available in free commerce in certain countries, is derived from strong peppers. Although very irritating to the eyes and airways, it seems not to be very toxic except for some cases of laryngospasm. Treatment consists of irrigation of the eyes and skin.

Incapacitating agents

The aim of these agents is to render the military or civilian population into a state where they are unable to act in a coordinated manner for several hours or days. They are essentially psychotropics or inducers of gastrointestinal disturbances ('vomiting agents').

LSD

LSD has three characteristic types of symptoms, according to whether they are *somatic* (vertigo, debility, trembling, nausea, somnolence, paresthesias, visual disturbances), *perceptual* (alterations of shapes and colors, accommodation disturbances, exacerbation of hearing), or *psychosomatic* (mood alterations, alterations of time perception, difficulty with expression of thoughts, depersonalization, a dreamlike state, visual hallucinations).

Agent BZ (quinuclinidyl benzylate; antichlorinergic psychotropic agent)

This product was conceived to be utilized in aerosols as a combat gas. Following inhalation of high concentrations, the poisoning progresses as follows:

- In 1–4 hours: tachycardia, vertigo, ataxia, vomiting, dryness of the month, visual disturbances, confusion, apathy leading to stupor, urinary retention.

- In 4–12 hours: incapacity to react effectively to environmental stimuli or to walk around.

- In 12–96 hours: increasing activity, unforeseeable behavior, progressive return to normal in 2–4 days after exposure.

The treatment is symptomatic. A urinary catheter can prevent or treat possible urinary retention.

Other psychotropic agents

For some time the use of tranquilizers (benzodiazepines) has been proposed during the hijacking of airplanes, where they could be delivered with the food demanded by the hostage takers. In fact, hostages are forced to consume the food before the terrorists and modification of their behavior, or if they fell asleep, would be immediately suspect in the eyes of the hostage takers. Anesthetics or narcotics certainly have a future in assault operations for freeing hostages and neutralizing the terrorists. Their handling would be difficult and risky.

Gastrointestinal incapacitants ('vomiting agents')

These include emetics (e.g. apomorphine, which provokes vomiting) and inducers of diarrhea (e.g. ingested ricin oil). All others consist of the injection or inhalation of ricin, a systemic toxin. In the liquid or crystalline forms, which are prepared relatively easily, this alkaloid of ricin seed induces gastrointestinal disturbances and also necrosis of the liver, spleen, kidneys, and muscles. Death can also follow from respiratory distress (interstitial pneumonitis). The mortality is dose-dependent. There is no antidote, but symptomatic treatment can limit the toxicity. Identification of the specific antigen in the serum and in the tissues by immunohistochemisty is possible.

Gas masks, as is well known, only protect against inhalation. Some vaccines are being studied. This systemic toxicant, in our analysis, marks the transition to lethal products.

Lethal agents with predominantly local or regional toxicity

Choking agents

These have exclusively respiratory toxicity (Table 3.4). The majority are chlorine-containing compounds. They provoke lesions of acute non-cardiogenic pulmonary edema. Phosgene is the most dangerous agent of this group and the most likely to be employed for military purposes. In the presence of water, phosgene is rapidly hydrolyzed with the formation of hydrochloric acid, but the mechanism by which it attacks the alveolar-capillary membrane has not been completely elucidated. The clinical presentation evolves in three phases:

- *Exposure phase* with irritation of the eyes and upper airways (tearing, pharyngeal irritation, cough, chest tightness): this irritation disappears at the end of the exposure.
- *Asymptomatic period* of 2–6 hours.
- *Phase of non-cardiogenic pulmonary edema.* Following a lethal exposure, death occurs in 12–48 hours in a clinical picture of asphyxia due to non-cardiogenic pulmonary edema. Beyond a critical period of 2–3 days, survival is possible at the price of respiratory sequelae (secondary infections, chronic bronchitis, pulmonary fibrosis).

Table 3.4 Choking agents

Common name	Chemical name	Chemical formula
Chlorine	Chlorine	Cl_2
Phosgene	Carbon oxychloride	Cl $\backslash$ $C=O$ $/$ Cl
Palite	Monochloromethyl- chloroformate	$Cl-C-O-CH_2Cl$ $\parallel$ O
Diphosgene surplicte	Trichloromethyl- chloroformate	$Cl-C-O-CCl_3$ $\parallel$ O
Chloropicrin	Trichloro-nitromethane	NO_2-CCl_3
Methyl isocyanate	Methyl isocyanate	$CN-CH_2-CO_2-CH_3$

There is no specific therapeutic management in common with other non-cardiogenic pulmonary edema cases treated in the intensive care unit. The NATO manual proposes, amongst other measures, inhaled corticosteroid therapy followed by intravenous administration as early as possible. The combination of DBcAMP (a cyclic AMP analog), aminophylline, terbutaline, and isoprenalol experimentally reduced the pulmonary edema caused by phosgene. The mechanisms of action are still poorly elucidated and necessitate more meticulous studies in humans [1].

Since the discovery of the neurotoxicants, choking agents have gradually been abandoned by military personnel because their physicochemical properties limit their use:

- High volatility: these are in fact fleeting agents, which only act at high concentrations, and are very dependent on weather conditions.
- Reliable toxicity with nearly total protection of personnel simply by wearing respiratory protection (gas mask).

The mortality due to the use of choking agents was on the order of 2% during World War I, that is, seven times less than that from firearms. Of the total losses of the various belligerent nations, combat gases were responsible for less than 1% of the deaths.

However, choking agents are intensively utilized in our time by industry and in domestic activities, which explains the relative frequency of civilian accidents and the numerous domestic poisonings from chlorine released by certain bathroom cleaning products and toilet bowl cleaners, or from tablets for the chlorination of swimming pools.

The most publicized example remains that of the 'Bhopal tragedy' in a factory that converted methyl isocyanate to make a pesticide. This is not a chlorine-containing compound, but rather an intermediate between phosgene and a carbamate pesticide (Sevin®). At high concentrations, the isocyanates behave like choking agents.

Vesicants

Sulfur mustard (diethylsulfur dichloride; Ypérite; mustard gas) If the choking agents were the first toxic chemicals used during World War I, in 1915, the efficacy of respiratory protection afforded by gas masks was rapidly demonstrated, leading the Germans to utilize, near the town of Ypres, diethylsulfur-dichloride, dubbed 'Ypérite'. This is a liquid that, when sprayed, is absorbed by the respiratory mucosa and penetrates through clothing and through the skin. It accumulates in intertrigonal areas. Sulfur mustard alters the structure of cellular membranes, enzymatic proteins, and nucleic acids. Once bound to the tissues, nothing can oppose its action. It is classified among the lethal agents, but its military and terrorist uses seek as much its incapacitant effects, as visually well demonstrated by its action on the eyes, skin and mucous membranes. The muco-cutaneous penetration is not painful. The latency period is usually 4–10 hours, but the extension of the lesions can vary from 1 hour to several days. The clinical presentation [7] consists of:

- *Ocular injury*: conjunctival irritation, photophobia, palpebral edema, blepharospasm, corneal lesions (delay to onset, 4 hours).

- *Tracheobronchial injury*: sulfur mustard causes lesions of the respiratory tract with a presentation of tracheobronchitis (delay to onset, 8 hours); inhalation of large amounts of vapor can cause extensive mucosal necrosis. Bronchial obstruction by pseudomembranes made up of desquamated epithelium and necrotic tissue debris can then lead to death in some days in a setting of mechanical asphyxia. Bacterial superinfections are frequent.

- *Cutaneous injury*: after a latent period of a dozen hours, erythema appears, with intense pain that becomes intolerable, as well as a dark brown hyperpigmentation centered in the hair follicles, characteristic of sulfur mustard and due to hyperactivity of the melanocytes. The moist areas of the body (axillae, inguinal folds, genital organs, perineum, feet, etc.) are preferentially injured. The cutaneous lesions evolve to vesication, with the formation of bullae and then necrosis. Although the appearance of these wounds resembles those of thermal burns, they are in fact a toxic dermatitis with epidermolysis, such as that observed in Lyell's syndrome. The cutaneous lesions from sulfur mustard are distinguished from thermal burns by a small exudation of plasma, by the absence of indications for surgical intervention, and by very slow healing (several weeks). The lesions can become superinfected and evolve towards maceration.

- *Systemic toxicology* of sulfur mustard can be expressed much later in survivors. Sulfur mustard exerts radiomimetic effects on tissues, particularly on hematopoietic tissue, with the possibility of medullary aplasia, and promotes the processes of teratogenesis and carcinogenesis. Analysis of karyotypes from the injured allows monitoring.

In five cases injured by sulfur mustard treated at the Fernad-Widal Hospital, Paris, sulfur mustard and its thiodigycol metabolite could be found in the wounded soldiers up to 15 days after the contamination. The melanoderma persisted for several weeks.

Treatment of sulfur mustard poisoning. Decontamination should be immediate: it is the only means of preventing sulfur mustard from penetrating the epidermis. It is preceded by disrobing, possibly by cutting off clothing, with storage of the contaminated clothing in waterproof trash bags. Decontamination works by means of an absorbent powder, and is best with powdered gloves having Fuller's earth on one side and a cotton sponge on the other side. The glove is patted on the surface to be decontaminated, without scrubbing, and only afterwards is the injured person showered. Ocular decontamination is done by rapid and copious lavage for at least 20 minutes with an isotonic solution of sodium bicarbonate or sodium chloride.

- *Ocular lesions.* If the lesion is superficial, an anesthetic with general rather than local action should be used (local anesthetics have been implicated in aggravating corneal lesions), combined with administration of an appropriate antibacterial ointment. If the lesion proves to be more serious (vesication of the eyelids, blepharospasm, etc.), it is necessary to continue the antibiotic ointment and to instill, once daily, one drop of 1% atropine sulfate to prevent adhesions between the iris and the cornea. If purulent secretions accumulate, it is necessary to carefully wash the eyes with sterile normal saline solution and apply sterile Vaseline between the eyelids to prevent matting. In all cases, never use an occlusive eye patch in order to prevent adhesions. When the eyelids can be opened without too much pain, evaluate the corneal lesions using the fluorescein test: the appearance of green staining confirms a corneal lesion. Treatment should then be pursued in a specialized setting.

- *Cutaneous lesions.* The aim of treatment, in mild and moderate injuries, is to attenuate the itching with soothing preparations such as anti-H1 powder, calamine lotion, and corticosteroid solutions. Ointments and creams should be avoided to prevent maceration, which can generate infections. The treatment of serious cases with blisters and necrosis appears to be the classical treatment for thermal burns. Antibiotics and opiates are generally necessary.

- *Respiratory lesions.* If the injury is mild, antitussives and gargles sooth the sore throat. If the injury is severe, mechanical ventilation may be required. Absorption of sulfur mustard is 30% by the respiratory route and 70% by the cutaneous route. It is evident that a gas mask does not protect exposed populations.

- *Bone marrow aplasia* is managed in a specialized setting. The treatment is non-specific.

Lewisite (2-chlorovinyl dichloro-arsine) This is another vesicant agent whose action, as opposed to nitrogen mustard, does not show a latent period: the symptoms are immediate. It increases capillary permeability and thus generates hypovolemia, shock, and tissue necrosis. Burns and stinging are immediate, with erythema in less than 30 minutes and formation of painful blisters of the skin and mucous membranes. The eyes are injured with blepharospasm, edema, then corneal blurring in several hours: blindness can follow if ocular decontamination has not been done in less than 1 minute. Systemic signs are a combination of diarrhea, agitation, debility, hypothermia, pulmonary edema, hypotension, hemolysis, hepatic necrosis, renal tubular necrosis, and necrosis of the gastrointestinal tract and respiratory tract.

Treatment of Lewisite poisoning. Alkaline solutions degrade Lewisite. A dilute solution of sodium hypochlorite (domestic Javel water) can thus be added to the standard decontamination with soap and water. 'British Anti-Lewisite' (BAL or dimercaprol) is the specific antidote, which acts as a chelator. The indication is the existence of pulmonary edema and/or cutaneous lesions involving more than 5% of the total body surface area which could not be decontaminated in less than 15 minutes. The initial dose is 2–4 mg/kg up to 400 mg, administered by the intramuscular (i.m.) route and repeated every 4–12 hours. The injection is painful. DMSA (succimer, or dimercaptosuccinic acid) administered orally has proved to be efficacious in animal studies.

Lethal agents with predominantly systemic toxicity

This group of agents includes the cyanides, which are discussed in Chapter 5, and the neurotoxic organophosphates.

Neurotoxic organophosphates

The organophosphate compounds are inhibitors of tissue and plasma cholinesterases and thus cause poisoning by accumulation of endogenous acetylcholine. These products have been utilized since 1935 on a large scale as insecticides and were substituted, little by little, for the organochlorines because they do not accumulate in the human body, despite a significant acute toxicity. Pesticides have caused 2–5 million poisonings world-wide in half a century; among these, 400 000 have been fatal [8].

The organophosphate compounds utilized as warfare agents are only slightly modified in comparison to those for agricultural use: they are more persistent and 'aging' of the phosphorylated enzyme, which renders it unable to be reactivated, occurs much more rapidly. They are colorless or pale yellow liquid agents. The term 'gas' is therefore, in the end, improper. Amongst these, those most often stockpiled are tabun, sarin, soman, and VX, in order of their known toxicity at identical concentrations (Table 3.5).

Their penetration strength is considerable: 30% is absorbed by inhalation and 70% by the cutaneous route. Hence gas masks alone do not protect against the anticholinesterases.

Table 3.5 Organophosphate chemical weapons: G and V agents

Code	Name	Formula
GA	Tabun (ethyl-*N*,*N*-dimethyl phosphoroamidocyanidate)	$(CH_3)_2N-\overset{\displaystyle O}{\underset{\displaystyle CN}{\overset{\|}{\underset{\|}{P}}}}-OCH_2CH_3$
GB	Sarin (isopropylmethyl phosphonofluoridate)	$F-\overset{\displaystyle CH_3}{\underset{\displaystyle O}{\overset{\|}{\underset{\|}{P}}}}-OCH(CH_3)_2$
GD	Soman (pinacolylmethyl phosphonofluoridate)	$H_3C-\overset{CH_3}{\underset{CH_3}{C}}-CH_3\ C-\overset{O}{\underset{CH_3}{P}}-F$
GE	Isopropylethyl phosphonofluoridate	$(CH_3)_2CHO-\overset{\displaystyle O}{\underset{\displaystyle F}{\overset{\|}{\underset{\|}{P}}}}-CH_2CH_3$
GF	Cyclosarin (cychohexylmethyl phosphonofluoridate)	cyclohexyl $-O-\overset{\displaystyle C}{\underset{\displaystyle F}{\overset{\|}{\underset{\|}{P}}}}-CH_2CH_3$
VE	*O*-ethyl-S-[2-(diethylamino) ethyl]ethyl phosphonothioate	$CH_3CH_2O-\overset{\displaystyle CH_2CH_3}{\underset{\displaystyle O}{\overset{\|}{\underset{\|}{P}}}}-S(CH_3)_2N\underset{CH_2CH_3}{\overset{CH_2CH_3}{<}}$
VG	*O*,*O*-Diethyl-S[2-(diethylamino) ethyl] phosphorothioate	$CH_3CH_2O-\overset{\displaystyle OCH_2CH_3}{\underset{\displaystyle O}{\overset{\|}{\underset{\|}{P}}}}-S(CH_2)_2N\underset{CH_2CH_3}{\overset{CH_2CH_3}{<}}$
VM	*O*-Ethyl-S-[2-(diethylomino)ethyl] methyl phosphonothioate	$CH_3CH_2O-\overset{\displaystyle CH_3}{\underset{\displaystyle O}{\overset{\|}{\underset{\|}{P}}}}-S(CH_2)_2N\underset{CH_2CH_3}{\overset{CH_2CH_3}{<}}$
VX	*O*-Ethyl-S-[2-(diisopropylamino)ethyl] methyl phosphonothioate	$CH_3CH_2O-\overset{\displaystyle CH_3}{\underset{\displaystyle O}{\overset{\|}{\underset{\|}{P}}}}-S(CH_2)_2N\underset{CH_2(CH_3)_2}{\overset{CH_2(CH_3)_2}{<}}$

Table 3.6   Effects of neurotoxic organophosphates

Muscarinic syndrome
  Bronchospasm
  Hypersecretion: excess sweating, tearing, nasal discharge, salivation, and especially bronchial hypersecretion
  Bronchial hypersecretion can present clinically as pulmonary edema
  Chest tightness
  Gastrointestinal spasm and colic
  Fecal and urinary incontinence
  Nausea and vomiting
  Hypotension and bradycardia

Nicotinic syndrome
  Represented essentially by the curare-like effects of the neurotoxicants with fasciculations and then muscular paresis and paralysis, in particular of the respiratory muscles
  Tachycardia is frequent

Central syndrome
  Seizures
  Coma with depression of the respiratory centers

Mechanism of action The major neurotransmitter, acetylcholine, acts at four levels:

- On the postganglionic fibers of the parasympathetic system: an action called 'muscarinic', specifically inhibited by atropine.

- On synaptic transmission in the ganglions of the autonomic nervous system: an action called 'nicotinic', inhibited by the ganglioplegics.

- On neuromuscular transmission at the motor end plate.

- On the central nervous system.

The clinical presentation of poisoning by acetylcholine accumulation (Table 3.6) includes the following features:

- *Muscarinic syndrome*: miosis (without relation to the severity of the poisoning), sinus bradycardia, involuntary micturation, diarrhea, bronchospasm, and bronchial hypersecretion.

- *Nicotinic syndrome*: muscle fasciculations and cramps, tachycardia and hypertension, and occasionally mydriasis (by excitation of the superior cervical ganglion), which appears later and represents an escalation of the poisoning. The effect on the motor end plate is expressed by weakness that rapidly progresses to paralysis with respiratory arrest.

- *Central syndrome:* behavioral disturbances and ataxia precede seizures and encephalopathy with coma, contemporaneously with respiratory paralysis.

The most recent descriptions are those regarding sarin in Tokyo by Nozaki [9] and for VX.

Prevention. The gas mask by itself is a sham, because there is a totally hermetically sealed military garment for protection against the neutotoxicants.

Treatment. Physicians are currently well-equipped to counteract anticholinesterase poisoning. Decontamination should precede all treatment, according to the principles described for sulfur mustard. Assisted ventilation is remarkably efficacious and, begun in a timely manner, can be life-saving for these patients. Naturally, on the battlefield or during a chemical attack on a concentrated civilian population, the administration of antidotes is the only large-scale intervention that can be envisioned. For this purpose there are autoinjection syringes, distributed to Western armies, which contain the following ingredients in separate chambers:

- *Atropine* at a dose of 2 mg (this rather large dose explains why, when it is used in the absence of poisoning, the atropine can be responsible for delirium states; this occurred during the Gulf War, for example, in the civilian population, with some fatal outcomes). This atropine dose should be repeated about every 30 minutes until the drying of the bronchial secretions, without considering mydriasis and tachycardia.

- *Diazepam* at a dose of 10 mg to prevent anxiety and possible seizures.

- *Cholinesterase re-activators*, also called *oximes*, should be administered, preferably starting less than 10 minutes after contact with the toxicant (because of the aging of phosohorylated acetylcholinesterase) and in large doses for several days. The two oximes accepted by the WHO (World Health Organization) are obidoxime and pralidoxime (Contrathion® in France).

Acetylcholine, under the action of acetylcholinesterase, is physiologically hydrolyzed into choline and acetic acid. In cases of cholinesterase inhibition by the organophosphates, this hydrolysis no longer occurs.

With anticholinesterases with a limited duration of action (such as eserine, prostigmine, pyridostigmine), the inhibition lasts several minutes and the cholinesterase is rapidly reconstituted. The brevity of this inhibition is the basis for *preventive* treatment with pyridostigmine of troops exposed to anticholinesterase organophosphates (proposed in 1991). We review this with regard to Gulf War syndrome [10] (see Chapter 7). In the case of organophosphates, only the oximes, utilized rapidly, allow this regeneration.

The preference between obidoxime and pralidoxime essentially involves the difference in osmolality: obidoxime is a bispyridium-di-oxime, a large molecule with two antidotal functional groups, while pralidoxime is a mono-pyridinium-mono-oxime, a small molecule with a single antidotal functional group (Figure 3.1).

Obidoxime, which has an osmolality equal to twice that of plasma, is thus more efficacious by the subcutaneous route and less painful than pralidoxime, whose osmolality is eight times greater. Clearly this inconvenience disappears with intravenous administration.

No conventional oximes have proven efficacy for soman. The Hagedorn group of Fribourg has synthesized some other oximes (H) whose strength of reactivation has been shown to be correct *in vitro* as well as experimentally. Unfortunately, this efficacy has not been found in human muscle (Table 3.7). Certain countries, especially South America, currently doubt the actual benefit of oximes during chemical terrorism operations and propose the use of sodium bicarbonate [11]. Chronic nervous sequelae after application of organophosphates in a bombing situation remain unproven and in all cases do not seem to have benefited from the use of oximes [11].

Chemical munitions and their delivery methods

The dispersion packaging of a chemical agent is clearly of primordial importance for its efficacy. It can thus be a matter of a spraying procedure from an airplane or helicopter, possibly on an aboriginal population. In the Tokyo subway, the simplicity of the dispersion devices (containers pierced with holes) without doubt contributed to the relatively benign mass sarin poisoning. It can be a matter of explosives, essentially artillery shells, rockets, missiles, possibly 'tactical', that is, with small ranges (about 600 km).

Long-range missiles, called 'strategic', apparently do not seem to merit the considerable expense that equipping them with chemical agents would necessitate: the efficacy:price ratio would certainly be mediocre, even given the dispersion of the products after an explosion. Aerial bombs also are rarely equipped with toxicants, among other reasons undoubtedly because of the difficulty of over-flying enemy airspace during a conflict. According to their protocols, strategic missiles pose a deterrent threat in all wars. The possibility of their detection, after the battle, allows them to be a retrospective threat to the victor.

Hand grenades can be chemical weapons. It is true that they could only be used for intervention in hand-to-hand combat or in enclosed spaces. The Soviets exposed their chemical arsenal in 1987 for purposes that seemed to be as much deterrent as political (Figure 3.2). The arsenal comprised all the dispersal devices/methods listed above (except for strategic missiles).

The majority of dispersion procedures thus utilize explosives as delivery systems. These are, by themselves, formidable for humans, responsible for the effects of overpressure injuries or blasts that cause barotraumas, for destruction of buildings with consequent human injuries, and for thermal and seismic effects, all of which certainly

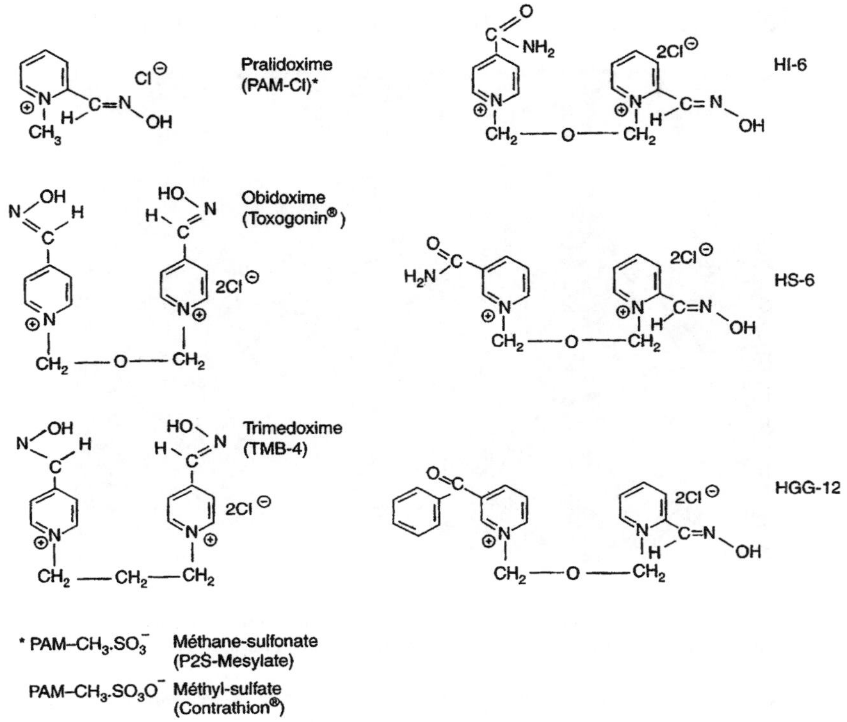

Figure 3.1 The various oximes

Table 3.7 Activity of pyridinium-aldoximes in soman poisoning in several animal models, including human

Preparation	Mouse or rat	Dog	Marmoset diaphragmatic muscle	Human erythrocytes	Human intercostal muscle
Obidoxime	0	0	0	0	0
Pralidoxime	0	0	+/±	0	0
HS-6	++	+	±/0	+	0
HI–6	++	+	±	++	0
HGG-12	+	++	–	±	0

The Soviets show their chemical weapons to the experts

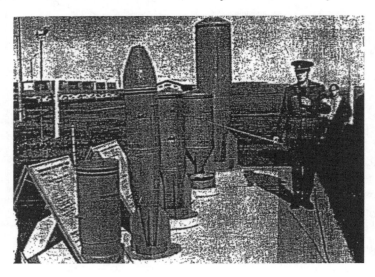

A soviet military representative explains the details of Russian chemical weapons deployed at the Shikhany military installation to participants of the Geneva talks on weapons. Photo, Reuter.

Moscow – The Soviet authorities have exhibited a military complex for chemical weapons on the Volga to military and diplomatic experts from 45 nations, insisting on the desire of the Kremlin for an accord for banning chemical weapons.

This unusual access to their military preparations came from an initiative of Mikhail Gorbachev, who last year had breached discussions on chemical weapons, which had commenced about 20 years earlier in 1968.

Three representatives from each of 40 nations represented in this colloquium at Geneva, plus some representatives from five observing countries, were allowed to view 19 specimens of chemical weapons at the Shikhony military camp on the Volga, according to the Tass news agency.

Of the deployed weapons, 10 were artillery shells and rockets, two were chemical warheads for tactical missiles, six were aerial bombs and spray products, and one represented a hand grenade.

Workers from the camp explained the nature of the toxic agents and responded to questions.

General Anatoly Kuntsevich, weapons expert from the Ministry of Defense, said that although the Soviet Union had shown its chemical weapons, 'the US authorities ostensibly adopted the decision to commence the production of binary weapons (made of two chemical products)'.

Last month, the Soviets allowed four members of the US government to observe a complex in Siberia that the Regan administration had declared in violation of the 1972 anti-ballistic missile treaty.

Figure 3.2 Exposition of chemical weapons by the Russian army in 1987. Adapted from Straight Time, Singapore, 1987

add to the panic of populations who become terrified by the eruption of unknown gases or liquids.

Workers in armament factories have sometimes been victims of occupational accidents during their work. It is by their description in Russian or American medical journals that physicians have been able to understand the actual toxicity of military chemical agents and to verify the efficacious treatments. With a view to protecting

Table 3.8 Stockpiles of chemical agents*

Chemical agent declared (in tons)	
Lewisite	6745
Sulfur mustard/Lewisite (mixture)	344
Sulfur mustard	13 839
Tabun	2
Sarin	15 048
Soman	9175
Agent VX	4032
Agent VR (or soman or VX)	15 548
Isopropyl alcohol, isopropylamine (binary weapon)	731
Methylphosphoryl difluoride (binary weapon)	444
Diisopropylamine ethyl methyl phosphonate (organophosphate)	46
Unknown	4
Chloroethanol	302
Thiodiglyol	51
Phosgene	5

*According to the Organization for the Prohibition of Chemical Weapons (OPCW) (2000).

this worker population in the USA, certain weapons have been supplied as 'binary munitions', made up of two elements which separately are neutral, and which become dangerous after they have been dropped and exploded. This is the case especially for weapons containing neurotoxic organophosphate gases.

Table 3.9 Comparison between chemical and biological agents

Factors	Chemical terrorism	Biological terrorism
Onset of signs	Several seconds to several hours	Several days to many weeks
Distribution of victims	Follow the direction(s) for leaving the dispersal site	Large dispersion
First aid	Pre-hospital emergency services	Hospitals and community physicians
Dispersion site	Rapidly known	Difficult to identify
Decontamination of victims	Frequently necessary	Generally secondary
Treatments	Symptomatic treatments: Assisted ventilation Re-hydration	Vaccines, antibiotics
Isolation/quarantine	Useless after decontamination	Crucial if contagious pathology

The dangers of the different toxic agents that could be utilized in terrorist actions are highly variable according to their intrinsic toxicity, as we have seen. They are thus also strongly dependent on the munition, its strength and load, its range, the chosen delivery method, and of its extensive possibilities. Table 3.8 lists the officially reported stockpiles of chemical weapons that exist today. This list is not exempt from manipulation: certain countries have an interest in exaggerating the threat of the weapons stockpiles. Others, on the contrary, wish to underestimate their potential. Table 3.9 schematically compares the evolution, the degree of urgency, and the treatment of chemical and biological aggressions, to make the transition with the chapter dedicated to biological agents (Chapter 11).

References

1. Bismuth C, Barriot P. Armes chimiques, dangerosité et prise en charge. *Encyclopédie Médecine, Chirurgie, Toxicologie. Paris: Éditions Techniques*, 1993; 16–650-A-10.
2. Official Iranian document, November, 1986.
3. Inns RH, Marrs TC. Prophylaxis against anticholinesterase poisoning. In Ballantyne B, Marrs TC (eds), *Clinical and Experimental Toxicology of Organophosphate and Carbamate*. Oxford: Butterworth-Heinemann, 1992: 602–610.
4. Karalliedde L, Meredith T. Socio-economics, health issues and pesticides. In Karalliedde L, Feldman S, Henry J, Marrs T (eds), *Organophosphates and Health*. London: Imperial College Press, 2001: 37–59.
5. Lachaux G, Delhomme P. *La Guerre des Gaz*. Paris: Hégide, 1985: 1–7.
6. Marrs TC, Maynard RL. Organophosphorus chemical warfare. In Karalliedde L, Feldman S, Henry J, Marrs T (eds), *Organophosphates and Health*. London: Imperial College Press, 2001: 83–108.
7. Nozaki H, Aikawa N, Fujishima S. *et al*. A case of VX poisoning and the difference from sarin. *Lancet*, 1995; 346: 698–699.
8. United Nations Agreement, April 1987.
9. Society for Medical Care of Chemical War Victims. Islamic Republic of Iran, November, 1987.
10. Sohaabpour H. Observation and clinical manifestations of patients injured with mustard gas. *Med J Islamic Republic Iran Rabiolaval*, 1987; 1408: 32–37.
11. Willems JL, Dons D. The United Nations and chemical disarmament. Role of medical experts in the verification of alleged use. *Ann Med Milit Belg*, 1999; 7: 157–175.

4

Chemical terrorism and cyanide

Arnaud Delahaye and Frédéric Baud

Hydrocyanic acid (HCN) and compounds that release cyanide ions are lethal agents. Hydrocyanic acid is rapidly absorbed by all routes (inhalation, percutaneous, ingestion). Hydrogen cyanide terrorism can be conceived either by direct utilization of a cyanogenic product, or by causing an industrial chemical accident (metallurgic, petrochemical, etc.) in an urban setting, or in the course of setting fires with combustion of natural (silk, wool, etc.) or synthetic (polyurethanes, polyamides, etc.) polymers containing nitrogen. War gases can be dispersed by low-altitude airborne spraying or by artillery munitions (missiles, rockets, artillery shells, etc.). The volatility of HCN, much lighter than air, is such that it is difficult to maintain high concentrations in an open and hot environment during spraying. Exposure to HCN must above all be feared in an enclosed setting. Contamination of water, food, and medications by cyanide is possible but very difficult.

The products and their effects on the body

HCN is a colorless gas with a characteristic odor of bitter almonds which, however, is not perceived by about half the population. All agents that release cyanide ions in the body can be utilized as chemical weapons.

Cyanogen chloride (CNCl) results from the reaction of a halogen (chloride) and HCN. It is a war gas that possesses the systemic toxic properties of HCN combined with the eye and pulmonary irritant properties of chlorine.

There are numerous salts of HCN [1]: sodium cyanide, potassium cyanide, gold cyanide, mercuric oxycyanide. These products are generally in the form of water-soluble powders which, when mixed with an acid solution, instantaneously release HCN gas.

The aliphatic nitriles [2] are in the form of volatile liquids. Intoxication is percutaneous, by inhalation after evaporation, or by ingestion. Release of cyanide ions in the course of hepatic metabolism of the nitriles explains the delayed appearance of the clinical signs, from minutes to several hours.

Cyanide causes dysfunction of cellular respiration by rapid binding to mitochondrial cytochrome oxidase. Inhibition of the respiratory chain and deviation of metabolism

Treating Victims of Mass Destsuction   Edited by Patrick Barriot and Chantal Bismuth
© 2008 John Wiley & Sons, Ltd

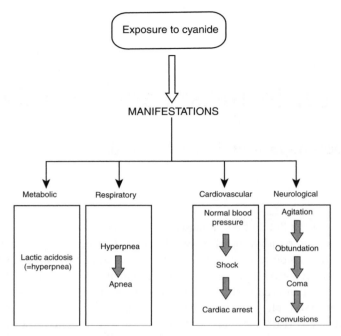

Figure 4.1   Clinical manifestations of cyanide exposure

to the anaerobic pathway is the origin of metabolic acidosis with increased plasma lactate levels.

Unfortunately, physiological detoxification is rapidly saturable. The biochemical mechanisms involved are: transformation of cyanide to thiocyanate by thiosulfate sulfur transferase (or rhodanese of Lang); binding to organic metal ions, such as the iron of methemoglobin or the cobalt of cobalamin; binding to carbonyl compounds; and unchanged elimination in the urine and by the respiratory route.

Clinical poisoning (Figure 4.1)

After inhalation, there rapidly follow: nasal and laryngeal irritation; dyspnea, with a feeling of suffocation and chest tightness; and air hunger and significant polypnea in response to metabolic acidosis. Systemic toxicity is a combination of cardiac, neurological, and respiratory effects.

The cardiovascular manifestations begin with shock with a preserved heart rate, followed by ventricular extrasystoles, and then asystolic cardiac arrest. In hyperacute forms, cardiac arrest occurs within seconds following inhalation.

The neurological manifestations begin in a deceptively non-specific fashion with headache, dizziness, anxiety, confusion, or paradoxical agitation. Symptomatology that rapidly becomes severe, with convulsive crises, profound and hypotonic coma, is the hallmark of hyperacute poisoning.

The respiratory effects of cyanide comprise an early phase with hyperventilation in response to metabolic acidosis, followed by inhibition of the central respiratory center that causes bradypnea and then respiratory arrest. Because of the impairment of oxygen consumption, cyanosis is absent and the skin and mucous membranes remain pink.

In ingestion cases, the delay before the appearance of these disturbances is much longer, on the order of 30 minutes or more. Similarly, with percutaneous absorption the asymptomatic latent interval can be several hours.

Diagnosis of cyanide poisoning

Exposure to a gas or liquid in an enclosed or open space, whether or not it follows an explosion, with development of neurological, cardiovascular, and respiratory signs, should lead to the suspicion of cyanide exposure. One of the differential diagnoses is intoxication with neurotoxic organophosphates, but mydriasis is a sign of cyanide poisoning, while miosis is a sign of organophosphate poisoning which also induces fasciculations and numerous muscarinic signs.

The presence of numerous deaths, which can include all the persons exposed, and the rapid evolution of symptoms aids in the diagnosis. At intervention sites, such as during fires, the presence of cyanide in ambient air can be detected by a colorimetric reaction. The threshold concentration considered to be dangerous is approximately 20 parts per million (ppm) and the lethal threshold is greater than 100 ppm.

Metabolic acidosis with elevation of plasma lactate is correlated with the severity of the poisoning [3]. In a context suggesting cyanide intoxication, a plasma lactate level ≥8 mmol/l (normal 1–2 mmol/l) is a sensitive and specific sign of severe intoxication, defined by a whole blood cyanide concentration greater than 40 μmol/l. In this manner, at intervention sites, biological measurements allow responders to identify victims of cyanide poisoning and to decide about the necessity to begin antidote treatment. The presence of metabolic acidosis with an elevated anion gap (≥16 mmol/l) has the same diagnostic value as elevated plasma lactate level.

Measurement of whole blood cyanide necessitates a blood sample in an anticoagulant tube. It is never done in plasma or serum. In the laboratory, HCN is measured in 90 minutes by gas chromatography or spectrophotometry. Its blood half-life of 60 minutes necessitates sampling as early as possible and preferably, except in emergencies, before antidote treatment. A concentration ≥40 μmol/l or about 1 mg/l (μmol/l × 0.027 = about mg/l) is considered toxic, and a concentration (≥100 μmol/l (2.7 mg/l) is considered to be potentially lethal. The biotransformation and detoxification of cyanide by thiosulfate leads to the formation of thiocyanate ions, which are measurable in serum or urine. Cyanocobalamin, product of the transformation with hydroxocobalamin, shows the presence of redistributed and bound cyanide. Its measurement in the plasma or urine retrospectively confirms cyanide poisoning.

For deceased victims, HCN can be measured by taking blood samples under the same conditions. Interpretation of the measurements should take into account the delay before sampling after the exposure and death, as well as the preservation procedures utilized.

Protection and victim decontamination

In the hospital setting, it is improbable that victims would arrive spontaneously and be so highly contaminated as to pose a risk to personnel. Hospital management does not require any particular protective measures.

Victim management (Figure 4.2)

Symptomatic treatment is essential to management and aims to correct the visceral adverse effects. It should be adapted to the severity of the clinical presentation. Direct mouth-to-mouth resuscitation is advised against in cyanide-poisoned patients because of the risk of poisoning to the rescuer. High-flow oxygen therapy or endotracheal intubation and ventilation with an inspired oxygen concentration (FiO2) of 100% should be done as soon as possible. Shock is corrected by intravascular volume expansion and/or utilization of catecholamines. Cardiocirculatory arrest, whose management is not specific, can require cardiorespiratory resuscitation of long duration. On the neurological level, seizures are usually managed with diazepam or clonazepam.

There are a number of specific treatments. They are all efficacious; the problems are their adverse effects and their cost. Oxygen is the first of these antidotes; among other effects, it causes reactivation of cytochrome oxidase.

Cobalt derivatives are the principal antidotes utilized during cyanide poisoning. Dicobalt EDTA (Kelocyanor®) is prescribed in adults in a direct intravenous dose of 300–600 mg without prior preparation. Its administration is followed by hypertonic glucose (30%) because of induced hypoglycemia. A second ampoule should be administered 15 minutes later in the absence of response to the first dose. Although cobalt is not devoid of adverse effects (shock or hypertension, tachycardia, intestinal upsets, and allergic reactions), its rapid utilization, immediate efficacy, and moderate cost allow large stockpiles to be kept. There is no pediatric dosing schedule, however.

Hydroxocobalamin (Cyanokit®) is infused at a dose of 5 g (70 mg/kg in children) over 15 minutes after reconstitution of the injectable solution in 100 ml normal saline. This initial dose can also be repeated. In our experience, utilization of high doses of hydroxocobalamin during severe cyanide poisoning allows immediate correction of circulatory shock. Hydroxocobalamin is devoid of adverse effects, except for a transitory reddish mucocutaneous coloration and production of reddish urine for 7 days, but its relatively high cost limits keeping large stockpiles that must be replaced.

Sodium thiosulfate, natural substrate of the rhodanese of Lang, is efficacious but its action is slow and it is therefore not an antidote of first resort for acute poisoning. It is administered in a slow intravenous dose of 12 g (over 15 minutes) following utilization of an immediately efficacious antidote (cobalt derivatives). Thiosulfate should not be mixed in the same bottle as hydroxocobalamin, with which it reacts.

Methemoglobin-inducing agents (amyl nitrite, sodium nitrite, etc.) are no longer utilized in France but are still proposed by the WHO as contingency antidotes. They form

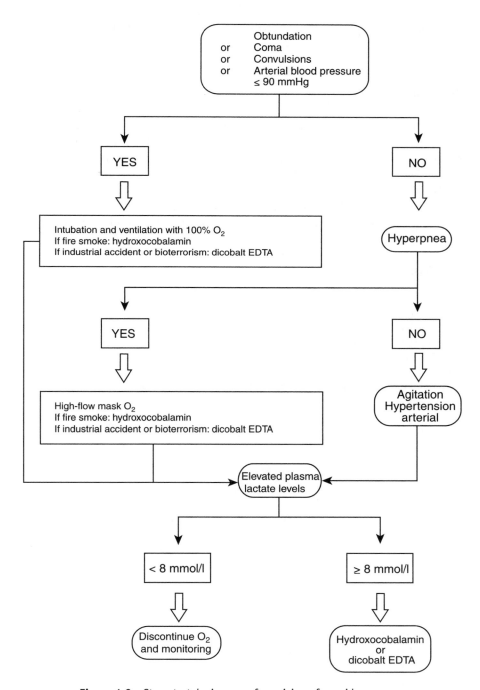

Figure 4.2 Steps to take in case of suspicion of cyanide exposure

non-toxic but reversible complexes (cyanmethemoglobin). Moreover, they decrease oxygen transport and aggravate toxicants such as carbon monoxide during exposure to fire smoke.

Conclusion

As with other toxicants, hydrocyanic acid exposure can be envisioned in terms of chemical terrorism [4]. It is certainly the most dangerous of the lethal toxicants, with a mortality close to 100% in an enclosed environment. The emergent therapeutic approach should be made on clinical grounds and a suggestive context; toxicological analysis confirms the poisoning later. Other than decontamination of the victims limited to the accident site, resuscitation of poisoned patients relies on symptomatic treatment and antidotes. Oxygen and the cobalt compounds should be preferred.

References

1. Benaissa L, Hantson P, Laforge M *et al.* Cyanures et toxiques cyanogéniques. *Encyclopédie Médecine, Chirurgie, Toxicologie.* Paris: Elsevier, 1999; 16–048-C-20, 7 pp.
2. Baud F, Benaissa L. Cyanures et nitrites. In Bismuth C *et al.* (eds), *Toxicologie Clinique.* Paris: Flammarion Médecine–Sciences, 2000: 907–918.
3. Baud F, Borron SW, Mégarbane B *et al.* Value of lactic acidosis in the assessment of the severity of acute cyanide poisoning. *Crit Care Med,* 2002; **30**: 2044–2050.
4. Bismuth C, Barriot B, Baud FJ. Le risqué chimique en situation de guerre. *Urgences,* 1993; **1**: 25–31.

5

Why chemical weapons were not used during World War II and the use of such weapons by terrorists

Robert L. Maynard and Timothy C. Marrs

Chemical weapons were used on a large scale during World War I and not at all during World War II, at least not in Europe. No satisfactory explanation has emerged for this general and unexpected reluctance to use such weapons. It is true that the effectiveness of chemical weapons declined significantly between 1915 and 1918: their use as a weapon of surprise against unprotected troops was certainly effective, although well-protected troops came to endure their use with comparatively little loss. It may be that it was realized that, except on a static battlefield, chemical weapons could produce little more than harassment of well-protected defensive formations; on a mobile battlefield they seemed ineffective. Development of chemical weapons had been rapid in the period 1915–1918 [1]. The first and very effective gas cloud attacks using chlorine were replaced by chemical shells fired by artillery. Although hundreds of different compounds were studied, the major weapons, phosgene as a lethal weapon and sulfur mustard as a casualty producer, were not surpassed. Irritants included a wide range of tear gases and compounds intended to break the protection afforded by respirators proved less effective than their developers had hoped. Contemporary accounts from late in the period do not pay great attention to these weapons [2]. Despite this, chemical weapons acquired a reputation for producing casualties and contemporary medical accounts provide eloquent testimony to the suffering of casualties. The War Poets recorded these effects and one German soldier, Adolf Hilter, left a detailed account of the effects of exposure to mustard gas [3,4] after the prolonged effects of damage to the respiratory system produced by chlorine were recorded after the war [5].

In the aftermath of World War I, chemical warfare was considered to be an egregious development, but some research into chemical weapons continued. There were few significant developments, although Lee Lewis's development of the arsenical vesicant Lewisite stands out [1]. Detailed account of chemicals developed after World War I can be found in Prentiss's classic account [1] and also in the first volume of the series of books produced by the Stockholm International Panel Research Institute (SIPRI)

Treating Victims of Mass Destsuction   Edited by Patrick Barriot and Chantal Bismuth
© 2008 John Wiley & Sons, Ltd

[6]. The account in the latter work of the rise of chemical and biological weapons is particularly well documented. Mustard gas was used by Italian forces in the Abyssinian campaign in the mid-1930s but this seems to have been an isolated incident.

It is now known that organophosphorus nerve agents were developed in Germany in the late 1930s. Schrader's work on insecticides revealed that fluorophosphorous compounds had marked mammalian toxicity, but the first nerve agent, tabun, was not a phosphorofluoridate and in fact is ethyl N,N-dimethylphosphosamido-cyanidate. This agent was apparently first prepared on December 23, 1936 [6]. Rapid production followed, with a production plant being established at Dyernfurth in Silesia (now Poland). Some 12 000 tons of tabun had been produced by 1945 but none was used. This was not due to difficulties in weaponization: a British report referenced in the SIPRI account by Perry-Robinson stated that 1200–1500 tons of tabun had been weaponized. Sarin was also produced, although in much smaller amounts, and soman, although developed, was not produced in quantity.

Work on chemical warfare agents in Allied countries also continued during World War II, although no compounds approaching nerve agents, in their extraordinary combination of toxicity and bulk production, were developed. Attention was focused on mustard gas, and in 1943 a US ship carrying 100 tons of mustard-filled bombs was blown up by German bombing in Bari harbour in Italy [6]. Eighty-one men died of mustard gas injuries. It is interesting that mustard gas contamination of casualties was not anticipated, and Perry-Robinson records that rescuers from another ship were so affected by secondary contamination produced by landing casualties that almost all the rescue crew were temporarily blinded and the rescue ship had difficulty reaching port. The author pointed out that almost an entire ship's crew had been incapacitated by exposure to perhaps 1 kg of mustard gas.

Towards the end of World War II, much of the nerve agent at the Dyernfurth plant was poured into the River Oder, and although the Germans tried to destroy the plant it appears that the plant was dismantled and sent to the USSR.

Willingness to use mustard gas and other weapons, including anthrax, was shown by Allied leaders. The official biography of Sir Winston Churchill records several occasions when the Prime Minister called for a close examination of mustard gas, as both a defensive and an offensive weapon [7], but no chemical warfare agent was used by the UK.

It may be that both sides overestimated the other's capacity to wage an effective chemical campaign. Such a campaign was certainly feared. In England the official handbook on Air Raid Precautions contains detailed descriptions of the effects of the compounds used in World War I and all citizens of the UK were provided with gas masks [8]. Little reluctance to attack civilian targets with high explosives without warning was shown by either side, and technical developments in ammunitions seem likely to have solved some of the problems encountered during World War I. There seems then, to be no clear answer as to why chemical weapons were not used during World War II: their absence continues to be an enigma.

Just as the reluctance to use chemical weapons during World War II remains unexplained, so does the very limited use of chemicals of all sorts by terrorists. Although attacks on military and civilian targets by well-organized terrorist groups have become common, the use of toxic chemicals in such incidents remains remarkably rare. The present authors are reluctant to speculate at length on the reasons for this – a sense of gratitude seems more appropriate. Contemporary and freely available accounts of chemical weapons list compounds that could be used [9]. These include classical chemical warfare agents and industrial compounds, which might offer the advantage of being easier to obtain. The authors are aware that details of how to produce chemicals that could be used are all too available but, again, we are reluctant to pursue these points.

Instead, we focus on incidents that occurred in Japan in the mid-1990s. These were extraordinary in that they involved the use of the nerve agent, sarin. Sarin, with its fluoride-leaving group, was generally regarded as one of the more difficult nerve agents to produce in bulk. Despite this, a well-organized religious terrorist group set up a small-scale production plant and produced enough sarin to mount two effective incidents. These are considered in detail. That such incidents could occur again is clear and some discussion of how casualties should be managed also seems appropriate.

The better known of the two major Japanese incidents occurred on March 20, 1995, when five subway trains were attacked in Tokyo [10]. About 600 g of sarin was placed in 11 plastic bags containing newspapers, and the bags sealed. These bags were then placed in five subway train carriages. Sarin was released by the simple process of piercing the plastic bags with umbrellas. Sarin is a comparatively volatile nerve agent (saturated vapor pressure at 20°C is 2–10 mmHg and the boiling point is 147°C) and sarin vapor would have been released from the plastic bags. As concentrations rose, the first effects–dimming of vision, pain in the eyes, running of the nose, and perhaps some tightening of the chest – would have been experienced. That an emergency had occurred was rapidly recognized. No detailed accounts have been published of the panic that may have occurred amongst people who staggered and collapsed. Details have, however, been produced of the casualties who appeared at hospitals. Thousands were affected: one estimate gives a figure of 4000. Sidell [11] reported that 984 people were moderately affected, 37 severely affected, 17 critically and 12 died: in all, 1050 were affected. He added that 4973 patients were seen at hospitals on the first day but not admitted. The much larger number seeking attention than were actually affected was stressed by Woodall [12]. It seems unlikely that as many people could have been directly affected by sarin released as described above, but the fear that they might have been exposed and that they would soon develop symptoms and perhaps collapse may well have driven them to hospital. Twelve people died: 11 passengers and 1 cleaner who attempted to remove contaminated material from a subway carriage. Some needed intensive care, involving the use of supported ventilation. The other casualties were less affected and the symptoms and clinical signs most commonly in need of treatment were eye pain and miosis [13].

The deduction that people had been exposed to some compound that led to an accumulation of acetylcholine seems to have been rapidly made. Miosis proved an excellent guide. It is difficult to think of anything other than exposure to a nerve agent that could render hundreds of people suddenly miotic. This is easy to say now, but doctors faced with the first few casualties, some walking, some collapsed, and some dead or dying, must have wondered what had happened. Bradycardia is a usual sign of nerve agent exposure: tachycardia was recorded. This was attributed to a nicotinic effect of acetylcholine at sympathetic ganglia [14].

Atropine and supported ventilation were the main therapeutic measures used. Eye pain produced by constrictor pupillary and cilary muscle spasm was relieved with atropine eye drops. This approach was effective [14].

Despite the fact that some casualties needed supported ventilation, no cases of the Intermediate Syndrome were recorded and no cases of delayed polyneuropathy have been recorded. It is believed that the Intermediate Syndrome could be produced by exposure to nerve agents, but delayed polyneuropathy, which is associated with and possibly caused by inhibition of the neuropathy target esterase enzyme (NTE), is very unlikely, given the much greater affinity of nerve agents such as sarin for acetylcholinesterase (AChE) than for NTE. In the authors' view, exposure to enough sarin to have a significant effect on NTE would be rapidly lethal, due to inhibition of AChE.

The other, but less effective, Japanese incident occurred before the attack on the Tokyo subway trains. A group of terrorists dispersed sarin from a lorry, using a heater to warm the liquid sarin and a fan to disperse the vapor [15]. The attack took place in a residential area of Matsumoto at midnight on June 27, 1994. The fact that the attack occurred at night, when few people were on the streets, limited its effectiveness, although some people living locally in apartment buildings were affected. Seven people were killed and 600 affected; 52 rescue workers were employed in the contaminated area and of these 18 were affected. Rescue workers exhibited the classical effects of exposure to nerve agent vapor: eye pain, darkening of the visual field, nausea, vomiting, running nose, fatigue, and shortness of breath. One rescuer was admitted to hospital and successfully treated with atropine and oxygen.

These, then were the two major Japanese incidents. A single report of an assassination attempt using VX has also been recorded: this appears to have been ineffective but details are lacking [16].

A number of lessons can be learnt from the Japanese incidents described above:

1. Nerve agents can be produced and deployed in significant quantities by well-funded and well-organized terrorist groups, the main difficulty probably being the acquisition of the reactive intermediates required for synthesis.

2. Nerve agents can be deployed effectively using simple technology.

3. Many casualties can be produced by releasing fairly small quantities of nerve agents in enclosed spaces.

4. Although the ratio of mildly affected to severely affected individuals is high, hospitals may be flooded with patients seeking treatment and reassurance.

5. Atropine and supported ventilation are the keys to the successful management of nerve agent casualties.

6. Delayed effects of moderate exposure to sarin are unlikely. The last point, regarding delayed effects, should perhaps be modified to take into account some effects reported. Hatta *et al.* reported the case of a 35 year-old man exposed to sarin in the Tokyo subway [17]. He was severely affected, experiencing convulsions and needing artificial respiration. He was treated with atropine and pralidoxime iodide. His plasma cholinesterase level returned to normal in 3 weeks and the red cell cholinesterase level in 3 months. Detailed neuropsychological testing at 6 months post-exposure revealed memory defects, in particular a difficulty in consolidating new learning and adding this to memory. Personality changes, including passivity and shallow affect, were also reported. Follow-up of casualties from the Matsumoto incident has been reported [18]. Among the 149 casualties selected on the basis of cholinesterase depression or miosis, four of six severely poisoned patients showed EEC changes at 1 or 2 years post-exposure, one patient developed sensory polyneuropathy 7 months post-exposure and showed a reduction in sensory nerve conduction velocity, and one patient showed visual field defects at 1 year follow-up, although these resolved completely by 17 months. A further study of those exposed in Tokyo revealed that in some subjects miosis was slow to resolve (up to 90 days), and that in some subjects visual evoked potentials were abnormal 6–8 months post-exposure [19]. These effects should be carefully noted: experience with sarin poisoning is very limited.

7. Identification of the compound used in a terrorist incident is as likely to depend upon deductions drawn from examination of casualties as from any physicochemical means of identifying the agents. Detectors that can identify nerve agents have been developed for use by military forces. These include the Chemical Agent Monitor (CAM), an instrument developed in the UK [20]. It seems unlikely that such devices could be made available at all possible targets of terrorist attack, the number of possible targets being vast. Being able to deduce the compound or class of compound used from clinical examination is thus likely to remain the most rapid form of identification.

As stated earlier, a wide range of compounds could be attractive to terrorists. Ricin received a good deal of publicity in early 2003 as a result of a police investigation of premises in London. Ricin, unlike nerve agents, cannot be readily synthesized in the laboratory but it can be extracted from castor oil seeds. The product is water-soluble and could be dispersed as an aerosol. Inhalation of ricin leads to a severe pneumonitis that is difficult to treat [21–23].

Planning to deal with terrorist incidents involving the release of toxic and perhaps lethal chemicals may engender a sense of despair. Launching an effective response will certainly be difficult but by no means impossible. It should be recalled that incidents involving the release of toxic chemicals occur frequently as a result of industrial accidents. Some, such as the release of methyl isocyanate and perhaps other compounds at Bhopal in India, may have devastating consequences [24]. Others, such as the release of dioxin compounds at Seveso in Italy, may have lesser immediate consequences in terms of loss of life, but greater long-term consequences in terms of possible delayed effects and, more importantly, fear that such effects may occur [25]. Most developed countries are prepared to deal with such incidents and it is from these preparations that we should learn how to deal with terrorist incidents involving the release of chemicals.

An essential first step in developing a plan for handling such casualties is to decide how soon after exposure to toxic chemicals therapy will be made available. In the case of exposure to nerve agents, the armed forces of many countries rely on a system of self-aid and buddy aid and troops are trained to both recognize the effects of nerve agents in themselves and in colleagues and to self-administer auto-injection devices or administer them to others. These generally contain atropine and an oxime and, in some cases, an anticonvulsant agent [26]. Such immediacy of treatment is not likely to be available in the civilian setting. Similarly, completely protected medical and paramedical staff are unlikely to be available in sufficient numbers to make rapid administration of therapy possible. It should be recalled that of all the chemicals that could be used by terrorists and which are likely to be lethal, only the effects of nerve agents are amenable to rapid and feasible antidotal therapy. Protection of rescue staff is critical: the experience of staff being secondarily affected by sarin in Matsumoto has already been described. Medical staff wearing satisfactory protective equipment will not find conducting a conventional medical examination easy: in fact, they may find it impossible. Thick protective gloves, a respirator and a hood deprive the doctor of his/her ability to feel a pulse or to listen to the heartbeat or breathing. The faculties of the doctor are thus reduced and only observation can be relied upon. Miosis, running noses, dribbling, cyanosis, twitching, semi-consciousness and coma may all be recognized by observation alone, and on the basis of such observations treatment should be commenced. In some cases, medical and paramedical staff may be held back until patients have been decontaminated and are safe to examine. This will cause a delay in giving antidotes. Training non-medical staff to recognise specific signs of poisoning is difficult but may have to be attempted, along with developing systems so that such staff can give antidotes at least intramuscularly. Atropine and oximes can be given intramuscularly, although this route produces less rapid effects than the intravenous route.

In all emergency patient care, it is essential to remember that the accepted rules apply.

Ensuring a satisfactory airway, maintaining respiration and, if possible, the functioning of the heart. Oro-pharyngeal airways and 'Ambu'-style bags should be used as close to the site of the incident as possible. Ambu bags should be protected with butyl rubber outer jackets and the air intake should be equipped with a canister filter, similar to that used in personal protective equipment. Portable ventilators should also be deployed [27].

Chemical casualties may need decontamination. This places an added strain on rescue workers: one-to-one care may be needed during decontamination and rescue workers themselves may need to pass through the mobile shower system that may have been provided. Decontamination in a mass casualty situation presents formidable problems and extensive rehearsals of procedures are necessary.

In any decontamination plan, an essential principle is simplicity. Warm water and detergent are the most useful decontaminants. The addition of low-concentration chlorinating agents, e.g. hypochlorite or bleach, may help but may also complicate matters. Concerns about achieving the correct concentration of bleach may lead to unacceptable delays. In an emergency, a fine warm water spray generated by fire tenders may be the best option. Even well-drilled decontamination teams cannot thoroughly decontaminate a casualty in less than about 10 minutes: triage will be essential to ensure that those most in need of care reach medical and paramedical staff first. In the case of casualties contaminated with liquids, removal of all clothing is the first priority. If this is done, up to 80% of contamination may be rapidly removed: clothing must be placed in sealed plastic bags. In the Tokyo subway incident, patients did not generally need decontamination: had mustard gas been used, the effects on attendants dealing with undecontaminated casualties would have been very different.

Decontamination close to the scene of an incident is critically important. Some casualties may, however, evade this process – deliberately or accidentally – and may make their way to hospital. Facilities for decontamination at Accident and Emergency Departments will thus also be important and should be established.

Handling a terrorist incident involving more than a trivial release of toxic chemicals will inevitably be difficult. Only a thorough examination of possible scenarios, the development of plans and the repeated exercise of such plans will provide any assurance of success. From a clinical point of view, doctors should be trained in the toxicology of compounds that might be used and in the management of casualties. If the effects of the chemicals used can be reversed by antidotes, these should be given as early as possible: in all cases supportive care should be provided.

References

1. Prentiss AM. *Chemicals in War*. New York: McGraw-Hill, 1937.
2. Graves R. *Goodbye to All That*. London: Jonathan Cape, 1929.
3. Hitler A. *Mein Kampf*, Vol. 1 [Transl. Murphy J]. London: Hurst and Blackett, 1939.
4. Owen W. Dulce et Decorum est., 1917, as cited in The Collected Poems of wilfred owen. New York, New Directions Publishers, 1965.
5. Vedder EB. *The Medical Aspects of Chemical Warfare*. Baltimore, MD: Williams and Wilkins, 1925.
6. Stockholm International Peace Research Institute (SIPRI). *The Problem of Chemical and Biological Warfare. Volume 1: The Rise of CB Weapons*. New York: Humanities Press, 1971.
7. Gilbert M. *Churchill: A Life*. London: Heinemann, 1991.
8. Home Office. *Air Raid Precautions. Personal Protection Against Gas*. Handbook No. 1, 2nd edn. London: HMSO, 1939.
9. North Atlantic Treaty Organization (NATO). *Handbook on the Medical Aspects of NBC Defensive Operations*. AmedP-6(b), Part III. Chemical Annex C, Brussels, NATO, 1996.
10. Nagao M, Takatori T, Matsuda Y. *et al.* Definitive evidence for the acute sarin poisoning diagnosis in the Tokyo subway. *Toxicol Appl Pharmacol*, 1997; **144**: 198–203.
11. Sidell R. *Proceedings of Seminar Responding to the Consequences of Chemical and Biological Terrorism*. USPHS/OEP. Washington, DC: Government Printing Office, 1995; 232–233.

12. Wordall J. Protect and survive. *Lancet*, 1997; **349**: 1332–1333.
13. Masuda N, Takatsu M, Morinari H *et al.* Sarin poisoning in Tokyo subway. *Lancet*, 1995; **345**: 1446.
14. Nozaki H, Aikawa N. Sarin poisoning in Tokyo subway. *Lancet*, 1995; **345**: 1446–1447.
15. Nakajima T, Sato S, Morita H *et al.* Sarin poisoning of a rescue team in the Matsumoto sarin incident in Japan. *Occup Environ Med*, 1997; **54**: 697–701.
16. Nozaki H, Aikawa N, Fijishima S *et al.* A case of VX poisoning and the difference with sarin. *Lancet*, 1995; **346**: 698–699.
17. Hatta K, Miura Y, Asukai N *et al.* Amnesia from sarin poisoning. *Lancet*, 1996; **347**: 1343–1344.
18. Sekijama Y, Morita H, Yanagisawa N. Follow-up of sarin poisoning in Matsumoto. *Ann Int Med*, 1997; **127**: 1042.
19. Murata K, Araki S, Yokoyama K *et al.* Asymptomatic sequelae to acute sarin poisoning in the central and autonomic nervous system 6 months after the Tokyo subway attack. *J Neurol*, 1997; **244**: 601–606.
20. NBC Defenses Horizon. Chemical agent detector has long life. *Nuclear Biol Chem Defense Technol Int*, 1986; **1**: 47–55.
21. Balint GA. Ricin: the toxic protein of castor oil seeds. *Toxicology*, 1974; **2**: 77–102.
22. Brown RFR, White DE. Ultrastructure of rat lung following inhalation of ricin aerosol. *Int J Exp Pathol*, 1997; **78**: 267–276.
23. Griffiths GD, Lindsay CD, Allenby AC *et al.* Protection against inhalation toxicity of ricin and abrin by immunization. *Human Exp Toxicol*, 1995; **14**: 155–164.
24. Mehta PS, Mehta AS, Mehta SG *et al.* Bhopal tragedy's health aspects: a review of methyl isocyanate toxicity. *J Am Med Assoc*, 1990; **264**: 2781–2787.
25. Barbieri S, Pirovano C, Scarlato G *et al.* Long-term effects of 2,3,7,8-tetrachorodibenzo-p-dioxin on the peripheral nervous system. Clinical and neurophysiological controlled study on subjects with clhoracne from the Seveso area. Neurophysiology, 1988; **7**: 29–37.
26. Marrs TC, Maynard R, Sidell FR. *Chemical Warfare Agents: Toxicology and Treatment*. Chichester: Wiley, 1996.
27. Baker DJ. Management of casualties from terrorist chemical and biological attack: a key role for the anaesthetist. *Br J Anaesth*, 2002; **89**: 211–214.

6

Toxins

Patrick Barriot

According to the terms of the 1972 Convention, toxins are classified amongst the biological agents. In effect, this convention prohibits 'the development, production, stockpiling, or transfer of biological agents or toxins'. However, unlike the biological agents, toxins cannot reproduce themselves and do not have a contagious character. In the future, the principal toxins likely to be used for aggressive ends could be industrially synthesized through biotechnology. For these reasons, they merit being ranked amongst the chemical agents.

Practically all toxins can be disseminated in the form of aerosols and instigate pulmonary symptomatology, which can evoke contamination by an infectious agent. They can also be poured into a potable water reservoir or onto a food product. Finally, they can be injected in a criminal manner. The toxins are largely considered to be lethal agents (ricin, botulinum toxin, mycotoxins, etc.) and rarely those, such as staphylococcal enterotoxin, which are likely to be intentionally utilized as incapacitating agents. It is classical to distinguish the peptide or protein toxins, such as botulinum toxin or ricin, from polycyclic toxins, which have a low molecular weight. Their mechanisms of action vary, e.g. inhibition of protein synthesis (ricin, trichothecene mycotoxins), disruption of the functioning of ion channels (saxitoxin), and inhibition of the liberation of a neurotransmitter such as acetylcholine (botulinum toxin). The clinical symptomatology guides diagnosis (Table 6.1).

Ricin

Ricin is a bush that grows in all tropical and subtropical regions and whose beans are collected in thorny indentations. Two products can be extracted from ricin beans: ricin oil and ricin. Ricin oil does not contain the toxin, but ricinoleic acid is endowed with some drastic laxative properties. Ricinoleic acid alters the intestinal membrane and provokes a major loss of fluids and electrolytes. In the fascist Italy of Mussolini, the Black Shirts made their opponents drink large glasses of ricin oil to provoke uncontrollable diarrhea. Ricin, a glycoprotein present in the beans and resistant to heat, is a

Treating Victims of Mass Destsuction   Edited by Patrick Barriot and Chantal Bismuth
© 2008 John Wiley & Sons, Ltd

Table 6.1 Guiding clinical signs concerning the toxins

Signs	Respiratory	Neurological	Cutaneous	Gastrointestinal
Ricin	+++			+++
Botulinum toxin		+++		
Mycotoxins	+++		+++	+++
SEB	+++			+++

dangerous toxin that is not soluble in ricin oil. It exerts its toxicity on the majority of body tissues and causes cellular death by blocking protein synthesis. The toxicity is maximal by inhalation and variable by ingestion. Some cases of death from consumption of the beans have been described. Without danger when it is placed on healthy skin, the toxin is mortal when injected. In September 1978, the Bulgarian secret service assassinated Georgi Markov in London by pricking him with an umbrella whose point was coated with ricin, while an attempt to poison some FBI agents by means of doorknobs coated with ricin failed, due to the absence of toxicity on intact skin. Ansar Al-Islam, an Islamic group similar to Al-Qaida and based in Iraq near the Iranian border, had tested ricin in view of terrorist actions. Some samples of ricin were discovered on January 5, 2003, in a London apartment. On the other hand, some suspect samples discovered on March 20, 2003, in a baggage room at the Gare de Lyon (Lyon train station) did not contain ricin, contrary to the initial announcements.

The clinical signs of poisoning are few or non-specific, and vary according to the absorbed dose and route of entry. The first signs generally develop in 4–8 hours. In cases of penetration by the respiratory route, one observes a picture of febrile bronchopneumonitis that evolves to acute respiratory distress syndrome (ARDS) with refractory hypoxemia. Treatment essentially consists of controlled ventilation and treatment of the acute lesion of pulmonary edema. Despite this therapy, death can follow in 2–3 days. In cases of penetration by the gastrointestinal or percutaneous routes, the clinical picture combines fever, abdominal pain, hemorrhagic diarrhea, anuria, and a state of shock. A cutaneous lesion with an inflammatory reaction and surrounding adenopathy can reveal a puncture lesion, signaling criminal inoculation. Confirmation of the diagnosis is done by immunodetection with an antibody capable of specific recognition. The treatment essentially remains symptomatic – resuscitation with fluids, electrolytes, and blood products replacement. Gastrointestinal decontamination by administration of activated charcoal has been proposed if one suspects poisoning by the gastrointestinal route.

Botulinum toxins

The botulinum toxins are amongst the most toxic substances currently known [1]. They consist of neurotoxins secreted by anaerobic bacteria of the genus *Clostridium* (essentially *Clostridium botulinum*). There are seven serotypes of botulinum toxin

(A, B, C, D, E, F, and G). Botulism is associated with serotypes A (the most toxic), B and E. The site of action of the toxin is the motor end plate, where it blocks neuromuscular transmission by preventing release of acetylcholine in a specific and irreversible manner. The toxin does not penetrate the blood–brain barrier, which explains the absence of central nervous system injury. It is relatively easy to procure this toxin, which is used in low doses in the cosmetic industry to make products for the treatment of wrinkles. In the context of aggression with botulinum toxin, the route of entry can be respiratory, gastrointestinal, or percutaneous (inoculation). The Aum sect carried out some studies on spraying of botulinum toxin, trying to disperse it by the aerial route. The toxin can be directly ingested from contaminated water or food. Ingestion of *C. botulinum* toxin contained in spoiled pork products or poorly-prepared canned food is the origin of several cases observed each year in France. Contamination of distribution systems for drinking water is prevented in part by increasing the level of chlorination. A mechanism of inoculation can also be envisioned because botulinum toxin poisoning is described in parenteral drug abusers; the toxin can pass directly into the general circulation from non-intact skin. Finally, contamination due to development of an intestinal focus of *C. botulinum*, secreting its toxin *in situ*, cannot be excluded because it has been observed in infants. The gene that codes for botulinum toxin could also be inserted into the genomes of other bacteria, such as *Escherichia coli* or *Bacillus anthracis*, in order to trigger endogenous poisonings. To date, there have been no confirmed cases of terrorist or warfare utilization of botulinum toxin. Iraq, under the regime of Saddam Hussein, had available large quantities of botulinum toxin and means for their dispersion. Some terrorist organizations, such as the Aum Sect and the Red Army Faction, have had this toxin in their possession with the manifest intention of using it.

The clinical signs result from blockage of the release of acetylcholine, principally at the neuromuscular junction. The symptoms are identical, regardless of the route of entry, whether respiratory, gastrointestinal, or percutaneous (inoculation). The delay to the appearance of the initial symptoms can vary from several hours to many days, according to the amount of toxin absorbed and the route of entry. Bulbar signs appear first. Initially this involves ocular signs, such as difficulty in accommodation, diplopia, mydriasis, ptosis, photophobia, and a decrease of lachrymal secretions, producing a 'dry eye syndrome'. However, involvement of the ENT area also occurs, with dysarthria, dysphonia, dysphagia, and dryness of the buccal mucosa responsible for difficult and painful swallowing. These ENT disturbances may be responsible for pulmonary aspiration and pneumonitis from difficulty in swallowing. The muscular lesion is manifested by symmetrical, progressive, and descending flaccid paralysis, which may lead to acutely fatal respiratory insufficiency. Development of cardiac rhythm abnormalities characterizes the severe forms. It is important to emphasize that botulinum toxin poisoning provokes neither fever nor alteration of consciousness. It should thus be considered systematically when there are bulbar signs with descending paralysis in a patient who presents with neither fever nor alteration of consciousness. Confirmation of the diagnosis is by immunological techniques that allow identification and serotyping (A, B, E) of the toxin.

Treatment is primarily symptomatic. It consists of ventilatory resuscitation in cases of distress due to paralysis of the respiratory muscles. Immunological treatment, with the purpose of neutralizing circulating toxin with specific antibodies, is proposed in the severe forms. Moreover, guanidine can oppose the action of the toxin at the neuromuscular junction. Guanidine chlorhydrate syrup (30 mg/kg/day, in three doses by mouth) is prescribed for this indication.

Other toxins

Aflatoxin is a carcinogenic substance isolated from mold fungus of the type *Aspergillus flavus*. It can induce cancers of the liver after a latent period. Under the regime of Saddam Hussein, Iraq produced large quantities of aflatoxin (2200 liters) that could have been dispersed by Al-Hussein ballistic missiles and R-400 aerial bombs.

The trichothecenes are formidable mycotoxins, produced by *Fusarium*-type molds, and cause severe inhibition of the synthesis of nucleic acids and proteins. They can be dispersed in the form of aerosols and easily penetrate across the skin and mucous membranes [2]. The clinical picture suggests radiomimetic effects, with injury to the hematopoietic tissues, gastrointestinal mucosa, and skin. It combines early vomiting, ulcerative lesions of the gastrointestinal mucosa, and bloody diarrhea, as well as bullous or necrotic–hemorrhagic cutaneous lesions. Syndromes of respiratory distress with bloody sputum have also been described. Cutaneous lesions of the necrotic type, with epidermolysis and petechiae, are suggestive of myotoxins. Death follows from respiratory distress, hemorrhagic syndrome, or superinfection. Treatment consists of symptomatic measures: assisted ventilation, replacement of hemorrhagic losses, treatment of cutaneous lesions, and administration of activated charcoal. The Soviet armed forces were suspected of having dispersed aerosols of mycotoxins, described as 'yellow rain' [3] or 'red rain', in south-east Asia (Laos and Cambodia). In fact, further analysis much later showed that insect excrement, particularly during prolific reproductive years, was responsible for these colored rains.

Staphylococcus enterotoxin B (SEB) is a protein toxin produced by certain strains of *Staphylococcus aureus*. This exotoxin, responsible for mass food poisonings, is more an incapitating agent than a lethal agent. It can be disseminated by the aerial route in the form of an aerosol or by the gastrointestinal route by means of contaminated foods or beverages. The clinical picture is variable, according to the route of penetration. Ingestion of SEB causes a cholera-like syndrome, with vomiting, abdominal pain, and profuse diarrhea. Inhalation of SEB causes a pseudo-influenza syndrome with fever, chills, headaches, myalgias, cough, and dyspnea. Exposure to high levels of the toxin can cause toxic shock syndrome. The evolution is generally favorable over 1–2 weeks. The treatment is purely symptomatic. The diagnosis is confirmed by immunodetection of the toxin.

Until the last few years, it has been relatively difficult to obtain large quantities of weaponizable toxins from bacteria, molds, or plants [4,5]. Extraction and purification of toxins from the primary materials necessitated long, costly, and complex procedures.

The development of genetic engineering techniques offers the possibility of producing toxins in an industrial fashion from now on. Creation of transgenic bacteria, equipped with a foreign gene coding for the synthesis of a protein toxin, allows collection in the culture medium and then purification of significant quantities of toxins. A Russian institute recently proposed to sell purified toxins from *Shigella* and *Pseudomonas*, as well as staphylococcal enterotoxins. It is also possible to amplify the virulence of certain microorganisms by inserting one or more genes coding for lethal toxins into their genomes. These pathogenic agents, if they are contagious, could propagate from person to person and secrete their dangerous toxins directly into the human body.

References

1. Arnon S, Schechter R, Inglesby T *et al*. Botulinum toxin as a biological weapon: medical and public health management. Working Group on Civilian Biodefense. *J Am Med Assoc,* 2001; **285**: 1059–1070.
2. Vidal PCC (Coordinateur). Mémento médical pour la protection contre les armes biologiques. Centre de Recherches du Service de Santé des Armées, École d'Application du Service de Santé des Armées, September 2002.
3. Seeley T, Nowicke J, Meselson M *et al*. Yellow rain. *Sci Am*, 1985; **253**: 128–137.
4. Lepick O. *Les Armes Chimiques*. Paris: Presses Universitaires de France, 'Que sais-je?', 1999.
5. Lepick O, Daguzan JF. *Le Terrorisme Non-conventionnel*. Paris: Presses Universitaires de France, 2003.

7

Gulf war syndrome

Chantal Bismuth and Andreas Schaper

Between the invasion of Kuwait by the Iraqi army on August 2, 1990 and the end of the Gulf war in March, 1991, the USA sent 697 000 volunteers or career military personnel into this region of the Persian Gulf, accompanied by troops from the UK and Canada. The Gulf war, which lasted 1 month (January–February, 1991), was the war with the fewest casualties that had been experienced by the USA. The different armies registered 219 casualties, of which 65 deaths occurred during combat, even though in the collective mentality it was expected to be a bloody war, taking into account the threats of utilization of chemical and biological weapons.

During the war itself, acute psychiatric problems were considered rare: only 400 amongst 6000 soldiers were invalided out of the war. On the other hand, since their return from the Gulf war, more than 180 000 veterans have complained of a variety of symptoms, including chronic fatigue, muscle and joint pain, cutaneous rashes, gastrointestinal disturbances, respiratory disturbances, headaches, difficulty in concentrating, memory loss, irritability, and depression. Such a diversity of complaints has led to numerous epidemiological, clinical, and experimental studies in order to determine the prevalence, distribution, etiologic factors and attribution criteria of what has been dubbed 'Gulf war syndrome'.

Risk factors

The working conditions of the troops engaged in the Gulf have been considered particularly laborious, often static, with long hours of waiting in position. The approaches remained secret and the troops were kept in ignorance of their movements. These working conditions were responsible for an intense psychological tension and led to an atmosphere of permanent stress.

The men were subjected to multiple preparatory vaccinations and medications, because of fear of contamination by insects, snakes, or rodents. The chemical contaminants they experienced were multiple: fires involving human and domestic waste, fuel and solvents, emissions of oil well fires during the re-taking of Kuwait, intense utilization of pesticides, and suspected exposure to chemical and biological weapons. Finally, the climate was hostile with temperature extremes and sand storms.

Treating Victims of Mass Destsuction   Edited by Patrick Barriot and Chantal Bismuth
© 2008 John Wiley & Sons, Ltd

Complaints and facts

Augmentation of the investigative process was rapid from 1992. Apart from a small number of cases of documented infectious diseases, directly attributable to the stay in the Gulf, and a small number of cases of post-traumatic sequelae, subjective complaints predominated; amongst these, neuropsychiatric symptoms appeared frequent. The symptoms commonly reported by the former Gulf war combatants were the following:

- Fatigue.

- Muscle and joint pain.

- Decreased attention and cognitive performance.

- Headaches.

- Various respiratory complaints.

- Various gastrointestinal complaints.

- Sleep disturbances.

- Rashes and other dermatological disturbances.

Epidemiological studies have established that this population complains of symptomatology identical to, but more numerous than, that of the general population [1] or of other combatants not deployed in this region during the same period. These signs are without specificity and resemble those observed in current medical practice in the general population [2].

If has not been possible to isolate a group of symptoms to justify calling the entity 'Gulf war syndrome', apart from the findings of Haley (see [5]), who proposed to distinguish: (a) a syndrome grouping sleep and memory disturbances; and (b) a more severe syndrome with symptoms such as mental confusion and vertigo – the affected individuals had objective injury of the nerve cells of the ganglions at the cerebral base, detected by magnetic resonance imaging (MRI). For other authors, pyridostigmine, a temporary anticholinesterase utilized in a preventive manner, and an eventual contamination by neurotoxic gas, were ideal suspect chemicals. These recent results require confirmation and interpretation [3].

In 1995, the US Department of Defense (DOD) established an important negative fact: the absence of a statistically significant increase of fetal malformations (for the moment) in the offspring of former combatants. This was one of the major concerns of this population. Moreover, the US DOD proposed that eligibility for medical care did not depend on a unique definition of 'Gulf war syndrome'. In effect, this new pathology has multiple clinical expressions.

Proven facts

Besides the strong predominance of neuropsychiatric symptoms, a high frequency of hypertension, low back pain, periodontal disease, and cancers (but not significant in large series) have been detected [4], as well as amyotrophic lateral sclerosis, with a two-fold increased risk in the veterans, recently reported by Hayley [5], alcohol or drug dependence, severe depression, and automobile accidents.

Infectious and parasitic pathologies

Two parasitic diseases, leishmaniasis and malaria, have been described in the veterans. Visceral or cutaneous leishmaniasis, a parasitic disease endemic in the Near East, has multiple expressions; the diagnosis is difficult, and has been confirmed and compensated for in 32 veterans. Seven cases of malaria, as well as some mycoplasma infections, have been detected.

Proposed toxic pathologies

Petroleum products

There existed a possibility of inhalation, but also of ingestion and cutaneous penetration. Petroleum products were heavily utilized in several operations: heating, incineration of wastes, suppression of dust and sand, and movement of vehicles. Exposure to petroleum products was above all caused during oil well fires, with release of inorganic gases (SO_2, NO_2, CO, CO_2, H_2S), aromatic, aliphatic, and aldehyde compounds, semi-volatile organic compounds, and releases of lead. In fact, gas monitoring was only begun in May, 1991, and the most severe exposures to ground troops in Kuwait were not evaluated. It is feared that the levels of benzene, toluene, ethyl benzene and xylene could have far exceeded 1 ppm. The concentrations of soot particles could have reached 500–2000 $\mu g/m^3$.

Desert dusts

During maneuvers, soluble particles could exceed several milligrams per cubic meter (mg/m^3), causing irritation of the upper airways. Pneumoconiosis, a consequence of long-term inhalation, remains improbable.

Uranium

Used as a coating for certain vehicles in an attempt to protect them, depleted uranium could be liberated during explosions or misfires. The radioactivity given off is very much lower than international standards. Surveillance for eventual delayed carcino-genesis could be done. Acute renal toxicity is known, as well as a risk of pulmonary accumulation (asymptomatic). There were no documented cases during the Gulf war.

Surfaces resistant to chemical agents

Vehicles and equipment were painted with protective materials with a toluene diisocyanate base, which is a pulmonary sensitizer. These surfaces could be the cause of the development of asthma or a syndrome of bronchial irritation in some veterans.

Vaccines

In addition to the usual vaccines, a vaccine against anthrax and another against botu-lism were administered to the soldiers. The two latter, products of the Michigan State Public Health Department, had been given to several thousand civilians and military personnel before the Gulf war. No long-term effects have been reported.

Pyridostigmine bromide

This was proposed for the prevention of possible organophosphate poisoning, in the form of 30 mg pills supplied in blister packs, to be taken every 8 hours in case of threat. The majority of US, UK, and Canadian soldiers were treated for the first 5 days of the aerial attack and during the first 5 days of the ground attack for prevention against pos-sible chemical weapons, such as soman.

Pyridostigmine produces a transient inhibition of cholinesterases, with a temporary accumulation of acetylcholine that is responsible for a very moderate muscarinic and nicotinic syndrome. Immediate side effects were noted in 5–50% of subjects (effects possibly increased by concomitant exposure to organophosphate insecticides). Elimination is renal, without passing the blood–brain barrier. The plasma half-life is 3.7 hours, without accumulation. This medication is utilized in myasthenia gravis at much higher doses, up to 6 grams/day, without reported long-term effects. However, other anticholinesterases that were used in combination in the Gulf war could explain its possible toxicity, mainly some organophosphate pesticides.

Pesticides

Those widely utilized include: pyrethroids, D-phenotrine, chlorpyrifos, presme-thrin, malathion, methonyl, lindane, azamethiphos, and insect repellents containing diethyl-m-toluamide. The pyrethroid insecticides have mainly nervous system effects and have been associated with hyperactivity, tremors, ataxia, convulsions, and eventually paralysis. The other insecticides utilized were above all the organophosphate insecticides, cholinesterase inhibitors that cause accumulation of acetylcholine in the poisoned organism (their acute effects are discussed in the chapter on chemical weapons). In the case of Gulf war syndrome, there has been concern about subacute effects at a distance from the initial cholinergic crisis; either the 'intermediate syndrome' (delayed muscular weakness with an onset after 1–4 days, with electromyographic abnormalities which can progress to respiratory distress), or 'delayed polyneuropathly' (onset after 1–3 weeks), also with electromyographic stigmata. These moderate- or long-term effects have not been observed in former Gulf war combatants.

Chemical and biological weapons

The Czechs detected sarin (a highly toxic and persistent anticholineterase) and sulfur mustard ('mustard gas'; with caustic effects on the skin and mucous membranes and a risk for bone marrow depression and aplasia) in two separate incidents. There has not been proven utilization of these weapons, but contamination during destruction of their storage depots has recently been described and involved several thousand troops. However, it must be emphasized that these weapons were supposedly not validated as active weapons. It is difficult to imagine that, in the absence of observed effects during acute exposure, one could presently link them with chronic manifestations. Certainly, some chronic effects exist in toxicology, but not after a single acute exposure where this has not caused any initial symptomatology. Current thinking has tended rather towards the responsibility of the additive effect of repeated exposure to different anticholinesterase agents.

In the civilian population of Kurdistan, physicians have reported an increased frequency of ischemic cardiac pathology, cancers, and congenital anomalies in subjects exposed to organophosphates without having developed symptoms after acute contamination. Moreover, it is known that possible chronic effects initiated after exposure to mustard gas (mainly respiratory, ocular, and malignant) were reported during World War I and in the Iran–Iraq conflict [6]. These diverse situations do not correspond to conditions observed during the Gulf war.

Data from previous wars

The morbidity of former combatants is greater in the number of reported cases, but identical in the range of causes to that of the general population. No epidemiological study has been able to isolate a strictly defined medical pathology.

One finds the same complaints in the situations of previous wars since the Crimean War [7] and the Civil War [8], with reports of numerous symptoms without objective lesions, in the two World Wars in all the belligerents, and during the Vietnam War. A multiplication of infectious pathologies was, of course, anticipated; in fact, the multitude of reported symptoms with identification is predictable and remarkably similar from one war to another. The sole act of sending soldiers into combat is sufficient to cause multiple somatic and psychological complaints.

Politico–economic factors

To numerous observers, Gulf war syndrome appears closely correlated in its unexpected occurrence and its demands:

- To media overstatements with dramatization of the threat of 'weapons of mass destruction'.

- To the greater and greater litigious nature of developed societies.

- To the obvious targeting and possible benefits represented by the recruiting administrations [9].

'Stressors'

This is a matter of manifestations, often muscular or psychological, initiated either by secretion of neuromediators during intense stress, or by generally olfactory exposures to chemical agents. In the case of former Gulf war combatants, 'post-traumatic stress disorder' can be authenticated in the face of certain abnormalities: chronic fatigue, myalgias that enter into the definition of this pathology, now recognized in the International Classification of Diseases. On the other hand, flash-backs and intellectual asthenia, while frequent in the former combatants, was not made part of the retained criteria.

These situations of stress with sequelae are sometimes assimilated as post-traumatic neurosis. In fact they go beyond this category and can generate anxiety, depressive states, and somatization. One of the effects of stress is amplification of commonplace bodily sensations, frequent in the total population, by the hypervigilance of a person placed in an unusual situation, resulting in endowing these sensations with emotional and cognitive overlay when the appearance of a new mysterious pathology is suspected, and above all if a responsible entity can be designated (environment, family, work-place, domestic or industrial chemical products, government). This situation, exacerbated by media spotlighting, preferentially affected the three armies most highly engaged: US, UK, and Canadian. Participants from other countries were less affected, perhaps because they had been involved in fewer deployments in dangerous actions, or perhaps because their societies are less litigious than the Anglo-Saxon countries.

It is possible that the Gulf war syndrome could be integrated into a phenomenon identified in occupational pathology as 'multiple chemical sensitivities' or 'idiopathic environmental intolerances', situations in which the tested subject cannot distinguish the application of the implicated chemical from that of a placebo [10].

In all cases (as in France, the suspicion of a Gulf war syndrome has been the study objective of a parliamentary commission since 2001), personalized medical management has been proven to be indispensable to avoid chronic debility.

Conclusion

Following a short war that aroused worldwide attention and numerous fears of chemical and biological exposures, a large number of former combatants developed diverse symptoms. These latter were easily described by the denomination 'Gulf war syndrome', characterized by multiple subjective symptoms and a paucity of individualized objective lesions, numerically significant, which remains a controversial and nebulous diagnosis. Currently, research of a specific morbid entity and a reproducible biological model has not been definitively established.

Wars have always affected the health of the combatants and it has never been possible to identify a unique organic illness [11].

References

1. Kang HK, Mahan CM, Lee KY *et al*. Illnesses among US veterans of the Gulf war. A population-based survey of 30 000 veterans. *J Occup Environ Med*, 2000; **42**: 491–501.
2. Fox DD *et al*. Base rate of post-concussive symptoms in health maintenance organization patients and controls. *Neuropsychology*, 1995; **9**: 606–611.
3. Haley RW, Meddrey AM, Gerschenfeld HK. Severely reduced functional status in veterans fitting a case definition of Gulf war syndrome. *Am J Public Health*, 2000; **92**: 46–47.
4. McCauley L, Lasarev M, Sticker D *et al*. Illness experience of Gulf war veterans possibly exposed to chemical warfare agents. *Am J Prevent Med*, 2002; **23**: 200–206.
5. Haley RW. Excess incidence of ALS in young Gult war veterans. *Neurology* 2003; **61**: 750–756.
6. Volans GN, Karalliedde L. Long-term effects of chemical weapons. *Lancet* (suppl), 2002; **360**: 135–136.
7. Da Costa JM. An irritable heart: a clinical study of a form of functional cardiac disorder and its consequences. *Am J Med Sci*, 1971; **61**: 17–52.
8. Hyams KC, Wignall FS, Roswell R. War syndromes and their evaluation from the US civil war to the Persian Gulf war. *Ann Intern Med*, 1996; **125**: 398–405.
9. Oumeish YO. Gulf war syndrome. *Clin Dermatol*, 2002; **20**: 401–412.
10. Brent J, Klein L. Gulf war syndrome, idiopathic environmental intolerance and organophosphate compounds: diseases in search of causal hypothesis. In Karalliedde L, Feldman S, Henry J, Marrs T (eds), *Organophosphates and Health*. London: Imperial College Press, 2001: 241–256.
11. Ferrari R, Russell AS. The problem of Gulf war syndrome. *Med Hypoth*, 2001; **56**: 697–701.

8

Organizational aspects of the management of large numbers of victims during a chemical or biological accident

David J. Baker, Caroline Telion and Pierre Carli

Massive destruction? The realities of managing victims from a chemcial or biological accident

Since the terrorist action against the World Trade Center in New York, there has been an increased concern within the general population about the risk of terrorist actions utilizing chemical or biological agents. This concern has been fed by broadcasts about several accidents of this nature that occurred in 1995 in Japan [1,2] and in 2001 in the USA [3]. This concern has been further increased by the constant evocation of 'weapons of mass destruction', a term used since the Cold War to describe chemical, biological, and nuclear agents. This fear has also been reinforced by the understanding of diverse programs for production of chemical and biological agents [4,5]. However, the term is used without any critical analysis concerning the reality of the poisoning which, from the medical point of view, has not been detected. It thus seems necessary to define the possibility of emergency medical responses to the effects that could be caused by chemical and biological agents. Whilst nuclear weapons have clearly demonstrated their responsibility for massive destruction of human life and property, a similar destruction (in terms of the number of victims) has never been described during the dispersion of chemical or biological weapons.

The objective of this chapter is therefore to describe the organization of the medical response during a chemical or biological attack on a civilian population. However, before describing the medical details, it is important to review some characteristics of chemical and biological agents.

First, there are significant differences in the effects that can be induced by chemical agents and those induced by viruses or bacteria. Chemical warfare is the equivalent of a deliberate release of chemical products. They are classified under the terms of

Treating Victims of Mass Destsuction   Edited by Patrick Barriot and Chantal Bismuth
© 2008 John Wiley & Sons, Ltd

'hazardous material release' (HAZMAT) [6]. The accidental release of chemical products can be responsible for various effects as well as deaths, such as in Bhopal in 1984 [7], where approximately 5000 persons died following poisoning with methyl isocyanate. Deliberate release of chemical agents was utilized during World War I [5], but also during the Iran–Iraq conflict in the 1980s. It must be clarified that the number of deaths caused by chemical weapons was much lower than that caused by the utilization of conventional weapons. Hence, during the Iran–Iraq war in the 1980s, where modern medical techniques were utilized, the number of victims with lesions due to mustard gas or neurotoxic agents only represented 1% amongst 27 000 victims [8]. Similarly, during World War II, air raids organized by the Allies against German cities caused thousands of victims and deaths amongst the victims: more than 60 000 victims at Dresden in February 1945, and more than 100 000 in Hamburg in 1943. In this fashion, the destruction in terms of loss of life or residential property has always been greater with conventional weapons than with chemical weapons.

When utilized for terrorist purposes, it has been shown that conventional weapons can be responsible for a large number of victims and can also cause fatalities, especially when they are utilized in enclosed spaces. In this fashion, the explosion that took place in 2002 in Bali was responsible for more than 200 deaths, which is equivalent to the total number of victims from various waves of terrorist attacks in England over a 30-year period. In contrast, the terrorist attack that took place in Japan in 1995 with the neurotoxic agent, sarin, caused only 12 deaths and a large number of victims who presented with effects that were treatable with antidotes and usual medical techniques [2].

Secondly, attacks carried out with biological agents will be different from attacks due to chemical agents. The dispersion of biological agents would above all be responsible for epidemic waves. The time required for the appearance of clinical signs can thus be considered as days to weeks, and not in seconds or minutes like those produced by chemical agents. The mechanism of action of bacterial and viral agents is different from that of chemical agents, of which the principle objective is damage to the respiratory system, leading to death from asphyxia in a few seconds or minutes. The patterns of lesions induced by chemical or biological agents are thus very different: chemical agents most often induce maximal lesions within a short time interval; in contrast, biological agents produce the same types of symptoms in patients, but at different times following dispersion of the agent, especially when an infectious agent is transmissible from one person to another.

The third important point regarding chemical and biological agents is to differentiate between risk and threat. These terms are often used without distinction, but they elicit different thoughts. In terms of chemical and biological warfare, a *risk* is an eventuality harmful to human life, while a *threat* elicits the idea that the *risk* can be extended and that the aggressor has the intention of incorporating it into a weapon. While many toxic chemicals can be true *threats* because they are incorporated into bombs, particles or clouds (aerosols) of biological agents are very unstable during dispersion and thus cannot infect a large population.

It is important to understand the real danger of chemical or biological terrorism in perspective in order to have a positive approach to management. In effect, the medical management of victims of this type of attack relies on the same principles as those for victims of attacks from explosives or firearms.

For medical responders, there is a known risk from toxic agents, which corresponds to the risk of terrorist utilization of a 'secondary bomb' designed to injure medical responders and victims still at the incident site. Nevertheless, emergency personnel must be trained to don and work in protective equipment and clothing in order to ensure their own protection.

Properties of chemical and biological toxicants

There are four properties of all chemical and biological agents that determine the appropriate type of patient management [9]. Each agent has:

- A *toxicity*, which can be defined as bodily lesions that develop in each patient.
- A latent period, which corresponds to the time interval between the time of exposure and the appearance of the first symptoms.
- A *persistence*, which is the time during which the toxic agent remains present in sufficient quantity to cause harm: this depends on the physicochemical properties of the toxicant.
- A *transmissibility*, which is the capacity for the toxicant to be passed from one person to another and thus to contaminate or infect another person.

The first two properties determine the type of medical management of patients, while the latter two should determine the measures that should be taken to assure decontamination of the patient and his surroundings in order to prevent secondary risks.

Practical response to a terrorist attack

Incident management

The response to a terrorist attack relies on the immediate establishment of three different zones, called the Hot Zone, the Warm Zone, and the Cold Zone [6,10] (Figure 8.1). The Hot Zone corresponds to the location where the toxicant is released; the concentration of the toxicant here is therefore maximal. If identification of the toxicant has not been accomplished, it must be considered to be persistent and transmissible and, in accordance with these suppositions, responders must be equipped with protective clothing and protective masks.

The mission of these responders is to evacuate the wounded from the zone of toxicant dispersion to a zone called the Warm Zone, where the concentration of the toxicant is lower. There, specially trained medical personnel can perform initial triage of the victims to discover those who have been exposed and those who require emergency medical assistance. Victims who can benefit from a decontaminating shower are then

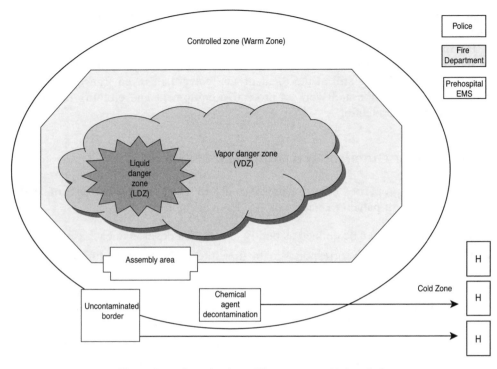

Figure 8.1   Organization of first response. H, hospital

taken to the Cold Zone before being transported to the hospital for continued therapeutic management.

Following the 1995 attack in Japan, numerous countries throughout the world have established response plans in the event of this type of attack. In France, response plans have been established to improve coordination between the Fire Department, First Aid, and the emergency medical services (EMS) [10]. The 'Piratox' plan anticipates the combined response of emergency services during a terrorist attack. Victim triage is based on the necessity for decontamination and the patient's medical condition. From the outset, arrangements for managing patients with respiratory distress in the decontamination zone must be anticipated, characteristics which other countries have been justified in adopting. Following the September 11, 2001, attack in New York, nearly all response plans have been revised and completed, emphasizing management of respiratory distress in the decontamination zone by special responder groups trained for intervention in a toxic environment. These plans also anticipate the organization of hospitals specifically dedicated to the management of contaminated victims. Another characteristic of this new planning is the purchase of small portable ventilators that can assure good quality ventilation on site or in hospitals that receive a large number of victims.

Resuscitation of chemical agent victims

In emergency medicine, resuscitation is classically qualified as either basic or specialized [11]. Resuscitation systems are based on management of the airway, respiration, and circulation (ABC management; where A = airway, B = breathing, C = circulation). The capabilities and equipment of the responders on site determines the significance of the resuscitation that can be accomplished. The best-known example of this type of resuscitation is represented by the response to cardiac arrest. Maintaining the head in a position to facilitate the passage of air, mouth-to-mouth respiration, and chest compressions are familiar actions to all who have taken a first aid course. In the context of lesions induced by toxic chemicals, the objectives are identical, but the methods employed to maintain an open airway and artificial ventilation are more sophisticated. In addition, in this situation cardiac arrest can be a consequence of respiratory arrest. To prevent cardiac arrest, it is therefore indispensable to maintain adequate respiratory function.

The necessity for simultaneous resuscitation of a large number of victims is more probable in case of a chemical attack than in case of a biological attack, because of a briefer delay of action. In the past, management of patients injured by chemical poisoning was traditionally based on the use of antidotes. There are, in effect, several specific antidotes for toxic chemicals, particularly neurotoxicants and cyanides. However, in recent years, the importance of resuscitation over utilization of antidotes has been recognized [10]. The majority of toxic chemical agents have an effect on the respiratory system; hence, having the means of airway management in place is essential. In effect, toxic chemicals induce respiratory depression, either by paralysis of the respiratory muscles, or by central nervous system effects, to which can be added upper airway obstruction. To overcome these different effects, the medical management must include maintaining an open upper airway but also the possibility of assuring artificial ventilation when respiratory distress or cardio-respiratory arrest occur. This response is currently well established and combines the management of both conventional and toxic lesions: it is called TOXALS [9].

If the toxic chemical is not persistent, the usual measures of resuscitation can be performed by the response services at the Assembly Point. However, problems occur when decontamination is necessary, since this inevitably produces a delay before the victim reaches the Cold Zone. All victims contaminated with persistent agents should benefit from decontamination concomitant with management of their vital distress. In this manner, only emergency care would be given by pre-hospital EMS responders, because working in a toxic environment presents difficulties in technical and logistical terms, particularly with regard to having available competent, trained, and properly protected personnel and obtaining a sufficient supply of oxygen.

Specific medical and supply problems during management of vital distress during a toxic attack

The different zones are generally delimited in an arbitrary fashion while waiting to determine the nature of the toxic agent(s). Entries and exits from the different zones are carefully controlled: this presents significant operational problems in terms of personnel and the supply and re-supply of equipment. It must include a certain porosity. Groups entering the decontamination zone must carry protective equipment, including a large supply of oxygen, indispensable for their own protection, but also a supply of oxygen for the patients who require ventilatory assistance with high concentrations of oxygen.

Victim triage

Patients presenting with respiratory distress require both the establshment of an open airway and artificial ventilation. Victim triage is based on a rapid medical evaluation in order to select those patients who would benefit from emergency medical care.

If the victims are contaminated, they should benefit from concomitant management of their vital distress and decontamination.

Management of vital distress in the decontamination zone

Personnel protection

All personnel working in the decontamination zone must be protected against toxic agents, but the necessity for protective clothing and a protective mask causes difficulties with vision and difficulty in performing precise actions. It is thus imperative that the responders have practiced and that they are accustomed to the proper level of protection before any incidents occur. This type of training has been very well developed by the military, but much less so for civilian responders. Following the introduction of the Bioteox plan in the pre-hospital medical response squads (SAMU) in France, personnel were supplied with equipment and received training including utilization of protective clothing and masks, in order to be prepared to work safety in the contaminated area.

Airway management

Rescuers must keep maintenance of an open airway in victims as a priority by removing secretions and foreign bodies which could prevent the passage of oxygen through the lungs. This requires maintaining the head in the proper position and utilization of a manual aspirator. If the patient is unconscious, a nasal or oral airway, as usually utilized in emergency medicine and anesthesia, is placed in such a way as to maintain an open upper airway and keep the tongue in a good position. More specific respiratory resuscitation can be instituted by placing an esophageal obturator device (positioned behind the epiglottis, below the throat) or by performing endotracheal intubation, another technique commonly utilized in anesthesiology. Pre-hospital paramedical personnel are all trained in the utilization of these techniques for airway management.

Ventilatory management

Artificial ventilation can be assured with either a resuscitation bag (of the Ambu type) or a portable oxygen-powered ventilator. Bag ventilation is a familiar technique in hospitals. However, it is necessary to mobilize two persons to be efficacious when the airways are severely injured by lesions of toxic origin. Portable respirators are part of the standard equipment for the SAMU in France. These devices are frequently powered by oxygen, and allow reliable ventilation that can easily be regulated following simple parameters. Despite their simplicity, they can deliver reliable ventilation that is comparable to that of more complex respirators usually found in intensive care services. As such, they are efficacious in an emergency situation and usually permit delivery of oxygen at either 50% or 100% concentration. Lower oxygen concentrations can be obtained with ambient air-powered systems, which allow lesser oxygen consumption for functioning. In a contaminated environment; however, these devices should not be utilized and only 100% oxygen-powered respirators are used. This limits the amount of assisted ventilation that can be accomplished, due to the increased consumption of oxygen and the difficulty of its re-supply.

Oxygen supply

Supplying oxygen is critical in the management of victims in the decontamination zone. Oxygen is usually liberally used in hospitals, but must be considered to be a rare commodity in the field and must be conserved as much as possible. The re-supply of oxygen in the field can pose problems in terms of the number of cylinders that can be transported by responders. Large reserves of liquid oxygen could be stocked in the Cold Zone and some smaller units in ambulances. Fire Services may also have at their disposal a large number of 'J'-size cylinders that can be placed in the decontamination zone if necessary. The 'D'-size cylinders utilized by the majority of the pre-hospital emergency services contain 340 liters of compressed oxygen. An increase of the volume of oxygen corresponds to an increase in the weight of the cylinder. In order to compensate for this inconvenience, steel cylinders have been replaced by aluminum cylinders, for which a 3 kg weight allows having 540 liters of oxygen. The recent introduction of Kevlar cylinders allows increasing the pressure of the compressed oxygen: thus, a weight of 1.9 kg corresponds to 821 liters of oxygen. The quantity of oxygen carried by each responder group must always be in proportion to the type and duration of the mission. It is important to consider whether re-supply of oxygen is available in the Cold Zone; the response groups who will work in the decontamination zone cannot depend only on the oxygen they carry themselves.

What amount of oxygen is useful for resuscitation?

The simplest means of administering oxygen to a patient with spontaneous respiration is to utilize a high-flow oxygen mask at a rate of 8–10 liters per minute. While this is the classic method of administering oxygen in the hospital setting, it consumes large amounts of oxygen.

If a self-filling resuscitation bag is utilized, it is imperative that it is attached to a protective filter: the patient is thus ventilated with oxygenated ambient air. This permits the use of a low oxygen flow rate while there is a high concentration in the mask. Portable respirators consume oxygen at a rate of 10–20 ml of gas per minute. The majority of portable respirators only function for 1 hour with a standard oxygen cylinder. If the patient presents only moderate respiratory distress but nevertheless requires assisted ventilation, only some portable respirators allow ventilatory support when this patient is breathing. In such cases, oxygen is delivered only when it is needed, which allows a significant economy in oxygen use. These functions can only be utilized for patients who are still breathing.

Filtration of ventilation air

An alterative to the use of compressed air for powering the respirator is the utilization of ambient air, which it is necessary to filter. This constraint also imposes the use of a filter to ensure the safety of the responders. Certain filters can be attached to the resuscitation bag (such as the Ambu MK3) and this can be used in the contamination zone. This approach has been applied to portable ventilators that can be powered not by oxygen but by filtered ambient air. The 'CompPAC' respirator, which is anticipated in the French plan, utilizes this technique. It has a common gas-powered motor that can be operated with filtered and compressed air under battery power. The respirator is thus capable of ventilating the patient with oxygen-enriched air. The 'CompPAC' respirator can function autonomously for 8 hours, and for 4 hours by utilizing a 'B'-type Kevlar oxygen cylinder with a fraction of inspired oxygen (FiO_2) of 50%. This represents a considerable improvement in comparison to use of the same cylinder with a conventional respirator that is limited to 1 hour.

Management and handling of victims in the decontamination zone

Organization

Having anticipated the need for personnel protection and the number of victims to be treated in a simultaneous fashion is indispensable. The widely expressed opinion has been that, generally, the utilization of chemical or biological weapons of mass destruction produces such a large number of victims that any action would be impossible. This opinion has since been somewhat disputed by the hypothesis that terrorist chemical attacks can generate only a limited number of victims requiring resuscitation in the decontamination zone (if this remains necessary). This hypothesis of a limited number of victims is supported by experience of managing toxic accidents and by study of the Japanese experience [2]. Thus, only intervention by equipped and trained fire service and civil defense responders is utilized in the Hot Zone. The necessity for medical groups in the decontamination zone is limited. For example, for the Paris SAMU, a single resuscitation group consisting of two persons, a physician and a nurse, is anticipated to be needed in the decontamination zone. The majority of other groups from Paris or the Paris region are either kept in the Cold Zone, close to the incident site, or would be sent to reinforce the medical groups at receiving hospitals. Equipment including respirators and low-weight oxygen cylinders can allow intervention in the contamination zone for about 6 hours. Victims requiring resuscitation are prioritized for decontamination and are then under the surveillance of the medical group. The patient is finally moved to the Cold Zone, where resuscitation can be pursued with the assembled resources that have been dispatched to the incident site.

How many victims can be managed in the decontamination zone?

The number of victims who can benefit from resuscitation depends upon the means possessed by the intervention groups. The medical groups of the Paris SAMU are made up of an ambulance driver, a physician, and a nurse capable of rapidly managing all cases of respiratory distress. Once the airway is secured, the patient can be placed on a respirator and entrusted to clinical surveillance. In this type of circumstance, a single medical responder group can take charge of different patients, assuring the management of vital distress. In practice, the number of these victims requiring specialized management before decontamination remains small. The majority of victims only require management by first-aid groups, who can when necessary assure mask oxygen therapy. Rapid triage allows identifying the most severely affected victims, who require immediate medical management and decontamination before they are transported to the designated hospital service.

Conclusion

A terrorist attack with biological or chemical weapons is completely possible and could generate a large number of victims. Evidence from previous attacks has allowed recognition of the small number of severely affected victims. With prior preparation, responder groups should be capable of operatiing in such an eventuality. Key factors are the problem of supplying oxygen and the necessity for training responder groups. The use of recently developed methods should allow extension of the initial management phase. The early use of antidotes combined with specialized resuscitation has radically changed the prognosis of victims exposed to chemical or biological agents, and the term 'weapons of mass destruction' to describe these situations seems inappropriate.

Planning, equipping, and training responder services are the best responses to the dispersion of chemical and biological agents.

References

1. Kaplan DE, Marshall A. *The Cult at the End of the World.* New York: Crown, 1996.
2. Matsuda N, Takatsu M, Morinari H, Ozawa T. Sarin poisoning in the Tokyo subway. *Lancet,* 1995; **345**: 1446–1447.
3. Borio L, Frank D, Mani V. Death due to bioterrorism-related anthrax. Report of two patients. *J Am Med Assoc,* 2001; **286**: 2554–2559.
4. Alibek K, Handelman S. *Biohazard.* London: Arrow Books, 2000; 319 pp.
5. Harris R, Paxman J. *A Higher Form of Killing.* London: Chatto and Windus, 1982; 272 pp.
6. Borak J, Callan M, Abbot W. Hazardous materials exposure: emergency response and patient care. Englewood Cliffs, NJ: Prentice-Hall, 1991.
7. Mehta PS, Mehta AS, Mehta SJ *et al.* Bhopal tragedy's health effects: a review of methyl isocyanate toxicity. *J Am Med Assoc,* 1990; **264**: 2781–2787.
8. United Nations. Report of the mission dispatched by the Secretary General to investigate allegations of the use of chemical weapons in the conflict between the Islamic Republic of Iran and Iraq, May 8, 1987. UN Document S/18852. New York: United Nations.
9. Baker DJ. Advanced life support for toxic injuries (TOXALS). *Eur J Emerg Med,* 1996; **3:** 327–348.
10. Baker DJ. Toxic substances. *Resuscitation,* 1999; **42**(special edn): 101–159.
11. The International Liaison Committee on Resuscitation. Guidelines for adult basic life support. *Resuscitation,* 2000; **46**: 29–71.

9

Hospital management of chemical incident victims

Frédéric Baud and Bruno Mégarbane

Chemical risk resulting from an accident or criminal activity does not seem very probable, but it carries significant consequences for the populace and the environment. Chemical risk poses medical problems for pre-hospital management, which are discussed in Chapter 8, and for hospital management, which form the focus of this chapter.

The potential severity of a chemical incident in the civilian setting must be emphasized, because of the diversity of the chemical products that can be involved. In effect, we are concerned not only with chemical weapons but also, as history has shown, with acute industrial poisonings with chlorine, ammonia, and methyl isocyanate (sadly well-known from the Bhopal catastrophe) and exposures to metals such as mercury, arsenic, or thallium, or to numerous and varied pesticides. Risks also exist in the domestic environment: lead is the cause of childhood saturnism, and threatens cities with old housing, while carbon monoxide remains the principle cause of domestic toxic deaths from fire smoke, a complex mixture of toxic gases including cyanide, which provokes incapacitation and then kills the victims before they have even been burned.

The unique properties of a chemical incident in the civilian setting are also characterized by the diversity of possible contamination routes, which determine the rapidity with which symptoms appear. If air contaminated with gases or similar products (aerosols, products with a high vapor pressure) is the exposure route of greatest concern, it should not lead to underestimation of the potential risk of contamination of drinking water, foodstuffs, or medications. Historically, amongst other incidents that have been documented are: adulterated cooking oil in Spain, which caused hundreds if not thousands of exposures; wines contaminated with methanol in Italy or ethylene glycol in Austria; capsules of over-the-counter analgesics adulterated with cyanide; and incidents or criminal activities implicating phenol or ricin in the UK.

There are two types of incidents in relation to the presentation of victims as a function of time:

Treating Victims of Mass Destsuction   Edited by Patrick Barriot and Chantal Bismuth
© 2008 John Wiley & Sons, Ltd

- Acute incidents characterized by hospital emergency department arrival of a large number of exposed persons over a short period of time.

- Incidents involving the contamination of drinking water or foodstuffs, which can cause additional subacute incidents that bring about a relatively rapid and progressive increase in the number of victims over a time period lasting up to several weeks. The incidents are similar to infectious epidemics, which form the main differential diagnosis.

The unique features of chemical incidents in the civilian setting are also characterized by the diversity of the civilian population, which can be affected by:

- Cultural diversity, with a large range of languages spoken in large metropolitan areas. It is evident that in such a setting some persons who are involved in a chemical incident may not understand orders, recommendations, and directions, which are generally given in the native language of the country.

- The particular population involved, notably children, the elderly, women of reproductive age, pregnant women, nursing mothers, and persons with pre-existing illnesses or allergies.

- Differences from the military setting, where personnel are prepared for such incidents. Civilian populations are neither prepared nor equipped to face such threats.

There is a radical difference between civilian and military hospitals. Response to chemical warfare response is among the missions assigned to military hospitals. Having thus been made an integral part of their possible role, military hospitals also train the combatants of the Army health services for this eventuality. To respond to this mission, military hospitals have reserves of beds and medications, but this is not the case for civilian hospitals, where chemical risks have only recently been integrated into their missions and, as yet, only for referral hospitals. There exists neither the infrastructure nor the reserve of beds to deal with this risk if these are not freed by suspension of normal activities, which could not be done without posing problems. If stockpiles of medications have been established, the question then arises as to their availability and who has the authority to order them to be dispensed. This vision should not lead to the belief that military hospitals are exempt from problems. The numerous closures of entire hospitals and their associated bed capacity is a grave crisis for the demographics of military physicians, demonstrating, if it is needed, that the health services of the Armed Forces are also confronted with major problems.

All these characteristics, moreover, draw attention to the differences between the civilian population and civilian hospitals and the military population and military hospitals. In effect, the military population is selected, trained, and equipped to confront the risks of chemical warfare. These major differences prevent simple transposition of military procedures to the civilian setting and necessitate rethinking concerning the management of civilian populations in civilian hospitals that are not prepared for this eventuality.

In France, ministerial directives have instituted referral hospitals. This appears to be an interesting initiative, but the missions of referral hospitals have yet to be defined. It must not be forgotten that in practice civilian victims are always taken to the nearest hospital. The role of the nearest hospital must be emphasized for highly acute incidents, such as the Tokyo subway sarin attack, as the chronology of the progression of events following the attack demonstrates. The first ambulatory patient presented himself to the nearest emergency department, St. Luke's Hospital, with only a brief delay, although the first ambulance arrived only after this first ambulatory victim. Thereafter, the flow of victims was very large, as 500 victims arrived at this hospital in 1 hour. One thing that should be remarked is the dispersion of management. In total, this attack involved 5000 victims, including persons only exposed or actually poisoned, who were managed at more than 100 hospitals and clinics. It would be wrong and dangerous to believe that the care of victims of chemical accidents only involves the administration of antidotes and that such nearby hospitals lack the capacity to confront the management of chemical accident victims. For a very large number of toxic chemicals, including some chemical weapons, no antidotes exist. Symptomatic treatments, among the first rank oxygen and the means for its administration, are of great efficacy for treating the respiratory, neurological, cardiac, and hematological failure that numerous chemical products can cause. The real problem is the availability of oxygen in sufficient quantities. The choice of antidotes and their place in chemical catastrophes remains to be clarified in the future.

For confronting acute or hyperacute accidents, consideration was made at the Lariboisière Hospital of the Public Assistance Hospitals of Paris and a management procedure has been proposed: it is available on the Internet site of the regional poison center. The hospital management of chemical accident victims is based on the points described below.

1. *Emergency recognition of a chemical accident.* The example of Tokyo demonstrated the need for this with ambulatory victims who were taken to the hospital before the health authorities had identified the chemical involved. The principle problem during acute accidents is represented by victim triage at the hospital doors. Triage is clearly the cornerstone of hospital management, because it separates patients at risk or poisoned from those who have only been exposed, in order to adapt treatment to poisoning severity. This has the triple purpose of decontamination and application of symptomatic and specific measures. This allows adaptation of the medical response to the individual problem and assures good utilization of the health care system. It is carried out by one or two trained and mobilized physicians and, as a function of the number of chemical accident victims, several nurses, nurses' aides, and hospital orderlies. The problem resides in the fact that a good triage physician is a trained physician and that in the realm of medical toxicology such physicians with clinical experience are rather few. The locations where these persons should be stationed, as well as their respective roles, should be determined in advance, a process that also determines the necessary numbers for each hospital.

2. *Definition of the necessity for protection of health care personnel.* It seems to us that in this field a certain extremism currently presides as to the choice of methods and materials. If optimal personal protection to bring about intervention at disaster sites appears absolutely necessary, its utilization in hospitals remains 'feasible'. It is a good bet that highly contaminated and probably incapacitated patients (e.g. victims of neurotoxic gases) will remain at the site and will be managed by specialized and protected teams. Contaminated but ambulatory patients (e.g. victims of sulfur mustard) can without problems be directed to decontamination lines.

   The methods and materials for 'heavy' decontamination require initial training and then regular practice, which the normal rapid rotation of personnel renders extremely difficult in the general hospital setting, even though it can be done for specialized pre-hospital emergency responders. The materials have a shelf-life and stockpiling them assumes that the problem of replacements has been resolved. It is probable that some simple remedials that can be rapidly deployed will be much more efficacious than 'heavy' ones that are difficult to put in place. The corollary with the protection of health care personnel is presented in the next section.

3. *Activation of a decontamination line that, however, is only of interest for a small number of strongly feared toxicants necessitating decontamination.* Decontamination procedures are now well standardized. They have two goals: (a) to limit absorption by the victim; and (b) to reduce the risks of poisoning response personnel during rescue and medical care of the victims. The principle of a decontamination line is based on the establishment of an open and unidirectional circuit, where the victims pass from a contaminated zone to a clean zone (marked out in advance) after undressing and showering. The complexity of such a decontamination line must not be underestimated. It calls upon personnel who are posted at different places along the chain for ambulatory persons: (a) reception and explanation of decontamination; (b) undressing; (c) accompaniment and monitoring of showering; (d) concomitant decontamination of valuable objects. Then, in passing to the uncontaminated zone with (e) reception, drying, and clothing the decontaminated persons to whom their valuable objects have been restored, and then (f) orientation towards an accommodation zone and medical examination. Decontamination is founded on a shower with soap for all toxicants of concern. The real problem is that of subsequent management of private persons and their dwellings, and that they must be housed and certain ones treated. Cutaneous and mucous membrane decontamination is easy to accomplish with water and soap, provided that conditions have been prepared, that is, a circuit has been defined, a tent or other place for showering has been set up, and shelter provided for victims who have been undressed, especially in the winter time. A slower process, in a parallel circuit, should be included when decontamination involves stretcher patients or frankly poisoned patients, who necessitate third-party assistants and many more personnel who must also be protected. The civilian setting poses the particular problem of the decontamination and preservation of victim's personal goods, administrative documents, and credit cards. This can be assured by passing

these effects through a dilute hypochlorite solution. All contaminated clothing is placed in sealed plastic sacks.

4. *Collection of pertinent medical data that permit an initial toxicological orientation and communication of this information to the poison center, in order to propose a probable toxicological diagnosis.* Data collection can be carried out by research on the initial victims' symptoms and signs, which have an orientation value. It involves collaboration between physicians and nurses. The toxic syndromes identified allow the evocation of a class of toxicants as the probable origin of the poisoning, by proposing the 'compatibility' of the clinical picture with a class of toxicants. We recommend taking urine samples (at least 10 ml) from all symptomatic and asymptomatic persons, after decontamination, in a closed and labeled container that can be stored as 'urotech'. Blood sampling should only be done in symptomatic patients admitted to hospital for monitoring, or in those who have received specific care or treatments. Usually, about 5 ml of blood in an anticoagulated tube is sufficient for toxicological analyses that can be done to better evaluate the reality of exposure of different victims to the incriminated toxicant. WARNING! Do not freeze whole blood.

5. *Thereafter, there can be an adaptation of personal protective measures and making use of prepared individual guides for management adapted to risk.* In effect, protective gear and decontamination are only of interest for a small number of chemical weapons and also a small number of currently utilized chemical products. The guides we have developed have been for exposures to asphyxiant gases, cyanide and its derivatives, organophosphates, and fire smoke.

   The advantages of individual therapeutic guides are to free the physician, who must manage the patients in accordance with information sources which in these circumstances can be difficult to consult, to give a medical response adapted to each victim, and to furnish a personal medical record which allows follow-up and tracking of what has been done. This initial management should in effect assure patient tracking and begin the follow-up of exposed and poisoned persons.

   The inconvenience of such guides resides in the necessity to regularly keep them up to date, adaptation of the medical responders on site to use these guides, the choice of proper therapeutics proposed, and the necessity of having available the medications recommended by the guides.

6. Immediately following the initial management, the aim of which is to correct the symptoms or oxygen system failures, follow-up is established. In effect, these acute poisonings can be the etiology of a chronic illness. They can be the sources of physiological or psychological sequelae. It is also necessary to define the agents of long-term risk to women of reproductive age and pregnant women, and to respond to the questions such women ask. Such medical monitoring can only be done through a multidisciplinary approach continued over a prolonged time period.

While hyperacute accidents are currently of most interest, we must not forget that subacute or chronic poisonings may occur. There are many examples in the medical literature of such risks. These incidents are characterized by the diversity of clinical manifestations that can affect the nervous system, lungs, and gastrointestinal and hematopoietic systems, among others. The insidious character of these factors and the confusing number of victims must be emphasized. As an example, during the toxic oil epidemic in Spain, it was the Spanish General Practitioners who alerted the public health authorities because of the occurrence of numerous suspect cases in a short period of time. In France, the French National Institute of Public Health (www.inrs.sante.fr) undoubtedly has an essential role to play in giving such alerts, complementing the role of the Poison Center. Prolonged patient follow-up is implicit in these cases.

The spontaneous or provoked chemical risk assumes varied forms. It is rare, but not completely exceptional. It strikes without warning. It is the etiology of human and environmental catastrophes (where a 'catastrophe' is taken to mean a situation that is unmanageable, except with enormous resources, permanently exceeding an efficacy–risk relationship supportable by the country). This risk is unforeseeable, such that hospitals can only organize themselves simply and for the duration.

Civilian populations wait for the public services to devise:

- The structure of an efficacious health care system, not only pre-hospital but also hospital-based, which allows an immediate management response.

- A precise toxicological diagnosis.

- Transparent information regarding the middle- and long-term risks.

- Follow-up to appreciate the actual damage and the not exceptional sequelae.

Appendix: hospital management of chemical risk

A chemical incident can result not only from exposure to products currently utilized in industrial, agricultural, or domestic settings, but also from the deployment of chemical weapons. This particular chemical risk, especially in unprepared civilian hospitals, requires having procedures in place that can allow them to fulfill their public service mission while protecting their personnel.

In the case of a chemical incident, the hospital should be alerted by the local authorities, the pre-hospital medical response services, or the Poison Center, to avoid the probable presentation to unwarned hospital emergency services of persons who have been exposed in such an incident. The purpose of the procedure we present below is for response to a situation where victims of a chemical incident present to the hospital emergency department when the hospital has not been alerted.

The hospital management of chemical risks is based on the following procedure:

- Recognition of a chemical incident at the hospital emergency department allowing a given alert.

- Definition of the necessity for personnel protection.

- Its corollary: activation of a decontamination line.

- Proposal of a probable toxicological diagnosis, which is based on: (a) the collection of pertinent medical data allowing a toxicological orientation, which must be carried out by the first responders present in the emergency department; (b) communication of these data to the regional poison center, which will eventually make a probable diagnosis.

From these, under the advice of the poison center:

- Adoption of personnel protective measures.

- Institution of individual management guidelines adapted to the risk. The individual guidelines are the following: (a) asphyxiant gases; (b) neurotoxicants (for cyanide, see Chapter 4).

These guidelines allow:

- Definition of the criteria for immediate hospitalization in the intensive care unit, initial monitoring, and discharge.

- Definition of symptomatic and antidotal treatment in relation to the severity of symptoms.

- Definition of monitoring parameters for the initial evaluation.

- Commencement of medical follow-up of patients.

- Assurance of data-tracking of symptoms and treatments applied, as well as medical and administrative decisions that have been undertaken.

Websites for more information, sample forms, etc.

http://www.premierinc.com/.../topics/disaster_readiness/downloads/aha_disaster_readiness_advisory_101601.doc
Useful tables on chemical/biological agents, their diagnosis, and treatment.
http://www.bt.cdc.gov

Centers for Disease Control and Prevention (CDC) Emergency Preparedness and Response website, with a large amount of information on bioterrorism, chemical emergencies, radiation emergencies, mass casualties, etc. Includes information on preparation and planning, training and education, and recent outbreaks and incidents, as well as related links.

http://www.atsdr.cdc.gov/hazmat-emergency-preparedness.html
Agency for Toxic Substances and Disease Registry, HazMat Emergency Preparedness Training and Tools for Responders website, with a large amount of information relating to hazardous chemical incidents, including training issues.

http://www.facs.org/civiliandisasters/trauma.html
American College of Surgeons reports on unconventional civilian disasters. Mainly intended for surgeons, but has a good discussion of chemical and biological disasters and useful links to other related sites.

http://www.ahrq.gov/clinic/epcsums/hospmcisum.htm
Evidence Report/Technology Assessment No. 95; Training of Hospital Staff to Respond to a Mass Casualty Incident, from the Agency for Healthcare Research and Quality (AHRQ).

http://www.gao.gov/new.items/d03924.pdf
A report from the General Accounting Office (GAO) on hospital preparedness.

http://www.nlm.nih.gov
The home page of the US National Library of Medicine. A search in Pubmed on 'hospital chemical disaster plans' returns 24 useful reference citations.

http://www.google.com
A search on 'hospital chemical disaster plans' returns over 2 million hits. The first 20 seem to be the most useful.

10

Non-conventional counter-terrorism

Chantal Bismuth and Stephen W. Borron

In October 2002, the liberation of hostages from a Moscow theater was accomplished, after a managed assault, not with firearms but with the aid of a gas infiltrated into the air-conditioning (HVAC) system, causing the deaths of 117 of the 800 hostages, but in conditions that had lasted for several days – the absence of replenishment of oxygen, sleep deprivation, anxiety, thirst, and hunger.

Today, the nature of the gas still remains conjectural. Shevchenko, the Minister of Public Health, clearly declared that it was an aerosol based on Fentanyl®, a strong opioid with a rapid action, utilized in anesthesia and analgesia. He added that no product prohibited by the Convention on Chemical Weapons had been utilized and that the first aid teams were supplied with the antidote naloxone, specific for opioids. The Fentanyl was without doubt part of a medication mixture. A toxicologist colleague, Zilker, could detect the presence of Halothane on the third day in two German hostages (without, however, finding traces of Fentanyl, no doubt due to the rapidly of its metabolism over several hours without accumulation in the body).

Utilizing rapidly-acting anesthetics in such an operation is always a high-risk proposal. Fentanyl, like Halothane, has a narrow therapeutic window, implicating some possibly lethal secondary effects, such as respiratory depression, at doses slightly higher than those required for its medical action. It is not, in fact, utilizable in slightly higher doses than those used in the operating room or intensive care unit, where there are immediate possibilities for assisted ventilation.

The assailants of the Moscow Theater have been blamed by certain professionals. Others have been more indulgent. 'I am stunned that they have succeeded in this,' said a consulting anesthesiologist for the American government, with regard to the medical risks of chemical weapons. 'The relative success of the raid indicates that the Russians have invested a great deal of time, effort, and money in this non-lethal chemical' [1].

Treating Victims of Mass Destsuction   Edited by Patrick Barriot and Chantal Bismuth
© 2008 John Wiley & Sons, Ltd

Is it legitimate for counter-terrorism to conduct an assault with non-conventional weapons?

In the case of hostage taking, the responsible parties are precluded from utilizing lethal non-conventional weapons, such as cyanides, organophosphates, sulfur mustard ('mustard gas'), or asphyxiants, against their own populace. The use of incapacitating agents, such as BZ, is generally disapproved. Neutralizing agents, such as the lacrimators, do not modify consciousness and thus immediately increase the aggressivity of the terrorists to take action against the hostages. Medication products are therefore the first line to use: during airplane hijackings in the past there have already been studies on ways of introducing tranquilizers, such as benzodiazepines (Valium®), or antidepressants, such as serotonin reuptake inhibitors like Prozac® or sertraline (Zoloft®), and even convulsant drugs or products that have been militarized [2] for inclusion in foods demanded by the airplane pirates. However, these various products act too slowly to assure rapid neutralization of the terrorists.

In fact, militarization of Valium or Prozac undermines the spirit of the treaty against chemical weapons, which:

'... interdicts the development and usage of all chemical agents which can cause incapacity or permanent damage' [1].

In effect:

'Targeted medications such as sedatives, and including those having a large therapeutic window, such as Valium®, can result in a mortality of 5 percent if utilized in sufficient quantities for neutralizing terrorists' [3].

This dilemma of dosage and the proscription of chemical weapons has currently led the USA to propose other technologies for the deterrence of terrorists, including microwaves and acoustical weapons [1]. The 'painful rays' are delivered as salvos of unbearable heating microwaves, without apparent damage to the body: volunteers have declared that it feels like 'being wound around a light bulb'. Another non-lethal prototype consists of an 'acoustic weapon', made of very precise acoustic energy waves that vibrate the internal organs, temporarily incapacitating these targets. The advantage of these two new approaches is the uniformity of their effects throughout the entire population, reducing the risks of overdose, as opposed to gas, and their ease of being interrupted instantaneously during their application.

The armed forces of the USA maintain specific chemical research programs. The Joint Non-Lethal Weapons Program has the intention of developing an anti-materiél and anti-personnel weapon that can hamper the movement of terrorists or demonstrators. These chemical products would then be liberated by pressure, dispersion, or encapsulated carriers [4].

Lakoski et al. from Pennsylvania State University have prepared a report for the US armed forces entitled 'Advantages and limitations of sedatives in technical non-lethal usage' (in which the term 'sedatives' is a US neologism, refusing identification with a chemical weapon). The authors concluded that there is a need for specific non-lethal techniques, selective and reversible, which avoid the occurrence of long-term side-effects for the users and their targets. The utilization of 'sedatives' as non-lethal weapons is both adequate and justified. The authors define 'sedative' as a pharmaceutical compound capable of inducing non-reactive behavior. They propose several classes of compounds with a 'high potential for utilization': benzodiazepines, alpha-2-adrenergic agonists, dopaminergic D_3 agnonists, serotonin re-uptake inhibitors, antagonists of the liberating factor for corticotropin, and cholecystokinin B receptor antagonists [5].

It is not excluded that the USA also maintains secret chemical research. Their experts understand the discretion of Russian officials:

'If the situation recurs, it is not to be hoped for that the terrorists know how to take appropriate counter-measures or can themselves utilize their weapons' [1].

Lewer and Feakin [6] have examined the perspectives and the implications of the proliferation of non-lethal weapons. They emphasize the difficulty of depriving countries or groups likely to use them of such weapons as means of torture or punishment (they give the example of a judge who delivered a 50 000 Volt electric shock to a criminal wearing an electric belt, because he howled in the courtroom). More worrisome yet, they note that:

'... non-proliferation measures are difficult to establish because of the techniques and equipment risk not being limited to non-lethal technologies.' [6]

Finally, the problems of packaging of weapons, of penetration to invested sites, of possible sanctions incurred *a posteriori*, for the moment considerably complicate anti-terrorist actions managed by unconventional means. Military assaults with firearms or blades, conducted for freeing hostages, themselves have their own risks and limitations. Perhaps the new technologies will prove themselves, in the end, to be more of the same, all for saving the hostages, for suppressing ongoing terrorist action, without incurring international condemnation [7].

References

1. A softer touch. The US is developing weapons that would subdue, not kill. *US News and World Report*, November 11, 2002; 32.
2. Stone A. US research on sedatives in combat sets off alarms. *Science*, 2002; **297**: 754.
3. Schiermeier Q. Hostage deaths put gas weapons in spotlight. *Nature*, 2002; **420**: 7.
4. Joint NLWP 2000 Annual Report: www.inlwd.usmc.mil
5. Lakowski JM, Murray WV, Kenny JM. The advantages and limitations of calmatives for use as a non-lethal technique: www.sunshine-project.org
6. Lewer N, Feakin T. Perspectives and implications for the proliferation of non-lethal weapons in the context of contemporary conflict, security interests and arms control. *Med Conflict Survival*, 2001; **17**: 272–286.
7. Wax PM, Becker CE, Curry SC. Unexpected 'gas' casualties in Moscow: a medical toxicology perspective. *Ann Emerg Med*, 2003; **41**: 700–705.

11

Introduction to biological weapons

Patrick Barriot and Chantal Bismuth

On April 10, 1972, a convention prohibiting the development, fabrication, and stock-piling of biological weapons was signed in London, Washington, and Moscow. It came into force on March 26, 1975, and was ratified by France in 1984. The arrangements of this convention apply not only to natural biological agents, but also to all agents result-ing from synthesis operations or genetic manipulation. Unfortunately, this convention does not establish any verification procedures and otherwise allows signatory countries to pursue research of a 'defensive character'. However, the mixed or dual character of this type of research, both civilian and military, carries the potential for diversion from defensive to offensive development. This was pointed out by Ivan Amoto in a recent in a recent article in Chemical and Engineering News [1]: "There are no bad molecules, only bad human beings."

It is important to emphasize that the nuclear powers (USA, former Soviet Union, and UK) were the originators of the 1972 Convention, which was not conceived for the purpose of eradicating biological weapons but rather for prohibiting their access by potential enemies. In this sense, it inscribes more of a counter-proliferation strategy than an eradication project. The proliferation of formidable low-cost weapons in effect threatens the supremacy of the possessors of nuclear weapons. The Convention must then prevent States that cannot attain atomic status because of technological obstacles from equipping themselves with the means of mass destruction. Nevertheless, despite the 1972 Convention, the list of countries conducting biological weapons research pro-grams, mostly for defence, now includes: South Africa, Bulgaria, China, North Korea, Cuba, Egypt, the USA, India, Iraq, Iran, Israel, Laos, Libya, Pakistan, Romania, Rus-sia, Sudan, Syria, Taiwan, and Vietnam.

In 1996 the director of the US Arms Control and Disarmament Agency declared:

"There are today in the world two times more States having an offensive military bio-logical program than during the entry into force of the prohibition of biological weapons Convention in 1975."

Treating Victims of Mass Destsuction   Edited by Patrick Barriot and Chantal Bismuth
© 2008 John Wiley & Sons, Ltd

While it may be possible for a country possessing nuclear weapons to dissuade a State from employing biological weapons, it is totally illusory to hope to dissuade a terrorist group engaged in 'asymmetrical' combat.

Utilization of pathogenic agents for hostile ends

In antiquity, it was usual in times of war to contaminate the enemy's water supplies by means of animal carcasses. The Scythian archers soaked their arrow points in putrefied cadavers in order to infect the wounded. Catapulting contaminated cadavers over the ramparts of cities under siege is mentioned many times in the historical record. In 1346, the Tartars laid siege to the town of Kaffa on the shores of the Black Sea, in which Genoese merchants had established a commercial trading centre. The besieging forces, victims of a plague epidemic, catapulted the bodies of victims into the interior of the city, which was taken some time later. In October, 1347, the Genoese merchants brought back the plague from the Black Sea region to the city of Messina in Sicily. This episode could have been the origin of the great epidemic of 1348 that spread throughout the ports of the Mediterranean, and then throughout all of Europe [2]. After 2 years, this disease, transmitted by the fleas of rats and by persons afflicted with the pulmonary form, had killed one-third, or perhaps nearly half, of the European population and more than 200 million persons had succumbed in the course of three pandemics.

It was with the aid of variola (smallpox) that Europeans conquered the Americas. In the sixteenth century, the Spanish conquistadors propagated smallpox among the Indians of South America. The most affected populations were those who suffered from malnutrition and lived in densely populated cities. The Indians of the Brazilian coast, who had abundant resources of fish for food and lived in isolated villages, were relatively spared. During the year 1763, British armed forces intentionally distributed blankets contaminated with smallpox to the tribes of the Ohio Valley, in order to provoke a devastating epidemic in the indigenous population, who were not immunized against this disease.

Unlike chemical weapons, biological weapons were not utilized during World War I. However, it is suitable to cite Dr. Anton Dilger, who in 1915 used cultures of *Bacillus anthracis and Burkholderia mallei,* furnished by the Imperial government of Germany, to contaminate horses and cattle destined for the Allied forces in Europe. On their part, the Allies attempted to contaminate the German cavalry horses by means of samples of *B. mallei.*

Between the two World Wars, Japan developed a significant program of biological warfare, which was entrusted to Unit 731 under the direction of Professors Shiro Ishii and Kitano Misaji. Numerous pathogenic agents, such as plague or anthrax, were tested in human beings, having been employed against the Chinese in Manchuria from 1932. Amongst other things, this infamous unit made an effort to disseminate plague by dropping porcelain bombs filled with fleas contaminated with *Yersinia pestis.* In September 1945, the Japanese Army considered bacteriological attacks on the west coast of the USA. This operation, code-named 'night of the blooming cherry trees', would have been carried out by seaplanes launched from submarines. After World War II, the USA recruited specialists who had served with the Japanese Unit 731 to begin their program of biological warfare research.

In 1941, the British government, suspecting Hitler of developing pathological agents for military purposes, decided to develop an anthrax bomb capable of annihilating German livestock and part of the population. In July, 1942, a bomb containing a wet anthrax culture was tested on the small Scottish island of Gruinard, resulting in the death of all the sheep there and causing long-lasting soil contamination. The British went on to be ready to respond to a biological attack and to this end stockpiled 5000 anthrax bombs. Hitler did not give them a reason to respond because he was reticent, if not hostile, to the use of biological weapons. These latter made no appearance on the battlefield during World War II.

Modern programs for offensive research

The Cold War was marked by intensive biological weapons research. In the days following signature of the 1972 Convention, the USSR created a gigantic unit charged with placing genetic engineering at the service of biological warfare [2,3,4]. Two facilities were in charge of the offensive biological program: the 15th Directorate of the Ministry of Defense and the Biopreparat civilian organization. This latter, created in 1973, comprised more than 50 installations, including the center for Virology and Biotechnology, 'Vektor', situated near Novossibirsk. This employed many tens of thousands of persons, including 9000 scientists. The experiments conceived in the Center for Studies of Biological Weapons were carried out on the island of Vosrozhdenje in the Aral Sea, near Kazakhstan and Uzbekistan. The major outlines of this offensive program were divulged by two defectors, formerly directors of the Biopreparat organization, Vladimir Pasechnik and Kanatjan Alibekov. The 'Enzyme' project, launched in 1972, was aimed at the militarization of a large number of pathogenic agents, such as smallpox (variola), plague, anthrax, tularemia, hemorrhagic fevers, and viral encephalopathies [5–10]. The Vektor Center for Molecular Virology worked on sequencing the genome of the smallpox virus as well as genetic recombinations between extremely virulent pathogenic agents. Two strains of anthrax bacilli were modified, the first for resistance to six classes of antibiotics, the second to attack erythrocytes. On Friday March 30, 1979, at 'Department 19' of the Sverdlovsk facility for production of biological weapons (Ekaterinburg, Urals), a negligent act caused the release of 50 grams of militarized anthrax spores [11]. These spores were spread throughout the atmosphere of Sverdlovsk, causing, according to the official report, contamination of 96 persons and the deaths of 66 persons; other sources have stated that there were 105–600 deaths. The facility was then transferred from Sverdlosk to Stepnogorsk (Kazakhstan). This accidental contamination of the population was not officially recognized until 1993, in a conversation attributed by Pravda to Boris Yeltsin. According to Ken Alibek, by the end of the 1970s the USSR had in its arsenal a permanent reserve of 20 tons of smallpox. Over the following decade, the Soviet forces adapted biological weapons to the warheads of SS-18 type intercontinental missiles. On April 11, 1992, President Boris Yeltsin announced that the Soviet Union had renounced all biological military programs and signed a decree prohibiting research programs contrary to the 1972 Convention. The former structures charged with studying 'special products' were renamed and reorganized within the Directorate for Nuclear, Biological, and Chemical Protection. As for the laboratories of the Biopreparat complex, they were charged with research of a 'defensive character'. The Vektor Molecular Virology and Biotechnology Centre, which had worked on the militarization of the smallpox virus, thus became one of the two laboratories in the world authorized by the World Health Organization (WHO) to preserve cultures of this virus.

The collapse of the USSR has probably favored the proliferation of biological weapons on the basis of a drastic reduction of budgets allocated to the thousands of scientists working on these types of program. With monthly salaries in the range 40–80, these specialists have been tempted to sell their knowledge to the highest bidder. A French parliamentary report written under the direction of Pierre Lellouche emphasized this peril:

'A GAO report estimates at 15 000 the number of underpaid scientists and researchers susceptible to present a risk of proliferation: 5000 persons represent a significant risk of proliferation in the biological area, while 10 000 others possess the aptitudes to adapt a biological agent to a military dispersal device.'

This uneasiness was shared by General Jean-Bernard Pinatel, who wrote in the journal *Défense Nationale:*

'The condition of destitution in which the decomposition of Russia has placed the scientists of Biopreparat, has pushed them very much to research as well as the means of their existence and gives thought to American experts that certain of them have responded to solicitations from Iraq, Iran and North Korea.'

The US research program, initiated in 1942, benefited from the expertise of biologists from the Japanese Unit 731. The majority of US biological weapons were developed during the 1950s at Camp Detrick. At the end of the 1960s, the USA had at its disposal a biological arsenal comprising the principal militarizable pathogenic agents. However, on November 25, 1969, President Richard Nixon announced:

'The United States renounces the utilization of fatal and incapacitating biological weapons … The American biological program will be limited to the research and development of materials for defense.'

The US Army Medical Research Institute of Infectious Diseases (USAMRIID), at Fort Detrick, Maryland, cultivated the Ames strain of anthrax bacillus and conducted work on inserting botulinum toxin genes into its genome. During exercises at the beginning of the 1970s, the Army diffused in some American cities aerosols charged with non-pathogenic biological agents, such as *Serratia marcesens and Bacillus globigii.* It seems, however, that these tests might have caused the deaths of some im-munosuppressed persons.

In the autumn of 1984, Casper Weinberger, US Secretary of Defense, announced to members of Congress that he was in possession of:

'... new proof that the Soviet Union had pursued its programs of offensive biological war-fare and that it exploited the methods of genetic engineering to expand its range.'

This threat apparently justified the pursuit of research programs on pathogenic agents, particularly in the area of molecular biology. In August 1986, Douglas J. Feith, Assistant Secretary of Defense, emphasized the dual character of this research and declared:

'It is possible in the future to produce by synthesis some pathogenic agents answering to very specific military criteria. The techniques which permit the fabrication of "custom-made medications" are equally applicable to custom-made pathogenic agents.'

In the name of biodefense, the Bush and Clinton administrations developed some pro-grams that could be construed by some to be to be contrary to the 1972 Convention. While the budget devoted to research on biological weapons was $15.1 million in 1981, it was increased to $90 million in 1986. During 2001, the USA declined to sign the international protocol responsible for strengthening the 1972 Convention in the endowment of means for verification and the structures for inspection. The grounds invoked were that this protocol was susceptible to place National Security at risk as well as industrial secrets, and confidential data of US biodefense laboratories. The US authorities equally asserted that the 1992 Convention allowed the development, production, and stockpiling of biological agents in limited quantities when they were intended for the development of vaccines, medications, or protection systems.

Using bioengineering techniques of gene amplification, sequencing, and inverse genet-ics, Jeffery Taunenberger's group was able to create in vitro the Spanish Influenza virus (an H1N1 virus originally of avian origin). The details were published in the journal Na-ture on October 6, 2005. An article published in the New York Times on October 17, 2005 was very critical of the open publication of the details of the re-creation of this pathogenic virus which was responsible for causing the deaths of somewhere between 20 and 40 mil-lion human beings. The other worrisome publication was that of a study of the genetic sequencing of the plague agent in Nature on October 4, 2001. These open publications, plus those on insertion of the gene coding for interleukin-4 into the rodent variola virus ("mousepox") by Australian researechers (interleukin-4 dramatically inhibits the immune system, thereby increasing the lethal potential of the virus), demonstrate the potential of these genetic engineering techniques to be used for development of efficacious counter-measures. [Mullbacher A, Lobigs M, Creation of a pox virus could have been predicted. J. Virol 2001; Sep 75(18):8357-5).]

The Iraqi biological weapons program was developed in the 1980s with the aid of Western powers hostile to Iran [12]. The program can be specified thanks to the defection of Saddam Hussein's son-in-law, General Kamel Hussein, in August, 1995. Under the direction of Ribab Taha, more than 8000 liters of anthrax bacillus were produced between 1988 and 1990, in particular in the Al-Hakam complex. The biological agents could have been dispersed by means of various carriers: aerial bombs, ballistic missiles, or dispersal devices. The Iraqi biological weapons were destroyed at the end of the first Gulf War in 1991. Under pressure from the USA, who accused Iraq of having preserved its stockpile of weapons of mass destruction, the United Nations Security Council voted in Resolution 1441, imposing a program of 'intrusive' inspections and complete disarmament of Iraq, on November 8, 2002.

While these arrangements were accepted by Baghdad, a US–UK coalition launched a war in March, 2002, to eliminate the weapons of mass destruction concealed, according to them, by the regime of Saddam Hussein. Such weapons, despite the presence of several thousand US experts in Iraqi territory, have never been discovered. Two suspicious trucks, which no independent expert could approach and that contained only suspicious traces, were presented as mobile laboratories intended for the production of biological weapons. They were, in fact, for material intended to produce hydrogen for weather balloons. The accusation against Iraq was based on estimations of what Baghdad could have fabricated; estimations performed in the 1990s from the quantities of precursors obtained during the Iran–Iraq war. The revelations of Kamel Hussein emphasized, however, that the biological weapons had been destroyed after the beginning of the inspections in 1991.

Political assassinations, terrorism, and counter-terrorism

In recent years, acts of terrorism utilizing pathogenic agents have increased. In January, 1972, two members of the Japanese 'Order of the Rising Sun' were arrested in possession of 40 kg of the agent causing typhoid fever (*Salmonella typhi*). In 1976, inhabitants in several cities in the USA received letters containing ticks that, according to the text of the enclosed letters, were carrying an infectious agent. In September 1984, members of a sect contaminated food in restaurants in Oregon in the USA with a liquid culture of S. *typhi,* causing illness in 600 persons [13]; the objective was to influence the outcome of a local election. An member of this sect had even coated his hand with the liquid culture before shaking hands with local politicians.

The most marked act of bioterrorism in recent years is undeniably the affair of letters booby-trapped with anthrax. On November 4, 2001, the US authorities announced that a man had been intentionally contaminated with anthrax contained in an envelope. On the east coast of the USA, a series of posted letters contaminated with anthrax spores caused the deaths of five persons among the 24 who developed this illness [14,15]. It was later proven that the strain utilized for this bioterrorist attack came not from the former USSR or an unknown rogue state, but from a US strain that was once utilized in a US biodefense and was first found in a natural anthrax animal incident in Texas.

Table 11.1 Non-exhaustive list of militarizable pathogenic agents

Bacteria, ricketsia, fungi
> *Bacillus anthracis (anthrax)*
> *Bartonella quintana (trench fever)*
> *Brucella militensis and Brucella suis (brucellosis)*
> *Burkholderia pseudo-mallei (meliodosis)*
> *Chlamydia psittaci (ornitho-psittacosis)*
> *Clostridium perfringens (gangrene)*
> *Coccidiomycetes (pulmonary mycoses)*
> *Coxiella burnetii (Q fever)*
> *Escherichia coli (transgenic bacteria)*
> *Francisella tularensis (tularemia)*
> *Listeria monocytogenes (listeriosis)*
> *Mycobacterium leprae (leprosy)*
> *Mycobacterium tuberculosis (tuberculosis)*
> *Orientia tsutsugamushi (Japanese river fever)*
> *Rickettsia prowazeckii (exanthematic typhus)*
> *Rickettsia rickettsii (Rocky Mountain spotted fever)*
> *Salmonella paratyphi and Salmonella typhimurium (salmonelloses)*
> *Shigella flexneri and Shigella dysenteriae (shigellosis)*
> *Vibrio cholerae (cholera)*
> *Yersinia pestis (bubonic plague and pulmonary plague)*

Viruses
> *Chikunguya virus*
> *Dengue virus*
> *Tick encephalitis virus*
> *Japanese encephalitis virus*
> *Venezuelan equine encephalomyelitis virus*
> *Yellow fever virus*
> *Rift valley fever virus*
> *Congo-Crimea hemorrhagic fever virus*
> *Korean fever virus*
> *Omsk hemorrhagic fever virus*
> *Argentinian hemorrhagic fever virus (Junin virus)*
> *Bolivian hemorrhagic fever virus (Machupo virus)*
> *Lassa fever virus*
> *Marburg fever virus*
> *Ebola illness virus*
> *Kyasanur forest illness virus*
> *Variola virus*

The different biological agents

The list of biological agents susceptible to be propagated intentionally for hostile ends is known not to be limited (Table 11.1), because the techniques of genetic engineering allow the creation of new virulent strains 'on the fly', as Jeremy Rifkin emphasized:

'One can program the germs in pathogenic micro-organisms to increase their virulence, their resistance to antibiotics, and their stability in the environment. One can insert fatal genes into inoffensive micro-organisms and obtain in this manner pathogenic agents that the human body perceives as harmless and against which there is no resistance. It is even possible to insert genes into some organisms affecting regulatory function that control the blood flow, behavior, or body temperature. Certain researchers claim to have the ability to clone selective toxins in order to eliminate certain racial or ethnic groups because their genotypic constitution predisposes them to certain illnesses. Genetic engineering could also serve to destroy certain species of cultivated plants or domestic animals to undermine the economy of a country.'

Production and dissemination of pathogenic agents

The success of a biological attack depends on numerous factors that are difficult to control, the first of which is the immune response in the exposed population. The militarization of pathogenic agents requires specialists in fields as varied as microbiology, epidemiology, molecular virology, physics of aerosols, explosives, and meteorology. Militarized anthrax is presented in the form of very concentrated spores, whose respiratory penetration is determined by a particle size of 2–3 microns and the addition of a product inhibiting the mechanism of electrostatic aggregation of the spores. Viruses are fragile organisms that are sensitive to heat, ultraviolet light, and abrupt temperature variations. Industrial production necessitates that it is 'good for dual usage' – in other words, civilian equipment can be utilized for military ends, such as fermentors, incubators, lyophilization apparatuses, micro-encapsulators, centrifuges, and air filters. The 'Australian Group', which unites the principal nations producing and exporting biological products, makes an effort to limit the diversion of these types of products. For all these reasons, the international diffusion of biological agents is very uncertain. It is, moreover, necessary to have available efficacious dispersion methods. This can be accomplished with more or less specific carriers:

1. Dispersion by explosion of munitions (e.g. artillery shells, bombs, missiles). The major problem is due to the fact that the detonation destroys part of the biological agent and can render the procedure inefficacious. The SS-18 missiles fielded by the Soviets, however, could be armed with warheads containing smallpox virus. Another agent, anthrax, possesses a major advantage because its spores are particularly resistant to mechanical forces; it is thus incontestably the biological agent best adaptable to explosive munitions. The Iraqi armed forces envisioned the dispersion of anthrax by means of R-400 aerial bombs and missiles derived from the Soviet Scud (Al-Hussein and Al-Samoud missiles). The Israeli offensive biological program anticipated being equipped with the Jericho rocket with a biological warhead.

2. Dissemination in the form of an aerosol by low-altitude aerial spraying. Spraying can be carried out by attack aircraft (e.g. Sukoi, Mirage, F-16) of the M-18 or L-29 type, or by drones such as the Hunter drone, equipped with special tanks for agricultural crop dusting. All light aircraft equipped for the spraying of insecticides

can be diverted by a terrorist to spread an aerosol of pathogenic agents below them, for example, on a sporting event or open air concert.

3. Dissemination in the form of an aerosol in an enclosed or semi-enclosed space, such as a subway, airplane, airport, shopping center, administrative office building, or theater. The aerosol could be dispersed by means of a home-made vaporizer or injected into a ventilation or heating/cooling system. The 'Top Off' exercise, conceived in May 1999 for the US government, envisioned the dispersion of the biological agent for pulmonary plague (Yersinia pestis) in the ventilation ductwork of a center in Denver. In an exercise for simulation of an attack with smallpox, 'Dark Winter', organized in June 2001 in the USA, clouds of aerosols were spread by fake gardeners in commercial centers in three large US cities.

4. The contamination of foodstuffs or drinking water with biological agents (e.g. cholera, typhoid fever, and gastroenteritis) represents a permanent risk in crisis situations. For terrorists groups, the sought-after effect is less that of killing a large number of persons than of setting off a panic reaction or ruining an economic network. Potable water distribution companies are sensitized to this problem and ensure that chlorination eliminates the effects of numerous pathogenic agents.

5. The transmission of infectious diseases by insects or arthropod vectors (e.g. fleas, lice, ticks) could also be envisioned, with examples mentioned above. In the USA, 37 persons recently contracted monkeypox, which was transmitted by prairie dogs kept as companion animals. Although the contamination of the prairie dogs seems to have been accidental, a terrorist group could utilize companion animals as vectors for a modified virus such as smallpox.

6. The transmission of pathogenic agents transported by passive media, such as a parcel or letter, proved its efficacy is the autumn of 2001 in the USA. It is known that the circulation of pathogenic cultures between laboratories, by mail, has been usual for a long time. Scientists who desire to exchange viral strains soak a filter paper in the culture and then let it dry under a hood. It is then wrapped up in a sealed plastic bag and simply sent by mail.

7. Finally, the human vector represents a particularly formidable mode of propagation of an infectious disease. An individual who voluntarily contracts a highly contagious infectious disease, such as smallpox, pulmonary plague, or a hemorrhagic fever of the Ebola type, before having contact with a dense population would constitute a veritable 'biological bomb'.

Biological warfare against livestock and crops

Recent epidemics of aphthous fever (hoof and mouth disease of cattle) and bird flu (avian influenza) emphasize the reality of concerns about infectious risk, accidental but also criminal, on breeding farms. Grain fields are equally threatened by devastating agents that could be intentionally propagated in the context of economic warfare. In reducing biodiversity and the natural means of resistance, current dissemination of genetically modified grains could favor mass contamination and assure the promotion of certain varieties of genetically modified organisms (GMOs).

From this point of view, an interesting example is the beetle *Diabrotica virgifera*. This is an organism of US origin that devastates corn, responsible each year for estimated losses of $1 million in the USA. This insect was inadvertently introduced into Europe by US military aircraft during the Balkans war. Since then, it has progressed across the continent. Curiously, firms such as Monsanto and Pioneer, who have transgenic corn resistant to *Diabrotica*, had proceeded to field tests in French territory even before this devastating insect was detected. This rapidity of reaction of large international firms seemed suspicious to Professor Gilles-Éric Séralini, who questioned the coincidence between the arrival of *Diabrotica* in the kit of a country's army and the proposition of GMO solutions to counter the devastating organism. Professor Séralini denounced 'a policy which consisted of introducing GMOs by a sort of ecological blackmail whose origins should be investigated'. Althought unproven, the beetle *Diabrotica* could constitute a tactical biological weapon on the economic battlefield.

The biological struggle against plantations of cocaine, marijuana, or opium poppies represents a 'legal' application of biotechnologies at high ecological risk. Washington admits to having invested $14 million for the development of biological agents capable of destroying toxic plants. One biotechnology firm from Montana has modified the genome of the mold Fusarium oxysporum in such a manner that it can destroy marijuana plantations. However, Fusarium molds are capable of rapidly propagating themselves and can attack other plants. Although proof is lacking, some Peruvian farmers have accused the USA of having spread a genetically modified mold in their cocaine fields that then attacked banana plantations. The utilization of such agents is envisioned in central Asia to destroy opium poppies. For want of a definition, a biological weapon that is capable of destroying 99% of the plants in a field is not covered under the 1972 convention.

Biological weapons: are they weapons of mass destruction?

It is very difficult to respond to this question with regard to several proven cases of biological warfare or terrorism [15–22]. Simulations and calculations, sometimes devoid of a scientific basis, too often take the place of analyses of real-life situations. According to a scenario of the US 'Dark Winter' smallpox attack simulation, 3 million persons would have been infected by a terrorist attack and 1 million persons could have died. The Secretary of Defense of the Clinton administration, William Cohen, declared in November, 1997, on the ABC television network, that 1 kg of Bacillus anthracis spores could annihilate half the population of Washington. To accentuate the dramatic effect, he appeared holding in his hand a packet of powdered sugar weighing 1 kg. In an edition of the journal Le Cahiers de Mars (The March

Papers), dedicated to the proliferation of weapons of mass destruction, Michel-Jean Allary wrote:

'It suffices to recall that a hundred kilos of the anthrax agent can kill 300 000 persons during spraying in good conditions, and with a lethality which could be maximal. In comparison, the nuclear bomb at Hiroshima killed 80 000 persons.'

With regard to Soviet doctrine, biological weapons were considered as strategic weapons, while chemical weapons represented tactical weapons. A Soviet SS-18 warhead charged with anthrax would have been capable of killing the equivalent of the population of New York City. Whatever its effects in terms of mortality, the use of biological weapons would have set in motion a severe destabilization of the national socioeconomic network, going on to become international. It is convenient to emphasize the very high cost of civilian protection measures and materials for biological risk, while relatively modest investments allow the fielding of these types of weapons [23–26]. On the strength of US simulations that measure the damage reported in proportion to the cost and the devastated area, a biological weapon is by far the most economical per square kilometer ravaged. In 1889, Albert Robida wrote in *Le Vingtième Siècle* [*The Twentieth Century*]:

'The times seem to me favorable for making medical war! … More than explosives as in former times, but only the artillery of putrescence, of microbes, of bacilli sent into the territory of the enemy.'

In fact, in the twenty-first century biological weapons could well play a role comparable to that played by nuclear weapons in the twentieth century. According to a document from the US Defense Threat Reduction Agency and disseminated by the NGO Sunshine Project, the most dangerous countries are not necessarily those that are regularly stigmatized. In a report dated July, 1999, and entitled 'Military Critical Technology', the experts classified the technical capability of different countries in four disciplines (production of biological agents, fielding of weapons for dispersion, detection of microbes, and defense systems) and according to four grades (from level 1 or 'limited' to level 4 or 'greater than a sufficient level'). It appeared that all the countries qualified as 'rogue' were for the four criteria at level 2 ('some knowledge') or lower. Only Iraq, and for a sole criterion ('production of biological material'), attained a level 3 in the 1990s, or 'sufficient level'. On the other hand, the USA, Russia, Israel, France, Germany, and the UK were at level 4 for all the categories.

References

1. Amoto I. Experiments of concern: Well-intentioned research in the wrong hands can become dangerous. *Chem. Engineer. News,* **July 30, 2007**: 51–53.

2. Derbes VJ. DeMussis and the great plague of 1348; a forgotten episode of bacteriological warfare. *J Am Med Assoc,* 1966; **196**: 59–62.

3. Rich V. Russia: anthrax in the Urals. *Lancet,* 1992; **339**: 419–420.

4. Wachtel C. Armes biologiques: le problème russe. *La Recherche,* June, 1998: 37–41.

5. Breman JG, Henderson DA. Poxvirus dilemmas: monkeypox, smallpox and biological terrorism. *N Engl J Med,* 1998; **339**: 556–559.

6. Dennis D, Inglesby T, Henderson D *et al.* Tularemia as a biological weapon: medical and public health management. Working Group on Civilian Biodefense. *J Am Med Assoc,* 2001; **285**: 2763–2773.

7. Henderson D, Inglesby T, Bartlett J et al. Smallpox as a biological weapon: medical and public health management. Working Group on Civilian Biodefense. *J Am Med Assoc,* 1999; **281**: 2127–2137.

8. Inglesby T, Dennis D, Henderson D *et al.* Plague as a biological weapon: medical and public health management. Working Group on Civilian Biodefense. *J Am Med Assoc,* 2000; **283**: 2281–2290.

9. Inglesby T, O'Toole T, Henderson D *et al.* Anthrax as a biological weapon: 2002 updated recommendations for management. *J Am Med Assoc,* 2002; **287**: 2236–2252.

10. Nowak M. Le spectre de la variole. *La Recherche*, 2003; **362**: 58–63.

11. Meselson M, Guillemin J, Hugh-Jones M *et al.* The Sverdlovsk anthrax outbreak of 1979. *Science,* 1994; **266**: 1202–1208.

12. Zilinskas RA. Iraq's biological weapons: the past as future? *J Am Med Assoc,* 1997; **278**: 418–424.

13. Török TJ, Tauxe RV, Wise RP et al. A large community outbreak of salmonellosis caused by international contamination of restaurant salad bars. *J Am Med Assoc,* 1997; **278**: 389–395.

14. Borio L, Frank D, Mani V et al. Death due to bioterrorism-related inhalational anthrax. *J Am Med Assoc,* 2001; **286**: 2554–2559.

15. Mayer TA, Bersoff-Matcha S, Murphy C *et al.* Clinical presentation of inhalational anthrax following bioterrorism exposure. *J Am Med Assoc,* 2001; **286**: 2549–2553.

16. Alibek K. *La Guerre des Germes.* Paris: Presses de la Cité, 2000.

17. Binder P, Lepick O. *Les Armes Biologiques.* Paris: Presses Universitaires de France, 'Que sais-je?', 2001.

18. Kohler P. *L'Ennemi Invisible.* Paris: Edns Balland, 2002; pp. 250

19. Leglu D. *Bioterrorisme: La Menace à Venir.* Paris: Éditions Robert Laffont, 2002; pp. 299

20. Lepick O, Daguzan JF. *Le Terrorisme Non-conventionnel.* Paris: Presses Universitaires de France, 2003.

21. Massey J. *Bioterrorisme, l'État d'Alerte.* Paris: Éditions de l'Archipel, 2003; pp 360.

22. Mollaret HH. *L'Arme Biologique.* Paris: Éditions Plon, 2002; pp. 214.

23. Postel-Vinay O. Le dossier du bioterrorisme. *La Recherche,* December, 2003: 70–77.

24. Christopher G, Cieslak T, Pavlin J, Eitzen E. Biological warfare: a historical perspective *J Am Med Assoc,* 1997; **278**: 412–417.

25. Khan AS, Morse S, Lillibridge S. Public-health preparedness for biological terrorism in the USA. *Lancet,* 2000; **356**: 1179–1182.

26. Simon JD. Biological terrorism: preparing to meet the threat. *J Am Med Assoc,* 1997; **278**:428–430.

27. Tucker JB. National health and medical services response to incidents of chemical and biological terrorism. *J Am Med Assoc,* 1997; **278**: 362–368.

12

Clinical approach to pathogenic agents

Patrick Barriot

In view of the very numerous pathogenic microorganisms that could be militarized by various terrorist groups, it would be impractical to attempt to describe them all. According to Ken Alibek, former head of the Biopreparat group, the Soviet Union had 52 militarizable biological agents available [1,2]. The infections caused by these agents are difficult to diagnose for several reasons. First, they are most often rare diseases, exotic or eradicated, that are seldom or not taught in the course of medical studies. The majority of physicians have never encountered these types of pathologies in their daily professional practice. Deputy Pierre Lellouche, member of the Defense Commission of the National Assembly, declared in 2001, regarding the biological risk:

> 'Are we prepared? The answer is no. The physicians are not trained, either for recognition of smallpox – since it has been eradicated, people do not learn to discern the symptoms – or to make the differential diagnosis between anthrax and bronchitis.'

Second, the first clinical signs are generally non-specific or unreliable. Finally, in the majority of cases, physicians do not routinely have available rapid and reliable biological tests that allow the diagnosis to be established when it is considered. There is thus a group of clinical, microbiological, and epidemiological arguements which probably evoke an intentional biological aggression [3–9].

Symptoms

There is little probability that the initial clinical signs of an atypical infection would immediately suggest a pathogenic agent which might have been spread intentionally [5,10]. It could be a matter of a common flu-like syndrome or of a devastating septicemic form that outpaces diagnostic measures. Moreover, the clinical picture

Treating Victims of Mass Destsuction   Edited by Patrick Barriot and Chantal Bismuth
© 2008 John Wiley & Sons, Ltd

varies according to the method of contamination. Anthrax, plague, and tularemia present different symptoms according to whether the portal of entry is cutaneous or pulmonary. All carry the belief that a biological attack aims at a human population having recourse to an agent penetrating by the respiratory route. Numerous illnesses can be transmitted by this route, in particular pulmonary anthrax, Ebola hemorrhagic fever, Q fever, pulmonary plague, tularemia, and smallpox. All these illnesses are not contagious, but certain among them can be propagated from person-to-person and set off an epidemic. This is above all the case with smallpox, pulmonary plague, Ebola hemorrhagic fever, and Q fever. The diagnosis will not be evoked before the simultaneous appearance of several cases of unusual pathology. Above all, it must not be concluded that the clinical examination is of little interest. It is on the contrary quite essential, as much for orienting the diagnosis as for evaluating the severity of the situation. Certain symptoms can evoke a microorganism with a respiratory, neurological, cutaneous, or gastrointestinal predilection, and guide the complementary examinations. In all cases, the appearance of severe respiratory, hemodynamic, or neurological signs imposes the admission of the patient to an intensive care service.

Pulmonary signs

They often are part of a flu-like illness combining: elevated fever, chills, general malaise, headaches, arthralgias, conjunctival and nasopharyngeal irritation, abdominal pain, and diarrhea. The appearance in this context of frank or progressive pulmonary symptomatology should evoke, most importantly, four diagnoses: virulent influenza, an emerging viral atypical pneumopathy, pulmonary anthrax, or pulmonary plague [7,8,11,12]. At all times, the development of respiratory distress syndrome necessitates care that must be understood and anticipated. All pulmonary symptomatology should evoke a risk of contamination by the respiratory route.

Endowed with an astounding genetic plasticity, the influenza virus can at any instant amplify its virulence and cross over the species barrier because of mutation or genetic recombination, natural or by human manipulation. The respiratory complications are represented by a primary viral pneumonia, which can cause cardiorespiratory failure, and secondary bacterial superinfection. The severe acute respiratory syndrome (SARS) or atypical pneumonia is due to an emerging virus of the corona virus type, of which we are still ignorant of its exact method of propagation. The mortality of this syndrome is about 20%. Some rapid diagnostic tests are in the course of being evaluated.

Pulmonary anthrax reveals itself in the form of afebrile bronchopneumonia, non-contagions, but this is a major alteration of the general state of health [8,10,13]. In the 2 to 5 days following the inhalation of spores, a dry cough appears, suddenly evolving to respiratory distress. The existence of stridor and acute sibilant rales are suggestive. Chest X-ray should be examined to look for characteristic mediastinal edema with enlargement of the mediastinum, sometimes associated with pleural effusions. A rapid test for detection is proposed shortly. To be efficacious, antibiotic treatment must be administered very early, before the bacteria can secrete its toxins.

The plague agent, *Yersinia pestis,* can be dispersed in the form of an aerosol causing a very contagious epidemic of pulmonary plague, transmissible from person-to-person by the respiratory route [5,7,14,15]. In this case, the incubation period is short; less than 48 hours. The clinical picture, of rapid onset, combines a severe infectious syndrome and a pneumonitis with rapid progression. The findings of bloody expectorations should suggest the diagnosis ('raspberry syrup' expectorations). Without early antibiotic treatment, death usually follows in 3 or 4 days.

The bubonic plague is transmitted by the fleas of rats. At the end of a 2–7 day incubation period, the onset is abrupt with the appearance of an infectious syndrome. Clinical examination most often allows finding of bubos in the inguinal, axillary, or cervical areas. In the absence of treatment, the evolution is towards death in several days in nearly two-thirds of cases, by septicemic dissemination of the organism. A pulmonary invasion of *Yersinia pestis* is possible in the septicemic phase. This form of plague is generally transmitted from person-to person by the intermediary, fleas, but pulmonary localization risks direct person-to-person contamination.

After having eliminated these three diagnoses, it must be understood to evoke a pneumonopathy due to mycoplasma, *Chlamydia* or *Legionella,* as well as certain pulmonary mycoses due to coccidomycetes (Table 12.1). Finally, it can be necessary to test for the following pathogens, also susceptible to provoke bronchopneumonia: *Brucella melitensis* (causative agent of brucellosis), *Burkholderia mallei* (causative agent of melloidosis), *Burkholderia pseudo-mallei* (causative agent of glanders), *Coxiella burnetii* (causative agent of Q fever) and *Francisella tularensis* (causative agent of tularemia). It must be emphasized that there is the possibility of human contamination by inhalation of an aerosol of *Francisella tularensis* leading to a primitive pulmonary form of this disease [4,16–18].

Table 12.1 Pneumopathies due to pathogenic agents

Influenza pneumonia
Severe acute respiratory syndrome (SARS)
Pulmonary anthrax
Pulmonary plague
Initial pulmonary form of tularemia (rabbit fever)
Pulmonary coccidiomycosis or 'desert fever'
Coxiella burnetii pneumonia (Q fever)
Burkholderia mallei (melloidosis) pneumonitis
Burkholderia pseudo-mallei (glanders) pneumonitis
Mycoplasma pneumonitis, *Chlamydia or Legionella*

Mucocutaneous signs

The mucocutaneous examination should be particularly meticulous. Inspection should include all areas of the body, without forgetting the scalp, the conjunctival mucosa and nose, mouth, and throat, and the palmar and plantar surfaces. It looks for in the first place extensive lesions such as a maculopapular or vesiculopustular rash, purpura or petechiae, and as well for icterus or beginning erythema. It also looks for isolated lesions such as ulceration, abscess, or signs of an insect or arthropod bite. Palpation of the lymph node areas can reveal adenopathies or plague bubos.

An atypical cutaneous eruption made up of maculopapular elements evolving in to vesicules and then into pustules should suggest a case of smallpox [3,6,9]. The cutaneous lesions predominate on the face, with involvement of the nasal and buccal mucosa, and the extremities, involving the palmar and plantar surfaces. The hemorrhagic form of smallpox is characterized by the intensity of generalized phenomena and a purpural rash. It leads to death in several days. A vesiculopustular rash can be observed in infections with *Burkholderia mallei* and *Burkholderia pseudo-mallei*.

The viral hemorrhagic fevers are accompanied by cutaneous lesions of the erythematous, petechial, or purpural types. Yellow fever is due to the yellow fever virus, transmitted by a mosquito. It is characterized by a sudden onset with fever to 40° C, violent pains, vomiting, facial congestion, and a thoracic rash. It classically evolves in two phases: a congestive red phase and an hepatorenal yellow phase in the course of which serious complications can occur: hematemasis (black vomit), hepatic and renal insufficiency. Complementary examinations should necessarily include a complete blood count and clotting panel with testing for coagulation disorders, as well liver and kidney function tests. Visceral lesions, particularly gastrointestinal, can be the origin of massive hemorrhaging with hypovolemic shock. The other hemorrhagic fevers (Table 12.2) should be considered when faced with petechiae or purpura in an infectious context, in particular Ebola viral fever, Marburg viral fever, and Lassa fever [19–21].

The exanthemous fevers combine a certain number of afflictions (Table 12.3) that combine on the chemical level, and exanthema and a thypus-like agent. The pathogenic agent is a *Rickettsia* or a *Coxiella* transmitted by a blood-eating arthropod (louse, flea, or tick). Exanthematous typhus or epidemic rickettsiosis is an illness due to *Rickettsia*

Table 12.2 Viral hemorrhagic fevers

Yellow fever
Dengue fever
Marburg viral fever
Lassa fever
Ebola viral fever
Hemorrhagic fever with renal syndrome
Korean fever
Omsk hemorrhagic fever
Kyasanur forest disease

Table 12.3 Exanthemous fevers

Exanthemous typhus
Murine typhus
Rocky Mountain spotted fever
Brazilian macular fever
Japanese river fever
Q fever
South African tick exanthamous fever

prowazeckii, transmitted by body lice and fleas. At the end of a 14-day incubation period, the onset is sudden with elevated fever, generalized maculopapular eruption, and neurological disturbances analogous to those of typhoid fever. In a general fashion, the rickettsial infections are responsible for a maculopapular eruption, sometimes presenting a marked rise (Spotted Fever), which involves the palmar and plantar surfaces. This eruption can take on a purpural aspect, in particular on the lower extremities [22]. It must be emphasized in conclusion that all serious infections in the septicemic phase can be accompanied by abnormalities of blood coagulation with mucocutaneous hemorrhagic lesions. In particular, the 'black plague' presents with diffuse hemorrhages of the mucosa and the skin.

When the lesion is isolated, it is necessary to consider cutaneous anthrax, tularemia, or an arthropod bite. Cutaneous anthrax is expressed by a pustule with an excoriated black center, evolving towards an edematous or necrotic ulcer. Tularemia is a zoonosis from game, due to *Francisella tularensis*, which can be transmitted to humans by simple contact with infected animals or by bites by arthropod vectors (ticks). *Francisella tularensis* easily passes through healthy skin and mucous membranes. The cutaneous lesion is a painful weeping ulceration, in the form of a chancre, with surrounding inflammatory adenopathy. The rickettsioses can be transmitted by tick bites. This bite, which is sometimes painless, can present in the form of an inoculation sore or 'blackmark' which can be located in the skin folds (groin, axillae) or on the scalp. With the possibility of being confused with a furuncle or an excoriation, it is generally drained by several enlarged lymph nodes. The discovery of a mark or bite should suggest a vectorial risk due to contamination of a vector (insect, arthropod, etc.). Faced with a cutaneous lesion that is difficult to diagnose; it is also understood that there is a need to test for *Clostridium perfringens*.

Neurological signs

The association of alterations of consciousness or neurological abnormalities in an infectious context should suggest an encephalitis [23]. The alterations of consciousness can range from simple obtundation to profound coma. They are sometimes preceded by behavioral changes. The neurological signs are essentially represented by generalized

Table 12.4   Viral encephalites

Yellow fever
Dengue fever
Venezuelan equine encephalitis
Japanese encephalitis
Tick encephalitis
West Nile viral encephalitis Chikunguya
Rift Valley fever

or focal convulsive crises and some varied signs of deficits (mono- or hemiplegia, paralysis of cranial nerves).

All the arboviruses have in common a predilection for the central nervous system. It must therefore systematically suggest yellow fever or dengue fever. The viruses responsible for encephalitis are divided into three principal groups: the equine encephalites (in particular Venezuelan equine encephalitis), Japanese encephalitis, and tick-borne encephalitis (Table 12.4). This does not, however, exclude the neurological manifestations that can be observed in the course of exanthemous typhus, or the rickettsias, typhus, brucellosis (meningo-encephalitic syndrome), anthrax, or plague.

Gastrointestinal signs

The presence of vomiting and diarrhea is often noted in the course of diverse infectious illnesses, such as brucellosis or the hemorrhagic fevers, as well as in the course of viral flu-like syndromes. However, certain infectious agents exert their pathogenic strength in a targeted fashion on the gastrointestinal mucosa, most often by secreting a toxin responsible for a severe gastroenteritis that can dominate the clinical picture. A Russian institute very recently proposed the sale of purified toxins from Shigella and *Pseudomonas,* as well as staphylococcus enterotoxins. The risk of diffusion of an infectious agent placed in contact with the stool or emesis of the patient should be systematically considered.

Cholera is an acute and contagious intestinal infection due to *Vibrio cholerae* variety *El Tor* that secretes a toxin that inhibits the absorption of sodium. Cholera is transmitted by water or food soiled by contaminated excrement. It can also be transmitted by person-to-person contact. Cholera is characterized by perfuse diarrhea, generally afebrile, and vomiting which leads to major fluid and electrolyte losses, responsible for a state of hypovolemic shock with anuria. The clinical course can be fatal in less than 3 days in the absence of treatment. Death can even occur before the appearance of diarrhea in the forms of 'dry cholera.' Some researchers have tried inserting the genes for cholera toxin into the genome of *Escherichia coli.* This bacterium, with a harmless appearance, eludes surveillance mechanisms and goes on to secrete in situ, in the human intestine, which makes the cholera toxin even more dangerous.

The salmonelloses are afflictions due to bacilli of the genus Salmonella responsible for typhoid fevers, epidemic gastroenteritis, and gastrointestinal toxic infections.

The shigelloses designate some intestinal infections of which the principal is bacillary dysentery or epidemic dysentery due to *Shigella dysenteriae* (Shiga bacillus). Certain sources suggest a number of attempts for militarization of rotaviruses to provoke severe diarrhea. The presence of diarrhea and vomiting in a severe infectious context should also provoke investigation of a case of plague, above all if there are associated respiratory signs. A flu-like diarrheal picture and plural-visceral injury can be signs of brucellosis.

The viral hemorrhagic fevers, as has been seen, can be the origin of febrile gastrointestinal hemorrhages responsible for a state of hypovolemic shock. A risk of person-to-person contamination exists by the intermediaries of secretions and bloody emesis or stools. A rare form of anthrax, gastrointestinal anthrax, is expressed by a lesion of the gastrointestinal mucosa provoking bloody diarrhea.

Preventive treatments

A certain number of vaccines are proposed in the battle against infectious diseases susceptible to be intentionally propagated. These are principally vaccines against smallpox, tularemia, yellow fever, exanthemous typhus, bubonic plague, Japanese encephalitis, tick-borne encephalitis, para-typhoid fever, and cholera. Certain of these vaccines can cause severe undesirable effects, even deaths, and their efficacy is inconstant. The Institute of Scientific Research for Microbiology of the Russian Ministry of Defense has finalized some vaccines against twenty infectious diseases, of which one is a vaccine against plague that can be administered in the form of tablets. Several vaccines of the second generation, called 'recombinant vaccines' coming from the techniques of genetic engineering, are recently in the clinical trials phase. Mass vaccination of armed forces or the civilian population poses numerous tactical, logistical, and health problems.

In certain cases, antibiotic prophylaxis can be envisioned for exposure to a pathogenic agent, even before the exposure. For example, in case of threat of use of *Bacillus anthracis;* preventive treatment with ciprofloxacin or doxycycline can be prescribed, as well as a specific vaccination, if however, it is available. The duration of antibiotic therapy is then based on the continuing threat. In case of proven exposure, the treatment should be continued for 8 weeks.

Urgent questions

Four essential questions should be immediately posed when a case of an infectious disease is detected.

1. *Is it a matter of an agent susceptible to be propagated by person-to-person contamination, and if yes, starting an epidemic?* From this point of view, it suggests it might be a virulent influenza, SARS, smallpox, pulmonary plague, or a hemorrhagic

fever of the Ebola type. The different methods of propagation of a pathogenic agent are thus taken into account: saliva droplets, biological fluids (blood, sweat, saliva, urine), stools, and emesis. When one only has clinical elements at one's disposal, the distinction between a contagious agent and a non-contagious agent is difficult, if not impossible, to distinguish in the initial phase. It is otherwise difficult to distinguish a respiratory injury by biological agents (virus, bacterial, yeast) from a respiratory injury by toxins. Staphylococcal enterotoxin B, certain mycotoxins, or ricin can provoke, when they are spread in the form of aerosols, some respiratory signs included in a general picture suggesting an infectious pathology.

2. *In the case where a positive response to the preceding question is envisioned, what are the health measures of premier urgency that are essential?* These measures essentially concern epidemiological alert, strict isolation of suspected cases and identification of primary contacts, protection of intervening parties (in particular medical personnel) by means of masks, goggles, gowns, and gloves, decontamination and disinfection measures, and destruction of wastes by incineration. The procedure for decontamination consists of undressing, showering with soap and water, rinsing, and drying. It is recommended to avoid scrubbing so as not to create cutaneous lesions that favor the penetration of the pathogenic agent.

3. *As for therapeutics, should urgent treatment be implemented?* (Table 12.5) The precocity of antibiotic treatment determines its efficacy, in particular in cases of the pulmonary form of anthrax, plague, or tularemia. These three bacteria are sensitive to fluoroquinolones, notably ciprofloxacin, as well as doxycycline. Ciprofloxacin and doxycycline allow treating the majority of bacterial afflictions susceptible to be intentionally propagated. Antiviral medications can attenuate the severity of severe viral pathologies, unreservedly with early administration [24]. These types of medications should be proposed in the cases of influenza syndromes, SARS, smallpox, and certain hemorrhagic fevers. In the case of smallpox, the injection of vaccine is only efficacious during the 4 days that follow exposure to the virus.

4. *What is the procedure for rapidly establishing the diagnosis?* The early implementation of therapeutics suggest a conflict as often as not with the problem of rapid diagnosis. In the majority of cases, physicians do not routinely have at their disposal biological tests that allow establishing the diagnosis as soon as it is is considered. The techniques developed are based on the early identification of the genome of the pathogenic agent after genetic amplification, from biological samples, or on the later appearance of specific IgM in the patient's blood. In abeyance, some 'biochips' allow identification in several hours of the genomes of the principal pathogenic agents. It is convenient to make contact with the reference laboratories in order for them to address the biological samples to be obtained in perfect conditions.

Table 12.5 Proposed urgent treatments

Antibiotic treatment with ciprofloxacin
1. Intravenous ciprofloxacin: 400 mg i.v. every 12 hours
2. Oral ciprofloxacin: 500 mg 2 or 3 times/day
3. Ciprofloxacin efficacy on:
    Bacillus anthracis (treatment duration, 60 days)
    Yersinia pestis (treatment duration, 10 days)
    Francisella tularensis (treatment duration, 14 days)
    Vibrio cholerae (treatment duration, 3 days)
    Burkholderia mallei (in association with cotrimoxazole; duration of treatment, 12–24 weeks)
    Burkholderia pseudo-mallei (in association with cotrimoxazole; duration of treatment, 12–24 weeks)

Antibiotic treatment with doxycycline
1. Intravenous doxycycline: 100 mg i.v. every 12 hours
2. Oral doxycycline: 100 mg twice daily
3. Doxycycline efficacy on:
    Bacillus anthracis (treatment duration, 60 days)
    Yersinia pestis (treatment duration, 10 days)
    Francisella tularensis (treatment duration, 14 days)
    Coxiella burnetii (treatment duration, 7 days)
    Brucella melitensis (in association with rifampicin; duration of treatment, 6 weeks)
    Vibrio cholerae (treatment duration: 3 days)
    Burkholderia mallei (in association with cotrimoxazole; treatment duration, 12–24 weeks)
    Burkholderia pseudo-mallei (in association with cotrimoxazole; treatment duration, 12–24 weeks)

Treatment with antiviral medications
1. Ribavirine (Rebetol®, Virazole®): efficacious for Lassa fever and Crimea-Congo hemorrhagic fever
2. Amantidine, rimantadine, zanamivir, oseltamivir: efficacious against influenza virus
3. Ciclofovir (Vistide®): probable efficacy on variola virus

Antivariola (smallpox) vaccination
Efficacious in the 4 days following exposure

References

1. Alibek K. La guerre des germes. Paris, Presses de la Cité, 2000.
2. Christopher G, Cieslak T, Pavlin J, Eitzen E. Biological warfare: a historical perspective. JAMA, 1997, 278: 412–417.
3. Breman J Henderson D. Poxvirus dilemmas: monkeypox, smallpox and biological terrorism. N Engl J Med, 1998, 339: 556–559.
4. Dennis D, Inglesby T, Henderson D *et al*. Tularemia as a biological weapon: medical and public health management. Working Group on Civilian Biodefense, JAMA, 2001, 285: 2763–2773.
5. Franz D, Jahrling P, Friedlander A *et al*. Clinical recognition and management of patients exposed to biological warfare agents. JAMA, 1997, 278: 399–411.
6. Henderson D, Inglesby T, Bartlett J *et al*. Smallpox as a biological weapon: medical and public health management. Working Group on Civilian Biodefense. JAMA, 1999, 281: 2127–2137.

7. Inglesby T, Dennis D, Henderson D *et al.* Plague as a biological weapon: medical and public health management. Working Group on Civilian Biodefense. JAMA, 2000, 283: 2281–2290.

8. Inglesby T, O'toole T, Henderson D *et al.* Anthrax as a biological weapon: 2002 updated recommendations for management. JAMA, 2002, 287: 2236–2252.

9. Nowak M. Le spectre de la variole. La Racherche, mars 2003, n°362: 58–63.

10. Mémento médical pour la protection contre les armes biologiques, coordinateur PCC Vidal, Centre de recherches du service de santé des Armées, Institut de médecine tropicale du service de santé des Armées, École d'application du service de santé des Armées, septembre 2002.

11. Nowak M. Pneumopathie, les lendemains d'une épidémie. La Recherche, juin 2003, n°365: 38–45.

12. Webster R, Walker E. La grippe. Pour la Science, édition française de *Scientific American,* mai 2003, n° 307: 30–33.

13. Bush L, Abrams B, Beall A, Johnson C. Index case of fatal inhalational anthrax due to bioterrorism in the United States. N Engl J Med, 2001, 345: 1607–1610.

14. Ratsitorahina M, Chanteau S, Rahalison L *et al.* Epidemiological and diagnostic aspects of the outbreak of pneumonic plague in Madagascar. Lancet, 2000, 355: 111–113.

15. Werner S, Weidmer C, Nelson B *et al.* Primary plague pneumonia contracted from a domestic cat in South Lake Tahoe, California. JAMA, 1984, 251: 929–931.

16. Francis E. Tularemia. JAMA, 1925, 84: 1243–1250.

17. Pullen R, Stuart B. Tularemia: an analysis of 225 cases. JAMA, 1945, 129: 495–500.

18. Teutsch S, Martone W, Brink E et al. Pneumonic tularemia on Martha's Vineyard. N Engl J Med, 1979, 301: 826–828.

19. Lisieux T, Coimbra T, Nassar E *et al.* New arenavirus isolated in Brazil. Lancet, 1994, 343: 391–392.

20. Martone W, Marshall L, Kaufmann A *et al.* Tularemia pneumonia in Washington, DC. A report of three cases with possible common-source exposures. JAMA, 1979, 242: 2315–2317.

21. Salas R, De Manzione N, Tesh R *et al.* Venezuelan haemorrhagic fever. Lancet, 1991, 338: 1033–1036.

22. Salmon M, Howells B, Glencross E *et al.* Q fever in an urban area. Lancet, 1982, 1: 1002–1004.

23. Deresiewicz R, Thaler S, Hsu L, Zamani A. Clinical and neuroradiographic manifestations of Eastern equine encephalitis. N Engl J Med, 1997, 336: 1867–1874.

24. McCormick J, King I, Webb P *et al.* Lassa fever: effective therapy with ribavirin. N Engl J Med, 1986, 314: 20–26.

13

Variola (smallpox)

Patrick Barriot

Smallpox (variola) is a severe illness, often fatal, against which no efficacious curative treatment is known. It is extremely contagious and can give rise to epidemics. Smallpox kills one patient in three and claimed 10–15 million victims each year in the middle of the 20th century. In France, the last epidemic in 1870 killed 500 000 persons over several months. At the end of a world-scale vaccination campaign, this illness was eradicated. In October 1977, a 23-year-old Somali was identified as the last human victim of smallpox. Smallpox eradication was proclaimed by the WHO in 1979.

Biological warfare and terrorism

The occurrence of a case of smallpox, 25 years after its definitive eradication in the world, could only result from a voluntary act of bioterrorism or an error of laboratory handling [4,8]. Militarization of the variola virus was made the object of offensive research, in particular in the former USSR [10]. According to Ken Alibek, former head of the Soviet program for biological weapons, the Soviet doctrine for the utilization of smallpox anticipated dispersion of 3 to 5 kg of the active product per square km, aiming for complete devastation of a given territory [1]. The agents of the KGB in 1967 had recovered, during an epidemic that had raged in India, a strain that was particularly virulent and resistant (India strain 1967). A bioterrorist attack could be carried out in two ways. The first consists of dispersing the virus by bombs, thus aerosolized in an area of high population density in a place such as an airport or a large office building. The second is based on propagation of the illness by suicidal terrorists who voluntarily allow themselves to be infected and who could attempt to transmit smallpox by going to commonly frequented places, such as subways. Otherwise, the risk lies in a failure of safety systems in a molecular virology laboratory, which should not be underestimated; the virus could escape from a P4 laboratory after a handling error.

Treating Victims of Mass Destsuction   Edited by Patrick Barriot and Chantal Bismuth
© 2008 John Wiley & Sons, Ltd

Human and animal viruses

Smallpox is caused by a virus belonging to the genus of orthopox viruses and the Family Poxviridea, DNA viruses responsible for pustular eruptions (*pox* in English) in humans [3]. In 1977, 18 laboratories still retained some strains. After having declared the eradication of smallpox, in 1984 the WHO decided to entrust to only two institutes the right to preserve cultures of this virus in order to have the ability at all times to conduct research on second generation vaccines. According to Ken Alibek, the Russian authorities continued to pursue works on the military uses of smallpox. Viral cultures were transferred from the Ivanovsky Institute in Moscow to Vektor (Novossbirsk) that had already carried out some research on the offensive uses of this virus. Destruction of the last remaining culture was scheduled by the WHO for June 1999 at the latest. It has finally been put back to an indeterminate date. The destruction of stocks of the virus is considered by military authorities to be a 'unilateral disarmament.' The CIA has accused several countries, such as Iraq, Iran, North Korea, and even France of retaining stocks of the virus, in violation of international accords. Ken Alibek affirmed that the USSR had tried in the past to produce a new smallpox virus by genetic engineering whose virulence would be increased and against which vaccines would be ineffective. Russian scientists had created some viral chimeras by recombination of the smallpox virus and viral genomes such as those of Ebola fever or Venezuelan equine encephalitis. Moreover, the genome of the smallpox virus having been sequenced, laboratories having it available may in future have available a 'plan for viral assembly' which could be synthesized *in vitro*, into a virus such as that of poliomyelitis.

Some minimal modifications suffice so that certain viruses responsible for animal poxes could contaminate humans. The pox viruses are distinguished by their extreme genetic instability. On the other hand, they spontaneously exchange between themselves some genetic material, forming natural hybrids. Numerous animal viruses arouse the interest of researchers, amongst others the virus responsible for the bovine vaccinia (*cowpox*) that is the basis for smallpox vaccine, and the camel variola virus (*camel pox*) or the monkey variola virus (*monkey pox*). At least 40 cases of the human form of monkey pox were recently reported in the United States (Wisconsin, Illinois, and Indiana). The virus had been transmitted to humans by prairie dogs, having been in contact with giant Gambian rats and sold as pets. Human contamination has been produced either by scratches or bites, or by the airborne route. The virus can then be transmitted from person-to-person. It was also susceptible to pass to other animal species, such as rabbits. In Africa, human monkey pox epidemics are striking with a 10% mortality. Prior smallpox vaccination carries some protection against this virus.

Professor Henry Bedson, who committed suicide in 1978 following an accident that occurred in his laboratory, conducted studies on the identification of animal pox viruses and on hybrids of human and animal viruses. In 1960, he had created, with Professor Dumbell of the Department of biology of St. Mary's Hospital Medical School (London), viral hybrids of cowpox virus and human smallpox virus. Recently, two Australian researchers, Ron Jackson and Ian Ramshow, have manipulated the genes of murine variola virus (*mousepox*) and have created by accident a virus more virulent than the common virus.

Contagiousness and method of propagation

Smallpox is transmitted by saliva droplets spread by victims, and the virus penetrates by the respiratory route. The patient is contagious from the appearance of signs of fever, before the skin eruption, and remains contagious throughout the illness. The transmission ability of the illness, evaluated by 'reproduction' factor is controversial. This factor expresses the number of persons that each sufferer is susceptible of infecting. If this number is low, less than or equal to two (either one or two persons infected), the progression of the illness is slow. If this number is on the order of about ten, the progression is exponential [7]. According to published studies, the 'reproduction' factor or transmission ability of smallpox varies from 1 to 38. Such disparities can be explained by the variable influence of population density, socio-economic conditions, or the quality of protective measures put in place in the hospitals. In optimal conditions for dissemination of the virus, one infected person could contaminate 20 others by simple contact. The development of air transport has rendered the world much more vulnerable to a viral attack: a patient infected in Asia could contaminate a Western City in several hours, before even having developed the clinical form of the disease. Transmission of the illness by contaminated objects must not be neglected. An article of clothing, bedding, or a soiled object could begin an epidemic. It was in this manner that the Spaniards and then the English decimated American Native populations who were not immunized during the conquest of the Americas between the 16th and the end of the 18th centuries.

The illness occurs in two forms

At the end of a two-week incubation period (10 to 17 days), the onset is sudden and in the form of a pseudo-influenza picture with hyperthermia to 40°C, chills, headaches, and vomiting. The phase of the condition is marked by the appearance, on the third day, of a cutaneous eruption that usually coincides with a temperature decrease. This exanthema, made up of maculopapular elements, begins on the face and upper areas of the trunk and then diffuses over 24 to 36 hours to the entire body, evolving into vesicles and then pustules. The palms and soles are not spared. Hemorrhagic evolution (black smallpox) has a poor prognosis. The pustules form crusts that permit healing with deep scars, depigmented and indelible. The major form of the illness results in the death of contaminated persons in 30% of cases. The majority of the survivors (75%) remain marked by the scars. The minor form of the illness, which is less common, presents with identical symptoms but without serious complications. Complete blood count shows leukopenia, thrombocytopenia, and numerous active lymphocytes. The confirmation of the diagnosis is based on detection by genetic amplification (PCR) of the viral DNA.

The battle against smallpox

There is no curative treatment efficacious against smallpox. The available antiviral medications allow an attenuation of the severity of the disease. Only vaccine administration within 4 days following exposure to the virus confers some immunity. Smallpox vaccination is no longer obligatory because of the global eradication of the disease. In France, vaccination has been abandoned since 1984 (Law of 05/30/1984). Thirty percent of the French population, those less than 23 years of age, have never been vaccinated against smallpox. The age group of persons aged 23 to 32 years have received a single vaccination and never had a booster. However, persons vaccinated against smallpox prior to 1984 are probably no longer immune. Amongst 621 American microbiologists vaccinated between 1994 and 2001, only about 40% are today still protected against the virus. It is probably not possible to count on any immunity 20 years after having been vaccinated.

Quarantine

The recent epidemic of atypical pneumonia showed the technical and logistical problems of placing thousands of persons in quarantine, since numerous cases were reported. In such a context of panic, of numerous persons placed in forced quarantine, some escaped from hospitals and assembly sites. In March 1998, at the request of President Bill Clinton, a group of experts was formed to study the scenario of an actual biological attack utilizing a pathogenic agent as contagious as smallpox. According to them, the military could be obliged to fire on citizens from their own country to make them respect quarantine orders aimed at preventing the dissemination of the infection.

Vaccination

Smallpox resulted in the invention of vaccination at the end of the 18th century (1796) by Edward Jenner who introduced pus from an infected with vaccinia (cowpox) woman as a vaccine into the arm of a child. Today, the virus serves for the fabrication of the vaccine against smallpox because there is a cross-immunity between these two illnesses. The vaccine comes from an original illness of cattle (*cowpox*), caused by an orthopoxvirus of the family Poxviridae. Human vaccination is invoked by inoculation of an attenuated live virus. An occlusive dressing is placed over the inoculation site. The vaccination causes formation of a vesicle evolving to a pustule, which reaches its maximal size 9 days after the injection. Healing leaves a circular scar. Possible complications are dermatological and neurological.

The 'first generation' vaccines were made from the vaccinia virus; the raw material came from secretions of infected cows before being purified. Some serious adverse effects, in particular fatal encephalitis, affected about 6 individuals per million persons vaccinated. France, at the time of the September 11th attacks, only had available a stockpile of 8 million doses of a first generation smallpox vaccine. This consisted of vaccines preserved for more than 20 years by the Army health service. Since then, France has reconstituted a stockpile of 72 million doses of vaccine: 55 million doses of Pourquier vaccine, retained by the military health authorities, and 17 million doses produced by the French multinational pharmaceutical firm Aventis-Pasteur. The supplies necessary for the injections consist of 'bifurcated' needles adapted for mass vaccination because they allow avoiding vaccination by scarification that requires much more vaccine product. The total amount is stored in two secure military sites, in the north and south of France. The Aventis-Pasteur firm could assure production of a second generation smallpox vaccine with a one-year delay if the public authorities were to establish a contract in this sense.

'Second generation' vaccines, such as the American vaccine, have the advantage of not inducing the adverse effects described with the first generation vaccines. The American vaccine is no longer produced from animals infected with vaccinia, but is made from mammalian cell cultures – from 'Vero' cells infected by the American *New York Board of Health* strain of vaccinia, after viral cloning. This vaccine will be efficacious in all cases with notably reduced risks of toxicity. The development of this vaccine resulted from a contract made between the CDC in Atlanta and the British basic research company Acambis. Industrial production and packaging are assured by the Baxter American Multinational Pharmaceutical Company. The United States had available 210 million doses from this source in the summer of 2003.

Smallpox vaccination is thus not without danger and the observed complications represent an obstacle to mass preventive vaccination. About one-third of persons vaccinated have minor signs, such as fever or malaise, leading to some lost work days. The risk is above all, severe vaccinial complications, sometimes fatal. Amongst one million persons vaccinated, about 15 or so suffer serious adverse effects that can lead to the deaths of one or two individuals. The most worrisome complication is the development of encephalitis, which leads to the death of the patient in 1 or 2 weeks in about 30% of cases. Recovery is, furthermore, often incomplete and sequelae of paralysis have been described. The other major complication is the development of severe cutaneous lesions such as eczema vaccination and above all 'generalized vaccinia,' a cutaneous illness provoked by the virus utilized for the vaccine. This latter can be fatal in immunosupressed subjects. Moreover, a vaccinated patient is susceptible to accidentally contaminate one of his close associates or family members despite the occlusive dressing placed over the inoculation site. Contraindications to vaccination should therefore exclude persons 'at risk,' but also take into account the entourage of vaccinated subjects (Table 13.1). Thus, vaccination of 60 million French citizens, with the current vaccine, might cause 90 cases of encephalitis (causing the deaths of about 20 persons) and more than 500 vaccinial eczemas (causing the deaths of a half-dozen persons).

Table 13.1 Contra-indications to smallpox vaccination

1. History of eczema or dermatologic illness (herpes, significant acne)
2. Immunosupression (treatment of cancer, organ transplantation, AIDS or HIV seropositive)
3. Pregnant or nursing women
4. Children less than 12 months old
5. Presence of a person presenting one of the above countra-indications in the entourage of the vaccinated subject

The United States and Israel have, however, recently opted for a campaign of preventive vaccination. Ten million persons had already been vaccinated in the United States by 2004, and, in 2004 each American who requested it could receive the vaccine. In Israel, 40 000 persons were in the process of being vaccinated. Amongst the first 15,000 persons vaccinated, 4 cases of severe complications were reported of which 2 did not concern the vaccinated subjects but rather members of their families. In France, in the context of the BIOTOX plan, 150 persons have been vaccinated in order to constitute *'a multidisciplinary group to lead the management of the first case(s) in French territory.'* A decree, published in the Journal Officiel [Official Journal] on Wednesday February 12, 2003 concerned this national group for initial intervention which combined civilian and military personnel: physicians, nurses, first aid providers, radio operators, laboratory personnel, firefighters, first responders, and ambulance personnel, but also law enforcement officers and members of the Ministry of Justice. A part of this group had been vaccinated beginning in April and the other half beginning in May 2003. It was also anticipated to vaccinate a group of 30 infectious disease physicians in the Provinces. Several persons expressed reticence to be vaccinated for fear of accidentally contaminating a member of their family. Jean-Phillipe Leroy, director of the vaccination center of the Rouen CHU, declared:

'If one comes to find these 150 persons, should they bear a vaccinial risk when, today, no information, neither from the Director General for Health, nor from the Minister of Defense, has not come to tell us the state of a real threat?'

The strategy of vaccination in response to an attack is relatively well-defined and graduated. In case of reappearance of the virus with slow progression of the illness, it is recommended to only vaccinate infected persons or those suspected of being infected, as well as their close family members and persons having been in contact with them. This strategy for targeted vaccination, called 'ring vaccination' or 'concentric vaccination,' aims to contain the epidemic around the foci while reducing the complications of vaccination. It would be applied, in particular, if a virus was released accidentally from a laboratory or in case of a single well-localized attack. On the other hand, if an attack occurred simultaneously in many locations or in case of large-scale attacks in airports, it would be necessary to vaccinate the entire population because it is unlikely that persistence of old immunity could protect the population. In France, in the case of a confirmed threat, a hospital group would provide vaccination in each of the seven defense zones that divide the territory (that is to say about 600 to 800 persons in addition to the primary intervention group). In the hypothesis of a case of smallpox occurring, no matter where in the world, vaccination should be extended to all the mobilizable responders by defense zone (this represents about 2 million persons for the health professionals and 2 million persons in addition to the health system). In case of occurrence of a case of smallpox being authenticated in France, all the 'contact subjects' and all those who could have potentially been exposed should be vaccinated within 4 days following the exposure, in order to prevent the illness or to attenuate the severity. In case it is impossible to control the epidemic by 'ring vaccination' and by quarantine, with vaccinations in large and larger circles, then going on to vaccinate the entire population should be done. It would require a maximum of 14 days to vaccinate the entire French population.

Interviewed by the newspaper *Le Monde* on the Biotox plan concerning smallpox, Professor Henri Mollaret stated on October 16, 2001:

'Bioterrorist threats impose the resumption of vaccination against smallpox, an illness which was eradicated thanks to a remarkable vaccination campaign which cost 300 million dollars. This measure, which was not anticipated in this plan, is according to me, essential. I understand the arguments advanced by those who are against this measure and who, possibly, are concerned about adverse effects, severe reactions are sometimes observed with the vaccine utilized. I have written […] that it is disappointing, disastrous, catastrophic that faced with an illness such as smallpox – for which there is no treatment, which kills greater than 40% and provokes blindness which effects between 10 and 15% of survivors – they forget to reveal the extreme contagiousness of this illness, which is in fact, precisely, all the military and terrorist interest. The strategy here consists of only initially involving a small number of persons assuring afterwards that they will themselves diffuse the virus and cause subsequent contaminations. We added to this an incubation period which is at minimum one week and that those who shed the virus can be protected by a vaccine that we no longer utilize. You can imagine without problems the difficulties that would confront the police services for identifying who were the initial sources of contamination. One such usage of smallpox virus would inevitably lead to – as various studies have proven – an epidemic of this illness, and I am obliged to observe that our health officials do not consider, as epidemiologists. But, we have available serious reasons to believe that non-official smallpox virus cultures exist, notably in Israel, Iran, and Iraq. I observed also that the health officials fear more and more legal actions that could be brought by those who might be victims of such vaccines. Imagine that this could be, in case of a resurgence of smallpox, the responsibility of those who have deliberately chosen to see to it that the population is not protected and directly exposed to risk which could be prevented … When does it pass here the precautionary principle? I add that, given the present stockpiles and the smallpox vaccines, we do not materially have the time to act fast enough to protect the population. I measure the complexity of the problem and I don't know if this protection should be imposed or offered, but I estimate that we must act now. This measure is essential and should be taken, even if, at the same time, we should work on improvement of the innocuousness of the vaccine.' [9]

Associated treatments

There is no efficacious curative treatment against smallpox. Available antiviral medications only allow attenuation of the severity of the illness. Ciclofovir (Vistide®), utilized in the treatment of cytomegalovirus infections, possesses an in vitro activity against smallpox virus. An anti-staphylococcal antibiotic should be systematically prescribed to avoid superinfection of cutaneous lesions (oxacillin: 3 g/day).

In a volume of the review Les Cahiers de Mars dedicated to the proliferation of weapons of mass destruction, Michel-John Allary emphasized the low cost of biological weapons, in relation to the square kilometers devastated:

'With a superior efficacy, the cost of biological weapons is low. This explains the choice made by certain parties. Classical weapons cost about 2000 dollars per square Kilometer. A nuclear weapon, about 800 dollars, a chemical weapon about 600 dollars per square Kilometer, and biological weapons about 1 dollar per square Kilometer.'

In review, protection of civilian populations against biological agents necessitates very heavy investments and sometimes taking risks. The example of smallpox is particularly demonstrative, as was emphasized by Jean-Francois Lacronique, President of the Administration Council of the Institute of Radioprotection and Nuclear Safety:

'It is true that all programs that fight against terrorism are costly and moreover represent unproductive expenses: re-vaccination against smallpox, for example, would cost several hundred million Euros, if it is necessary. It has not, moreover, any positive counterpart; on the contrary, it could have relatively frequent undesirable secondary effects.'

References

1. Alibek K. La guerre des germes. Paris, Presses de la Cité, 2000.
2. Binder P, Lepick O. Les armes biologiques. Paris, Presses Universitaires de France, 'Que sais-je?', 2001.
3. Breman JG, Henderson DA. Poxvirus dilemmas: monkeypox, smallpox and biological terrorism. N Engl J Med, 1998, **339**: 556–559.
4. Henderson D, Inglesby T, Bartlett J *et al*. Smallpox as a biological weapon: medical and public health management. Working Group on Civilian Biodefense. JAMA, 1999, **281**: 2127–2137.
5. Lepick O, Daguzan JF. Le terrorisme non conventionnel. Paris, Presses Universitaires de France, 2003.
6. Massey J. Bioterrorisme, l'état d'alerte. Paris, Éditions de l'Archipel, 2003, 360 pages.
7. Nowak M. Le spectre de la variole. La Recherche, mars 2003, **362**: 58–63.
8. Postel-Vinay O. Le dossier du bioterrorisme. La Recherche, décembre, **2003**: 70–77.
9. Propos du professeur Henri Mollaret recueillis par Jean-Yves Nau sous le titre 'Les menaces bioterroristes imposent de reprendre la vaccination contre la variole.' Le Monde, mardi 16 octobre 2001, p. 20.
10. Wachtel C. Armes biologiques: le problème russe. La Recherche, juin 1998, 37–41.

14

Influenza and pneumonitis

Patrick Barriot

Our societies are now frequently confronted with emerging viral illness caused by pathogenic agents harbored by animals. With a simple mutation, some of these viruses can jump the species barrier, contaminate humans, and sometimes propagate through person-to person contamination to launch an epidemic. Viruses with a respiratory predilection should be considered as agents capable of being employed for military or terrorist purposes and studied as such. On the one hand, one never knows, in the initial phase of an emerging viral illness, whether the cause stems from natural illness or is the result of a bioterrorist attack. The means of modern air transport allow worldwide propagation of a virus in the space of a few hours. On the other hand, analysis of national and international health countermeasures is richer in lessons than all the exercises for civil security regarding biological warfare or bioterrorism.

Influenza

Influenza is one of the great scourges of humanity, responsible for several tens of millions of deaths [5]. The influenza virus belongs to the family of Orthomyxoviridea (RNA Viruses) and is divided in to four types: A, B, C, and Thogoto. The Type A viruses, which infect humans and numerous animals (birds, horses, pigs), are closely watched because they are responsible for pandemics. The B viruses more often remain localized and provoke a less severe illness than those of the A viruses. The C viruses, which infect humans and pigs, are not very pathogenic and are responsible for sporadic infections. The Thogoto type is transmitted by ticks.

Type A viral influenza, originating from avian strains, are quasi-spherical particles of about 0.1 μm in diameter. A viral particle is surrounded by a protein capsule enclosed in a lipid membrane, into which are inserted some surface proteins: hemaglutinin, neuraminidase, and the M2 ionic channel. The virus is distinguished by the nature of two of the proteins, present on its surface: hemaglutinin and neuraminidase. These are glycoproteins which intervene in the phenomena of cellular penetration and disper-

Treating Victims of Mass Destsuction   Edited by Patrick Barriot and Chantal Bismuth
© 2008 John Wiley & Sons, Ltd

sal in the body. The hemaglutinin is indispensable for the penetration of the virus into human cells and the neuraminidase guarantees the dissemination of the viral particles, that is to say, the propagation of the infection in the body. Virologists have identified 15 types of hemaglutinin and 9 types of neuraminidase in avian viruses responsible for pandemics, on which are based the nomenclature of the Type A viruses. The genes coding for these two glycoproteins mutate regularly such that the proteins they produce are modified, and in this manner avoid the immune system of previously infected persons. The modifications of these two glycoproteins thus define the sub-type which appears by progressive mutation of one or the other protein, or by the appearance of novel variants. Once in the interior of the cell, the genome of the virus penetrates into the nucleus. It diverts the cellular machinery to its benefit, making numerous copies of its RNA. Contrary to the DNA viruses, RNA viruses such as that of influenza lack repair enzymes, so that errors in replication are not eliminated. The viral genome is made up of 8 distinct RNA segments that code for a total of 10 proteins: 8 code for structural proteins, including hemaglutinin and neuraminidase. Two RNA segments do not code for structural proteins.

The voyage of viral influenza begins in wild aquatic birds, notably ducks and wading birds that are the reservoirs for the virus. These migratory birds can propagate the viruses all over the world. The viruses harbored by wild birds generally reproduce in an intermediate host, most often a domestic fowl or a domestic pig, before passing to humans. Migratory birds can transmit the virus to captive breeding ducks that, by the intermediate of their excretions, transmit the viruses to domestic pigs. In these intermediate hosts, the virus is sometimes lethal. The poultry and domestic pigs in their turn infect the farmers, who contaminate citizens when they go to town to sell their products. In certain regions of Asia, numerous factors favor propagation towards the human species of influenza viruses in perpetual mutation: high population density and intensive pig and poultry breeding. Asia, in particular Hong Kong, with its markets for live poultry, will be the epicenter of influenza pandemics.

Endowed with an astonishing genetic plasticity, the virus can amplify its virulence and overcome the species barrier through mutation or a genetic recombination at any instant. Thus transformed, the virus can survive in a human host and be transmitted from person-to-person by the respiratory route. These frequent mutations result from a mechanism called antigenic shift. The RNA viruses, as we have seen, lack repair enzymes, so that errors of replication of their genomes are conserved. These mutations can modify the viral antigenic sites, notably the surface glycoproteins, in this way eluding immunological defenses. Besides antigenic shift, type A influenza viruses at regular intervals undergo a genetic break with important modifications to their genomes. The transfer of genetic material, or genetic recombination, between viruses of different species can also provoke the emergence of new pathogenic properties. The pig is the ideal crucible where these recombinations operate. In effect, pig cells possess some receptors for different viral strains which cohabitate in the pig's body: porcine strains, avian strains, and human strains. At the time of replication of the viral genomes, some genetic re-assortments can occur, leading to the creation of new strains against which humans do not possess any immune defense. The physiological proximity between humans and pigs favors human contamination. When one of these strains infects the human population, it is reproduced in the respiratory system and is spread by droplets emitted during coughing or sneezing.

Epidemic risk

The Spanish Influenza pandemic of 1918-1919 broke in three successive waves and infected about 500 million persons throughout the world, killing from 20 to 40 million human beings, according to estimates. In 10 months, the virus caused twice as many victims as the First World War. This pandemic was due to the H1N1 virus which also occurs as a porcine strain. Some other influenza pandemics took place in 1957-1958 (Asian Influenza) and in 1968-1969 (Hong Kong Influenza). During these two latter influenza pandemics, the genes of avian viruses and human viruses were recombined in the bodies of infected pigs to give rise to a very virulent agent.

In 1997, an A virus (H5N1), responsible for avian influenza, propagated in Hong Kong from poultry, to infect 18 persons, of whom 6 died, and it is the first proven case of direct transfer of influenza from poultry to human beings. This avian virus probably acquired its virulence during recombination of genes from viruses that were harbored by geese, quail, and Teal ducks. The Hong Kong live fowl markets, where numerous species of birds cohabit, represent a favorable environment for these genetic re-arrangements. A gene explaining the virulence of this H5N1 agent has been placed in evidence: it is a matter of an NS gene that codes for a protein that neutralizes cytokines. To stop an epidemic that could have threatened the planet, virologists immediately convinced the health authorities to destroy more than a million domesticated fowl harboring the virus. These rapid health measures limited the number of victims to 6, and the virus was eradicated before it had acquired the capacity to propagate from person-to-person. No human-to-human contagion was observed with the two avian influenza viruses (Hong Kong H5N1 and H9N2) that, these last years, have managed to cross the species barrier.

At the beginning of March 2003, the Dutch health authorities detected an avian influenza virus in several chicken farms in the Netherlands. The public authorities were immediately ordered to slaughter several million fowl near the Belgian border. The implicated virus, type A (H7N7), was reputed to be innocuous for humans until the death of a veterinarian on April 17, 2003 in a setting of pneumonitis. Only 2 cases of transmission to humans were found in the medical literature in the form of benign symptoms (conjunctivitis). Shortly after the onset of this chicken influenza, 82 cases of human infection were recorded. The majority of persons affected suffered from simple conjunctivitis, but 6 of them presented with some symptoms of influenza. The epidemiologists then looked at some cases of interhuman transmission of the illness. Three cases of contagion were in effect observed in persons who, living with the breeders, had no direct contact with the animals carrying the virus. It is, however, difficult to assert that the virus has effectively been transmitted directly by human beings carrying the germ. Boots soiled with animal excretions could have sufficed to carry the virus into the house. It is, however, feared that the H7N7 virus is better adapted to humans than its predecessors. Furthermore, analyses conducted at pig breeding farms have placed in evidence the presence of antibodies directed against the influenza virus in the bodies of numerous pigs. The fowl had thus transmitted the germ to the pigs, which play a decisive role in the launching of epidemics. A mutation of the 'chicken influenza' virus could lead to the emergence of a new human epidemic.

Clinical signs

At the conclusion of an incubation period from 24 hours to 5 days, the influenza syndrome begins suddenly, combining headaches, chills, dry cough, nasal congestion, high fever, myalgias, malaise, and anorexia. The evolution can be monophasic with attenuation of the signs and with coughing becoming productive, or biphasic with a return of the fever. The coughing and debility can persist for 1 or 2 weeks. The respiratory complications are above all represented by primary viral pneumonia, which can set in motion cardiorespiratory failure in elderly persons, and bacterial superinfection responsible for a secondary pneumonia. Some neurological complications, such as influenza encephalopathy, post-influenza encephalitis, or Reye's syndrome, are equally to be feared. Some muscular lesions can involve the myocardium: myocarditis associated with pericarditis has been described. In 1918, half the victims of the Spanish influenza pandemic were between 20 and 40 years old, and we are ignorant of how so many persons, previously in good health, could have succumbed. The diagnosis rests on isolation of the virus from the nasal secretions and above all the detection, in the patient's serum, of viral antigens and antibodies produced by the immune system.

Countermeasures and prevention

We have seen the critical importance of veterinary surveillance to guard against a virus most often transmitted by poultry or pigs. The measures of slaughtering millions of fowl in Hong Kong in 1997 and in The Netherlands in 2003 have probably avoided two pandemics. Epidemiologic surveillance of influenza cases is equally important. WHO has established a network for worldwide alert incorporating 110 surveillance centers distributed globally. In France, the propagation of the influenza virus is followed by sentinel networks. Physicians report regularly, to regional groups for the observation of influenza, the number of cases treated week by week.

Development of vaccines comes up against the plasticity of the influenza virus genome. The genes that code for the hemaglutinins and the neuraminidases mutate regularly, so that the proteins they produce are modified and thus elude the immune systems of previously infected persons. The antibodies fabricated during the initial infection do not activate the immune system. In this manner, a vaccine based on the active strain one year is an ineffective counter-measure against the strain which appears the following year. Each year, biologists from WHO identify two strains of Type

A and one strain of Type B susceptible to be responsible for epidemics in the coming season. The pharmaceutical industry produces vaccines from these three strains. The inactivated vaccine gives incomplete protection (60-80%), but allows a reduction of the severity and the number of infectious episodes.

First generation antiviral medications, such as amantadine and rimantadine, act by blocking the function of the M2 ion channel. They can reduce the severity and the duration of the symptoms. However, they are only efficacious against Type A influenza viruses, because Type B viruses lack M2 proteins. Moreover, the influenza viruses rapidly become resistant to these substances. Second generation medications, such as zanamivir and oseltamivir, are inhibitors of neuraminidase and also block viral replication. They cause problems of adherence to the surface of the infected cell, such that the infection cannot propagate itself and they are efficacious against both Type A and Type B influenza viruses. Administered as curative treatment less than 48 hours after the onset of symptoms, they permit a reduction of the duration and intensity of symptoms. When they are administered in a prophylactic manner, these antivirals are capable of preventing the appearance of the influenza syndrome. Oseltamivir has a prophylactic efficacy of 74%, and zanamivir has an 84% prophylactic efficacy, but the actual indications for these compounds remain to be precisely defined. Moreover, they seem less inclined to result in resistance and are better tolerated than medications against the M2 protein.

Avian influenza ('bird flu'): the 20 key points

1. The epizootic of avian influenza, which has raged for two years in an endemic fashion in Southeast Asia and in China, has reached Europe and Africa.

2. The H5N1 virus, for the moment, is only transmissible to humans from close contact with contaminated fowl. Persons are contaminated by inhalation of dust or droppings infected by the virus, in the course of close contact with a sick animal (in particular, during plucking the feathers of poultry). It is thus essentially a matter of contamination by the respiratory route.

3. Human contamination by consumption of meat from a chicken carrying the H5N1 virus has not been established. The virus does not seem to cross through the gastrointestinal barrier. It is, however, strongly recommended to cook meat from poultry well and to avoid the consumption of raw eggs.

4. In comparison with classical influenza, avian influenza presents a rapid and severe evolution with fever, diffuse aching, and severe respiratory signs. In Africa, human cases of avian influenza can be difficult to distinguish from other infectious diseases. Moreover, contamination of immunodepressed persons (AIDS) by the H5N1 virus can have severe health consequences. The H5N1 virus has infected at least 176 persons (of whom 90 have died in Asia and Turkey) since 2003. The level of

mortality of contaminated persons is on the order of 50%, which seems very high on first glance. But the statistics do not take into account benign forms that do not necessitate hospitalization, or asymptomatic infections. In case of mutation of the H5N1 virus favoring person-to-person contamination, forecasts are based on the hypothesis of a 'humanized' virus of which the level of mortality would remain low, in the range of 1% to 2%. An influenza pandemic with the H5N1 virus would be susceptible, according to the French National Safety and Health Institute (INSR), to contaminate between 9 and 21 million persons in France (about 15 to 35% of the population) and to cause between 91,000 and 212,000 deaths. The number of hospitalizations could reach a million. Between 1917 and 1919, the Spanish influenza virus, a virus which was probably of avian origin and which contaminated a billion persons, caused the deaths of more than 20 million human beings.

5. There are not, for the moment, cases of person-to-person contamination: the virus is not transmitted from an ill person to a healthy person. The H5N1 virus has not yet accomplished the mutation that would allow it to propagate from person to person. The strains of the H5N1 virus found in the first two Turkish victims of the human form of avian influenza presented a mutation in their genetic makeup similar to that observed in 2003 in Hong Kong and in 2005 in Vietnam. It is the hemaglutinin gene, one of the surface proteins of the virus (the 'H5' of the H5N1 virus) that plays a particular role in the infection of cells, which is concerned. The precise effect of the mutation is still unknown. It seems to be a modification of the hemaglutinin that allows the virus to bind more easily to the receptors of human cells which it infects. There is no evidence that this mutation is directly responsible for deaths or that it could be the origin of person-to-person transmission of the viral infection. However, the accumulation over time of these type of mutations could be of a nature as to facilitate human contamination. A genetic combination of an avian virus and a human virus (seasonal influenza virus), or point mutations of the current avian epizootic H5N1 virus could produce a new viral strain. If such a mutation occurred, the danger of a global pandemic would be real. The alarm signal would be the appearance of outbreaks of numerous human cases (at present one observes, in countries where the infection is transmitted from animals to humans, outbreaks of two or three human cases).

6. The instructions to the populace are simple: respect the rules of hygiene; report all suspected poultry; keep children away from chickens; do not buy a dead fowl in an African market on the basis that it is sold at a low price; thoroughly cook poultry meat and avoid consuming raw eggs.

7. Masks of the type called 'FFP2' or of the type 'N95' (English name) assure efficacious respiratory protection. The quality of a mask depends on the capacity of the filter material to resist penetration of solid and/or liquid contaminants present in the air flow that passes through it. A respiratory protection mask of the FFP2 or N95 type assures filtration of particles with a size less than 1 micron with a 95% level of efficacy.

8. Tamiflu® seems efficacious both for prevention and treatment of the influenza virus, which includes the avian influenza virus. For preventive treatment, the recommended dosing schedule is one 75 mg tablet per day during the period when the virus is circulating. For curative treatment, Tamiflu® is efficacious when administered early, from the first appearance of the initial symptoms. The dosing schedule for an adult is 150 mg per day (two 75 mg capsules). A recent publication concerning Tamiflu® mentioned the necessity of increasing the doses of this antiviral when it is prescribed as a curative treatment. This study suggests that the doses of this antiviral necessary to treat the severe influenza syndromes provoked by the H5N1 virus should be multiplied by two. In this fashion, it should not be 150 milligrams of Tamiflu per day to treat an adult, but rather 300 milligrams. However, recent information as reflected in the Package Insert for Tamiflu® notes under neuropsychiatric events (http:www.rocheusa.com/products/tamiflu/pi.pdf, accessed 11/15/06):

> There have been postmarketing reports (mostly from Japan) of self-injury and delirium with the use of Tamiflu® in patients with influenza. The reports were primarily among pediatric patients. Patients with influenza should be closely monitored for signs of abnormal behavior throughout the treatment period.

9. Cases of resistance of the H5N1 virus to antivirals belonging to the recent family of 'neuraminidase inhibitors' (Tamiflu® and Relenza®) remain rare because viral neuraminidase is not commonly subject to genetic mutations. The first cases of resistance to Tamiflu® have, however, been reported. The *New England Journal of Medicine* has reported two deaths in patients infected with a virus presenting some genetic mutations which rendered it resistant to Tamiflu®. The journal *Nature* has also published the case of a Vietnamese girl carrying an H5N1 virus resistant to Tamiflu®. This strain was, in review, sensitive to Relenza®, which should be encouraged for stockpiling as well as Tamiflu® for guarding against an eventual pandemic. However, a massive consumption of these medications could lead to a rapid loss of their efficacy and facilitate the emergence of resistance.

10. Concerning the adverse effects imputed to Tamiflu®, in particular behavioral disturbances and hallucinations, it is necessary to be extremely careful. Some fatal accidents have been reported in Japan in adolescents being treated with Tamiflu®: two adolescents died after having presented 'abnormal behavior.' A 17-year-old high school student threw himself under a truck and a boy fell from the 9th floor of his apartment building. However, as of today, the investigation has not allowed establishment of a cause-and effect link between taking Tamiflu® and fatal accidents in a country where 20 million doses of this antiviral were prescribed in 2004 for influenza syndromes.

11. The vaccine against classical seasonal influenza does not protect against the H5N1 virus.

12. A 'pre-pandemic' vaccine is a prototype vaccine directed against the H5N1 virus responsible for the current epizootic, a virus which is at present incapable of launching a pandemic. This vaccine therefore risks not being efficacious against the 'humanized' mutant strain which could launch the pandemic. Two studies judged as satisfactory have been performed up to this time with the French 'pre-pandemic' vaccine produced by Sanofi-Pasteur. The 'pandemic' vaccine, itself, can only be manufactured after the emergence of a new strain of H5N1 virus by genetic mutation, having acquired the capacity to be easily transmitted from person-to-person. In all cases, it would be necessary to wait for many months before having available initial stocks of pandemic vaccines. The major problems center around production capacity and delays in distribution of supplies.

13. The first 'pre-pandemic' vaccinations were aimed at developing industrial protocols and defining the manufacturing procedures for the future 'pandemic' vaccine: yield of viral cultures, speed of production, dose of antigen necessary for each vaccination, number of injections, addition of an adjuvant or not. All this should permit shortening the delay for manufacturing the 'pandemic' vaccine in case of emergence of a 'humanized' H5N1 virus. It is a matter of vaccines that are monovalent, directed against a single antigen (hemaglutinin), although the vaccine against seasonal influenza is trivalent. Studies were aimed at determining the adequate dose of antigenic protein (a classical influenza vaccine contains about 15 micrograms of antigenic protein). They were also aimed at deciding whether or not to add an adjuvant. An adjuvant is a molecule that allows stimulation of the immune reactions of the body and reduction of the antigen dose. The addition of an adjuvant, however, exposes the patient to the risk of undesirable side effects. Finally, studies should determine the number of injections (one or two) necessary for acquiring a satisfactory immunity. Many factors must thus be taken into consideration. On the one hand, a vaccine with a high dose of antigenic protein (between 60 and 90 micrograms) could not be produced in large quantities for logistical reasons. On the other hand, a low-dose vaccine or a vaccine without an adjuvant, risks provoking an insufficient immune response. The problem this poses is the following: should one efficaciously vaccinate a small portion of the popular with high-dose vaccines or should one vaccinate a large part of the population with a vaccine whose efficacy is limited? In these two cases, the decision is perhaps with significant consequences on the social and health levels.

14. Two studies judged sufficient have been performed to date with the French 'pre-pandemic' vaccine produced by Sanofi-Pasture: a study conducted in the United States in 400 persons in the month of August 2005 and a study conducted recently in France in 300 volunteers. The viral strain utilized for this vaccine came from a patient infected with H5N1 in Vietnam in 2004. This viral strain was submitted to genetic manipulation before being cultured in fertilized eggs. The volunteers were divided into two groups: one group received the vaccine with adjuvant (to stimu-

late immunity) and the other group received the vaccine without adjuvant. Some sub-groups received different doses of antigen: 7.5 micrograms, 15 micrograms, or 30 micrograms. Each volunteer received two doses of vaccine at three-week intervals. The results indicated that two doses were necessary to have good immunity and that the best responses were obtained with the highest dose (30 micrograms) combined with an adjuvant. At the highest doses and with an adjuvant, the majority of volunteers presented an effect of protective levels of antibodies. Some other firms have also prepared vaccines against the H5N1 virus, in the United States, The Netherlands, Australia, and China.

15. Global stockpiles of 'pandemic' vaccines produced in case of a crisis will only permit vaccination of a small percentage of the world's populace. After vaccination of health care personnel and security forces of the different countries, it will be necessary to evaluate the possibilities for mass vaccination. This poses ethical problems within each country, and also disparities between rich and poor countries. Some refugee movements in search of vaccines could be observed and a dose of vaccine could go for a considerable sum on the black market.

16. Conventional vaccines are made from the inactivated virus, cultivated in fertilized chicken eggs. In case of a human pandemic, it is estimated that 1.2 billion human beings would need to be vaccinated; this would necessitate nearly 4 billion fertilized eggs and would take approximately 6 months. Recently, some researchers have developed a new type of vaccine by genetic engineering, and by manipulating an adenovirus responsible for the common cold in humans. They have integrated into the genome of this adenovirus, the gene of the H5N1 virus which directs the synthesis of hemaglutinin, one of the proteins which allows the H5N1 virus to bind onto cells which it then goes on to infect. These researchers are sure that they could develop an efficacious vaccine by genetic engineering in only one month after having received the strain of the virus to combat.

17. Faced with the threat of a pandemic, the efficacy of all responses rests on a 'decision framework' and 'coordination authorities,' international and national. Coordination between international authorities concerns above all the United Nations Organization for Food and Agriculture (FAO), the World Organization for Animal Health (formerly the International Office for Epizootics, IOE), and the World Heath Organization (WHO). These authorities are charged with issuing recommendations. The coordination between the national authorities relies upon activation of an interagency crisis center.

18. In a crisis situation of this type, financial compensation for breeders should be immediate, particularly in poor countries. In effect, the economic consequences are very significant for breeders, who, in the absence of compensation, are tempted not to report sick poultry to avoid quarantine measures and to sell their dead poultry at low prices in the markets.

19. In a crisis situation, criminal acts multiply; these range from the absence of decla-
    ration of sick animals, productiont of false certificates, sale of counterfeit medica-
    tions or vaccines, or a black market. Beijing recently announced the arrest of an
    attending veterinarian who delivered, for payment, false certificates of good health
    to some breeding facilities affected by the virus. The Chinese Ministry of Health
    has also admitted that some counterfeit vaccines have played a role in the propaga-
    tion of the H5N1 virus.

20. The problems of society, infrequently involved in ethical issues, must not be un-
    derestimated: intervention of the armed forces to make persons respect isolation
    and quarantine procedures, limitation of travel, mandatory designation of priority
    beneficiaries for protective equipment, antiviral medications, and vaccines. In case
    of a pandemic, measures that appear to be 'fair and equitable' should be publicly
    discussed and clearly announced.

Because of the unpredictable nature of influenza viruses, the timing or severity of the
next pandemic cannot be predicted with any certainty. As international air travel could
be a means of widespread dissemination of an influenza virus with person-to-person
transmission, the International Civil Aviation Organization (ICAO) with assistance
from the International Air Transport Association (IATA), the World Health Organization (WHO), the Airports Council International, and other bodies have developed
preparedness guidelines, in accordance with WHO guidelines, but with specific focus
on international aviation aspects [2].

Effective communication between all stakeholders is an important aspect of these
guidelines. Communication with international airline passengers and those considering travel is important to make individuals aware of the risks associated with traveling
to various regions worldwide and to provide them with information on risk-reduction
measures they may be subjected to or could take themselves on aircraft or in airports.

As of September 2006, according to the WHO's Global Influenza Preparedness Plan
with 6 Phases, Phases 1 and 2 ('interpandemic period') have already passed and currently we are in Phase 3 (of Phases 3 through 5 'pandemic alert'). Phase 6 is the 'pandemic period' during which little or nothing can be done to prevent the spread of the
disease.

Based on experience gleaned from the SARS epidemic in 2003, ICAO and the other
organizations listed above have developed guidelines, which can be summarized as:

General preparedness – States Partners (countries)

Countries should establish a national plan in accordance with relevant guidance from
the WHO plan, including:
- Establish a defined contact point with an identified individual or individuals at the national aviation level for formulating policy and organizing operational preparedness

- This individual or individuals should be integrated into the national general preparedness plan

- Develop national and regional networks for sharing of expertise and resources

- Develop a national preparedness plan that includes and links all relevant aviation-related stakeholders

- Develop guidance for all communicable diseases, which can be readily adopted for specific communicable diseases

- Develop guidance based on WHO guidelines to ensure global information harmonization

- Develop methods to inform the traveling public at the point of trip planning and ticket booking of relevant personal and public health risks

- Give consistent advice by national public health authorities to passengers regarding postponement of travel or to when to seek medical advice based on signs and/or symptoms of a communicable disease with a public health risk potential

- Develop consistent health requirements for entry or denial of entry into a country, in accordance with WHO recommendations

- Develop a communication system to facilitate the above

Contact tracing and health declaration cards are currently problematic and require standardization. Also, the interrelationship between personal privacy data and personal/public health matters also needs further work at the international level. While the value of passenger health screening on departure and arrival has been questioned, it is recommended by the WHO when Phase 4 has been declared. Whether or not health screening has a beneficial deterrent action (some passengers declining to fly if they know they will be screened) is difficult to measure.

Epidemic of atypical pneumonia

The epidemic of atypical pneumonia, severe acute respiratory syndrome (SARS), was the first worldwide epidemic of the 21st Century [3, 4]. In 5 months, from November 2002 to February 2003, this illness was propagated in thirty countries. At the beginning of the month of May, there had been 6,914 cases of illness and 498 deaths. Some lessons should be learned from this experience because the SARS epidemic placed our health systems in a veritable situation of biological warfare. Doctor Arthur Slutsky,

Vice-president of the Saint-Michael Hospital of Toronto, stated in the newspaper, *Le Monde* on May 8, 2003:

> It must be evaluated, all that has been done, to review all the procedures. This epidemic has served as a practice exercise when faced with the dangers such as a mutant virus of H5N1 influenza or bioterrorist attacks.

History of the edpidemic

The history of severe acute respiratory syndrome (SARS) began in the south of China, in the providence of Guangdong, in November 2002, with large numbers of cases of atypical pneumonia. The city of Foshan was considered as the birthplace of the epidemic where the 'case zero' was reported. It involved a businessman who contaminated several nurses from a hospital in the city. A second man, a shrimp vendor, had carried the illness from Foshan to Canton. The first report from the province of Guangdong on the case of atypical pneumonia, sent to the central authorities, was concealed for 2 months. At the end of January 2003, although the epidemic was largely widespread in the province, the authorities refused to report the danger of propagation of the illness, for fear of decreasing the amount of tourism. In February 2003, the Chinese authorities assured that the situation was 'on the way to being controlled.' The health authorities announced having identified a type of *Chlamydia* bacteria sensitive to doxycycline in the patients and having formally eliminated an epidemic of influenza, anthrax, pulmonary plague, or hemorrhagic fever. The attitude of dissimulation of the Chinese authorities lost all chance of an early stoppage of the propagation of the illness. The Chinese media, manipulated by high-level functionaries and the party in power, favored the waiting game in the name of purely economic interests. On February 11th, the WHO distributed the first alert message via the ProMED network on a potentially fatal respiratory illness, but the WHO experts were not authorized by China to make a study in Canton province.

In the month of February, the epidemic was propagated outside of China. A nephrology physician, originally from Canton and carrying the illness, arrived at the Metropole Hotel in Hong Kong where he directly contaminated at least 12 persons of different nationalities who spread the virus. This physician was then hospitalized in the intensive care unit of a hospital in the city where he advised the medical service that he believed he had contracted a 'very virulent illness.' Despite this warning, some members of the hospital nursing staff did not protect themselves even with a mask and were contaminated. Hong Kong thus became the second center for propagation of the illness after Foshan. The clients of the Metropole Hotel, contaminated by the physician, then exported the illness to different countries, such as Canada which was the most affected country outside of Asia. An elderly woman took a flight and in several hours transported the virus from Hong Kong to Toronto, where she was considered as the 'index case' of the epidemic. Also in the month of February, a Chinese-American businessman traveling from Hong Kong was admitted to a French hospital in Hanoi. He was treated by a member of the WHO, Doctor Carlo Urbani, who died several weeks later of the illness. Doctor Urbani very quickly evoked a risk of an epidemic of avian influenza and alerted the WHO. Seven persons who had treated the businessman at the French hospital in Hanoi were contaminated with SARS and died. The Chinese authorities waited until March 10th to ask the assistance of WHO in order to attempt to discover the cause of the epidemic. On March 12, 2003 the WHO launched an international alert on '*a severe and atypical form of pneumonia in Vietnam, Hong Kong, and in the province of Canton.*' On March 15th, the WHO gave a name to this illness: SARS (severe acute respiratory syndrome). An Air China flight connecting from Hong Kong to Beijing on March 15th was the origin of a part of the epidemic in Asia. On board was a Chinese septuagenarian who died on March 20th in Beijing and contaminated several persons in the three hospitals to which he was admitted before dieing. Several passengers of this flight CA112 disseminated the virus. Despite the risks due to humans traveling and grouping together, the Chinese authorities did not cancel the National Congress of the People which took place in Beijing between March 5th and 18th, as well as the trade fair in Canton in mid-April. At this date, the Assistant Director of the Center for Disease Prevention again suggested to the Chinese to move the occasion of the First of May holidays.

On April 16, 2003, the network of laboratories working under the aegis of the WHO announced that '*a new pathogenic agent, a coronavirus never before observed in humans,*' was the origin of SARS. After having refused access to WHO inspectors, the Chinese authorities attempted to conceal the actual number of patients hospitalized from the experts. *Le Monde* of Tuesday April 22, 2003 related the cynicism of these concealments:

> In order to deceive the delegation of the World Health Organization (WHO), who had conducted an enquiry in Beijing at the beginning of last week, the management of the Sino-Japanese Friendship Hospital, informed at the last minute of the arrival of the experts - had hurriedly installed thirty patients ill with SARS in ambulances which were driven around the capital for several hours during the time when the embarrassing visit occurred. In the military hospital 'Number 309,' 46 patients ill with SARS were also transferred to a nearby hotel in order to shield them from the view of the WHO delegation.

In the month of May 2003, while the epidemic pursued its progression in China and Hong Kong, 7,600 cases of SARS and about 600 deaths were recorded in thirty countries.

The pathogenic agent and its detection

From the month of March 2003, under the aegis of WHO, a group of 13 research laboratories representing 10 countries was set up to identify the agent responsible for SARS. At first, a human metapneumovirus similar to paramyxovirus and *Chlamydia* was incriminated, but finally a coronavirus, not apparently any of the 13 species inventoried in the *Coronaviridea* family, was identified by the CDC (Center for Disease Control) in Atlanta and the Institute Pasteur in Paris. Among the 13 corona virus species listed, a single strain (HCoV) is responsible for quite commonplace respiratory infections in humans, even though some rare cases of pneumonia have been described in debilitated patients. The human coronavirus is in fact very poorly understood because it has aroused only a few research studies. On the other hand, veterinarians know well how the coronavirus spreads in the animal world where it has, as principal hosts, pigs, cows, and fowl. These agents are responsible, amongst others, for gastroenteritis transmitted by pigs, for avian infectious bronchitis, and for feline infectious peritonitis. There seems to exist a relationship between the virus called PRCV (*porcine respiratory coronavirus*), a respiratory virus affecting pig farms, and the virus called TGEV (*transmissible gastroenteritis virus*), causal agent of transmittable gastroenteritis in pigs which can be propagated by the airborne route. The factors for the propagation of this virus within pig and poultry breeding farms remain mysterious in large part. These agents are generally found in grazing animals. They have the reputation of remaining confined to their natural host and have difficulty jumping the species barrier, contrary to the paramyxoviruses. No example of a coronavirus responsible for a viral zoonosis, this to say infecting at the same time humans and animals, has been described to date. The atypical pneumonia is thus the first example of the passage from animals to humans. The species barrier having been breached, one can fear that the emergence of this virus in the human species could lead to its becoming endemic.

The voluminous genome of the RNA virus (30 kilobases) is enclosed within a characteristic envelope, studded with spicules forming a structure in the form of a crown. As with all RNA viruses, the coronaviruses are suspected of accumulating mutations because their mechanism of replication lacks an error correction system. The pathogenic agent may have suddenly acquired its virulence through mutations or genetic recombination within an animal species such as the pig. At the beginning of the month of April, WHO distributed on its internet site the sequences of characteristic fragments of the viral genome, named 'primings.' On April 12, 2003, some Canadian scientists announced having performed genetic amplification by PCR and the complete sequencing of the 30,000 base pairs of the virus genome, results that were confirmed several days later by American scientists from the CDC in Atlanta from a viral sample taken from a patient who died in Canada. On May 1st the journal *Science* published the genomes of two strains of coronavirus (SARS-CoV). Analysis of the variations of the common sequences allowed definition of two distinct genotypes of SARS-CoV: the first corresponds to the infections from the Metropole Hotel in Hong Kong and the second to the infections from Hong Kong, Canton, and Beijing without a relationship with the Metropole Hotel. One ignores for the moment whether these genetic differences, which translate to a process of selection, correspond to some differences in the clinical presentation or to the capacity of the virus to propagate itself. The genome of SARS-CoV was compared to the genomes of animal coronaviruses stored in different international databanks. The two groups having performed the sequencing confirmed that it was a matter of unknown forms of coronavirus and not mutations of a known form.

These comparisons have placed in evidence some common sequences with an avian bronchitis virus and with a murine hepatitis virus, but no relationship could be established with an already listed coronavirus. According to the authors of this study, the structure of the virus argues

> in favor of the hypothesis according to which it could be a matter of an animal virus which, from a currently unknown animal host, has recently mutated to develop the capacity to infect humans.

An unidentified animal is thus probably implicated in its transmission. If it is a matter of a non-domesticated species, its identification could be difficult. The Chinese have accused the pangolin, a mammal from the Indochinese peninsula, of being responsible for the SARS epidemic. Faced with the emergence of this new virus, there was no existing natural immunity in the human population and a large fringe of the population would thus be susceptible to be infected. A group of Dutch scientists have confirmed the virulence of this coronavirus by succeeding in infecting macaques by the nasal route.

The identification of the coronavirus by the classical methods of microbiology necessitates several days of delay. It was urgent to have rapid tests available for screening. A rapid test is, in effect, indispensable for hampering the epidemic, in order to rapidly distinguish those patients afflicted with SARS who must be isolated, from those suffering from another illness. It also reassures patients who are not infected with the coronavirus and requires surveillance of those who have been in contact with SARS patients. In the month of April, several pharmaceutical firms and the Institute Pasteur announced the development of tests giving a response in several hours from nasopharyngeal or tracheal samples taken from persons suspected of contamination. At the end of April, the Institute Pasture made its detection test available to 7 French hospital laboratories designated by the Director General for Health and to 22 institutes of the international network of the Institute Pasture. The majority of these tests were based on a technique which consisted of detecting some fragments of the virus genome and amplification by PCR (polymerase chain reaction). Once amplified, these fragments of the viral genome are placed in the presence of molecular probes capable of recognizing them by a matching mechanism. All laboratories mastering the PCR technique could thus put in operation this type of experimental test. These latter are never positive before the third day, starting from initial manifestations of the illness and having, moreover, a certain number of false negatives. Certain patients, in whom the initial test is negative, are submitted to a second test which is revealed to be positive. Three reasons can explain a negative test in an infected person: a defective sampling technique, a collection done at a time when the virus is undetectable, and the type of sampling done. The detection of the virus can depend on the stage of evolution of the illness as well as the site of sampling of the secretions. It seems, in effect, that the coronavirus is more easily retrieved from sampling in the lower airway (bronchi) than from the upper airway (nasopharynx). Some Canadian scientists have emphasized that the coronavirus is not detected in 60% of suspected or probable cases of SARS, although it is detected in 14% of persons unscathed by the illness. Some other less sophisticated tests, such as immumofluorescence, have also been developed. The diagnostic tests for SARS by testing for specific antibodies (seroconversion) become positive later, 10 to 24 days after the onset of the symptoms. They thus serve to confirm a probable diagnosis. An ideal test, capable of reacting at the beginning of contamination, without giving false negatives, is therefore not yet available. In the month of May 2003, WHO reminded that:

> At the present time there does not exist a test for the coronavirus of SARS which is valid and generally available.

The definition of suspected cases of SARS is, therefore, above all on a clinical and epidemiological basis: fever, cough or respiratory difficulties, the notion of contact with an ill patient or of travel in an area at risk. The abnormalities visible on chest radiographs and the presence of a positive biological test for the coronavirus confirm the suspicion. Professor Didier Sicard, who presides over the French National Consultative Committee for Ethics, has also declared:

> Soon a biological test for infection with coronavirus will be available. It will be expensive. We do not give in to the irresponsibility which consists of requesting this test every five minutes when faced with the most basic bronchitis or rhinopharyngitis. We do not allay our fear by demanding the proof of a negative. We do not confuse rigorous vigilance for an actually suspected patient with fanciful measures that are both costly and irresponsible.

Propagation of the virus

The only mode of transmission of SARS that is well documented is contamination by the respiratory route when face-to-face with an ill person. Droplets of saliva, containing the virus, which are emitted by a patient during coughing or sneezing, enter into contact with nasopharyngeal mucosa or ocular conjunctiva of a nearby person. The most exposed persons are those who have repeated contacts with contaminated persons, in practice the patient's family members and health care personnel. But it sometimes suffices to have only a brief contact with a patient to contract the virus. Certain patients, designed as 'supercontaminators,' have each infected several dozens of persons before the launching of the worldwide alert on March 12, 2003. It was probably a matter of very ill subjects who were excreting a large quantity of germs or of persons who transmitted the virus by the airborne route better than others. In the majority of cases, one enumerated one or two contaminations by persons ill with SARS, although for an illness which diffuses rapidly, such as measles, the ratio is 1 to 5. But slow dissemination does not prevent a pandemic. It seem that only the affected persons can transmit the illness; but this ignores vectors who appear to be healthy before the clinical signs appear or who present with delayed signs that can escape diagnosis. It seems that the respiratory route is the only mode of contamination. Contact with sweat, urine or feces from infected patients have been implicated, as well as contact with infected objects such as the buttons of an elevator, door knobs, stairwells, telephone receivers, or computer keyboards. The time of survival of an ordinary virus outside the body is a mean of 6 hours. In a communiqué dated May 5, 2003, WHO indicated that the coronavirus could survive in cells and urine at ambient temperatures for at least one or two days. The virus can survive for several hours in the cells of a 6-month-old baby and for 6 hours in the cells of an adult. On the other hand, it possesses a much greater stability (up to 4 days) in the cells of patients having diarrhoea, because these latter are less acidic. Contamination by means of fecal matter truly explains the great number of observed SARS cases, especially in the Amoy Gardens in Hong Kong. In this apartment complex, more than 300 persons were contaminated through the sewer system. Cockroaches were also implicated in the propagation of the infection. The virus can also survive for 48 hours on a dry inorganic surface such as plastic. Moreover, the presence of the virus does not necessarily signify that it has retained its infective ability. On May 15, 2003, some German researchers published a study in the *New England Journal of Medicine* establishing the presence of the coronavirus in the saliva of ill patients, in the feces, and also in the blood. Numerous uncertainties persist, in particular on the modes of transmission of SARS and the infectious virus dose.

Statisticians and biomathemeticians attempted to establish predictive models for the medium term of the evolution of the epidemic in order to evaluate the risk of a pandemic and the risk of establishing the virus endemically. The epidemiologists feared in effect that the epidemic would then take root in an endemic and seasonal form, as a function of the genetic evolution of the virus and of the immune response of contaminated persons. The human species would then confront a risk of SARS epidemics in a permanent fashion. The virus could also improve its mode of transmission as well as its dissemination, becoming more and more contagious. Jean-Claude Manuguerra stated on this subject:

> It must be expected that the virus, like all viruses, undergoes mutations and modifies itself. It is already very well adapted to humankind and is transmitted without apparent difficulty from one person to another. At this stage, it is however too soon to create a mutation which could then increase the aggression of the virus.

However, according to the results of a study published on May 9, 2003 on the internet site of the British journal, *The Lancet*, this coronavirus seemed to present a rather large genetic stability for an RNA virus. Two Canadian microbiologists had evoked in the month of May

> a remarkable genetic conservation of the virus since the epidemic was known, in February,

indicating moreover that

> one can conclude that in passing to human beings the SARS-CoV maintained its common basic genotype, and that it is in this manner well adapted to the human host.

This stability thus leaves the fear that the SARS virus has already adapted itself to the human species well.

Clinical aspects

SARS can develop both in a form with a favorable evolution as well as in a severe form, which can be fatal. One does not know all the pathophysiological mechanisms and the reasons which make it such that young persons in good health can die from the infection while 90% of patients survive without sequelae. The incubation period of SARS lasts from 3 to 10 days, with a mean of 5 to 8 days. These variations can be related to the amount of virus transmitted during the contamination. Patients generally consult a physician with a delay of 3 to 5 days after the appearance of the initial symptoms. One of the principle questions is to know if, during the incubation phase which precedes the appearance of clinical signs, infected persons are or are not capable of contaminating their immediate families. It seems that only persons presenting symptoms of the disease can transmit the virus. As of the month of May 2003, no cases of transmission of the virus by an asymptomatic person were recorded.

However, certain viruses with a respiratory predilection begin to be excreted in the days which precede the final phase of incubation, which justifies the wearing of protective masks. The first study analyzing the characteristics of 50 patients hospitalized with the diagnosis of SARS between February 26th and March 26th in China was published in *The Lancet* on April 28, 2003. The mean age of these 50 patients was 42 years. The clinical picture combined fever and some signs of influenza (chills, malaise, nasopharyngitis with sore throat, myalgias, headache, cough, and respiratory distress). The hospitalized patients arrived at the hospital in a mean of 5 days after the onset of the initial symptoms. The rate of patients requiring admission to the intensive care unit was 10% and the rate of those who died was 5%.

This level of deaths was revised to be higher in the course of subsequent studies, in particular in a study published in *The Lancet* on Tuesday May 6th, which analyzed the 1,425 initial cases and the 122 deaths reported in Hong Kong as of the date of April 28th. The mortality rate in this group was a mean of 20%, with variations according to the age of the patients. For those over 60 years old, the rate was increased to 43%. The existence of a pre-existing chronic affliction was, of course, a pejorative factor. Some variations of the mortality rate as a function of the affected region have also been noted at the beginning of the epidemic: 8% in Vietnam, 10% in Hong Kong, 19% in Canada. The mortality rate in Canada could be explained by the higher mean age of the patients. The aggravation, when it occurs, begins about 8 days after the onset of symptoms. The patient then presents a picture of acute respiratory insufficiency with crepitant rales on auscultation and white lung fields on radiography. The pulmonary lesions observed in these patients are not a direct consequence of the replication of the virus, but rather result from a violent inflammatory reaction such that one can observe non-cardiogenic pulmonary edema in certain cases. A modification of the modulation of cytokines could be the origin of the observed pathogenic effects.

It is emphasized that the illness which affected the inhabitants of the *Amoy Gardens* residence was more severe: about 20% of the patients from this residence were hospitalized in the intensive care unit, as contrasted with 10% of those having been contaminated elsewhere in the area during the same period. Moreover, approximately 66% of the *Amoy Gardens* patients suffered from diarrhoea, as contrasted with 7 to 26% of the other patients. It could be that these patients had been contaminated by a large dose of virus or a more virulent strain. Some clinicians from Hong Kong have reported cases of patients who, having been discharged well from the hospital, have presented a sudden recurrence with reappearance of symptoms. After investigation, it was proven that these patients had developed other illnesses which were not due to SARS. The authors of all studies published to date insist on the fact that the more rapid the hospital admission and patient isolation after the appearance of the initial symptoms, the greater were the chances of stopping the propagation of the epidemic.

The complementary examinations most often show evidence of neutropenia, lymphopenia, and thrombocytopenia. In addition, certain patients present an elevation of creatine phosphokinase (CPK) blood levels, probably a sign of lysis of muscle cells. Chest x-ray in the severe forms reveals a white lung fields appearance, such as are seen in acute non-cardiogenic pulmonary edema.

In China, the initial attitude of the authorities regarding SARS was in all points comparable to that adopted regarding the AIDS virus (HIV) in earlier years. A great number of persons were contaminated by HIV due to the negligence of the public health authorities who favored economic considerations to the detriment of measures for public health. Persons afflicted with AIDS are particularity vulnerable to pneumonias, in particular *Pneumocystis carinii* pneumonia, and they can be the target of this new virus. Moreover, the propagation of the epidemic was accentuated by the fact that the most handicapped social groups, living in poverty-stricken regions and totally deprived of medical infrastructure, were excluded from the system of care. Two peasants out of three needing hospital care could not obtain it because they couldn't afford it.

Treatment

The Hong Kong public health authorities proposed, even before the identification of the coronavirus, a treatment combining antivirals and steroid anti-inflammatories. Ribavirin was prescribed because of its efficacy against respiratory syncytial virus, similar to the metapneumovirus isolated for the first time in Hong Kong and which was thus initially thought to be responsible for SARS. It is a wide-spectrum antiviral which inhibits the replication of nucleic acids. Certain physicians have, however, estimated that this treatment is not only inefficacious but dangerous. According to them, prolonged administration of ribavirin could aggravate multiorgan failure. The utilization of the antiretroviral molecule, lopinavir, a protease inhibitor indicated in the treatment of HIV infection, seems to have given better results. The corticoid treatment (methylprednisolone) was aimed at reducing the inflammatory response. Antibiotic therapy with doxycline was systematically added at the beginning of the epidemic, from the isolation of bacteria of the *Chlamydia* type. In effect, some other infectious agents, viral and bacterial, can be associated with the coronavirus and aggravate the clinical picture.

Interferon, which is a modulator of the immune defenses, was also proposed. In severe forms, recourse to respiratory assistance is very evidently essential.

A group of German researchers have opened a path which could lead to development of an antiviral medication against the coronavirus. They are parties to a study of the structure of the protease type which is indispensable to the replication of already known coronaviruses. This enzyme in effect plays an essential role in the construction of new viral particles. The researchers have cloned the gene directing the synthesis of this protease in a coliform bacillus in order to better study it. The goal is to find some inhibitors, otherwise called antiproteases, capable of binding to the enzyme in order to neutralize it. After having studied different types of possible connections, they have calculateded the molecular structure of the antiprotease and have examined closely the data from a large number of medications to research the ideal candidate. In this fashion, they have discovered an inhibitor (AG 7088), developed by the Pfizer company against the rhinovirus responsible for the common cold, which could serve as a model for the elaboration of a medication that could neutralize the coronavirus protease.

The development of a vaccine against SARS comes up against several problems. It must in the first place assure that the coronavirus induces the synthesis of neutralizing antibodies by the human body which it infects and that the virus can be cultivated. If such is the case, one could envision development of a traditional vaccine from an inactivated or attenuated live virus. The sequencing of the genome of the coronavirus should also permit the development of vaccines by genetic engineering. Canadian researchers have already identified the genes of 4 proteins essential to the penetration of the coronavirus into the cells of the host and to its replication. The AlogNomics Company of Gand (Belgium) has developed software which researches the fragments of the viral envelope (the epitopes) suitable to serve for the elaboration of a vaccine by genetic engineering. The veterinary experience is, however, far more negative. After 40 years of work, all the vaccine trials against animal coronaviruses have not allowed the availability of vaccination methods whose efficacy and innocuousness could actually qualify as satisfactory. There is no efficacious vaccine against porcine gastroenteritis. The only efficacious vaccine is that against avian infectious bronchitis which affects chicken farms, but it must be modified regularly. Vaccines against coronaviruses affecting felines are actually capable of worsening the illness. However, the Merck Laboratory has launched an important research program, in collaboration with the American National Institutes of Health (NIH) to develop a vaccine against SARS.

Public health measures

The international alert constituted the first emergency measure. On February 11th, WHO disseminated the first alert message via the ProMed network. Specialists in infectious diseases could, in this manner, simply establish the relationship between the cases described in China, in Vietnam, or in Canada. A global alert was launched by WHO on March 12th with establishment of an international surveillance network comparable to that for influenza, combining clinicians, specialists in molecular virology, epidemiologists and industrialists from the entire world. Some recommendations were issued for the surveillance of travelers in airports and for the protection of hospital personnel. This international cooperation has allowed, amongst other things, to put together the chain of contamination from case to case. It must be emphasized on this occasion that the public health regulations of WHO are not adapted to emerging diseases. These regulations instituted in effect an obligation for notification in case of epidemics of three illnesses only: cholera, yellow fever, and plague.

Strengthening of public health measures within the population made up part of the emergency measures, based in view of limiting the propagation of the infectious agent. Careful and frequent hand washing with soap and water should be widely recommended. The popular statements in China were that it would be better from now on to avoid shaking hands as a greeting and to return to bowing in the Japanese manner. According to the location and the level of risk, it could be necessary to propose wearing a mask for respiratory protection. The dissemination of notes with information on the disease, the cleaning of public places, and the disinfection of means of transport were also part of the public health measures.

The early screening of ill patients by means of taking the temperature was rapidly imposed in different sites of crowd gathering. In the Chinese schools, the parents upon arising each morning took the temperature of their children and wrote it on a sheet to be returned to the teachers. At the University of Beijing, each student had instruction to take his or her temperature twice a day; all temperature elevations resulted in immediate isolation. In certain airports, such as those in Taiwan or Hong Kong, departing and arriving passengers were submitted to temperature monitoring with the obligation to submit to a medical examination for all temperature elevations greater than 37.5°C. Certain airports were even equipped with infrared body temperature detectors, signaling all passengers whose temperature was greater than 38°C. Clandestine passengers very evidently slipped through these screenings.

Isolation of ill patients, their close contacts, and of subjects entering into contact with them without protection is a crucial measure to prevent an explosive epidemic. Putting in place a voluntary quarantine, however, comes up against refusal by certain persons. In China, some panicked patients attempted to slip away from the hospital in the dark of night to escape from quarantine. According to a decision of the Supreme Court published on Thursday May 15th:

> Those who voluntarily spread pathogenic agents of contagious diseases, place the public safety in danger, or lead to severe injuries, to deaths, or significant material harm, are liable to be imprisoned for at least 10 years, to be imprisoned for life, or be under pain of death.

The dissemination of a virus by negligence carries a penalty of 3 to 7 years in prison. WHO on its part, expressed the fear that this disposition could be counter-productive and a spokesperson for the American Department of State declared that this type of sanction 'increases the reactions of fear and discrimination encountered by the victims of SARS.' The first person detained for 'criminal' action of this type was a physician afflicted with SARS who had left the hospital and had infected his family. In order to counter certain irresponsible behaviors, a French legal degree anticipated mandatory hospitalization for contagious illnesses. On April 16, 2003, Monsieur Jean-Louis Fousseret, Mayor of Besançon, addressed a letter to Jean-François Mattei and Dominique Perben, respectively Ministers of Health and Justice, requesting that the government inform the French National Ethics Committee on the possibility of involuntary hospitalization of a potentially contagious patient. A short time before; a patient visiting in the province from Hanoi and presenting with signs of atypical pneumonic had left the Besançon hospital after having signed a release. He was later hospitalized at the CHU in Strasbourg. In his letter, Monsieur Fousseret stated:

> The concerns of public health and those of protection of hospital agents demand according to me to prevail over the precautionary principle. I am astonished that this point of view is only in cases of psychiatric illnesses anticipating the possibility of recurring mandatory hospitalization. It seems to me that the appearance of severe infectious illnesses should allow personnel to proceed to mandatory hospitalization.

The Minister of Health, Jean-Francois Mattei, announced on April 22, 2003, the publication of a decree allowing 'mandatory hospitalization of patients' afflicted with contagious illnesses, under the order of the Prefect and in urgent and perfectly specified situations. Professor Didier Sicard, President of the French National Ethics Consultative Committee, declared in the daily newspaper, *Le Monde*, on May 6, 2003:

> The circumstances of the transmission of the coronavirus are now well identified; physicians have died after contact with patients afflicted with acute pulmonary infection; rigorous isolation measures should be taken, even under restraint, in anticipation of a suspected case.

Placing a preventive quarantine for 'populations at risk' of several thousand persons poses a whole other problem. According to some, it should be the major remedy for preventing the fulminate propagation of the virus. In Canada, some thousands of persons were placed in isolation, in some closed hospitals and some isolated apartment buildings. The example of Canada showed that even a good health system can be overwhelmed when the number of cases is too large. The authorities in Beijing decided to place more than a thousand persons in quarantine in the People's hospital. In Singapore, more than 2,400 persons who worked in the city vegetable and fruit markets were placed in quarantine for 10 days following contamination of these sites by a taxi driver and an employee. Jean-Claude Manuguerra, virologist at the Institute Pasteur in Paris, in an interview in the daily newspaper, *Le Monde*, on April 22, 2003, showed reservations on the utility of such measures:

> It is necessary to distinguish between two cases. Isolation is a useful preventive measure in countries which are not highly populated and where imported cases are very limited and when there has not been person-to-person transmission. This is notable in the case of France. But having exceeded a certain level of infection and contamination, placing persons in quarantine is neither useful nor even worth considering. The demonstration of

this was notably made during the Spanish Influenza epidemic at the beginning of the last century.

In China, numerous assembly sites were closed, such as markets, leisure establishments (bars, discotheques, swimming pools, and sports arenas), educational facilities, cultural sites, exhibition centers, or commercial centers. According to a decree of the municipality of Beijing published on April 24th, 2003, all buildings or public places where cases of SARS were discovered must be closed. Numerous international events were cancelled. In the same manner, travel to the interior of the country was limited in a drastic fashion, with prohibition of group excursions and cancellation of cultural and sporting events. The traditional vacation week of May 1st, during which several tens of millions of Chinese ordinarily travel throughout the country, was also cancelled. However, the closure of schools and universities set in motion a mass exodus because the school children and the university students wished to return to their home provinces and packed and filled the trains and buses. The decision to close the scholastic establishments thus could have favored the propagation of the virus into the countryside. Numerous migrant workers, fearing mandatory quarantine, fled the cities and were refugees in the rural regions to escape the screening.

Public health screening at the borders was rapidly imposed. Passengers on flights from areas at risk had to fill out a health questionnaire, retained for 2 weeks and mentioning the flight number, the passenger's seat in the airplane, the address and telephone number where the person could be reached. In France, all suspect persons were identified and isolated from their arrival in the country, then entrusted to a specialized group of pre-hospital ambulance emergency care providers (SAMU) charged with taking them directly to a designated hospital. On April 2nd, for the first time in its history, WHO broadcast a notice for restriction of travel and recommended not going to Hong Kong and into the providence of Canton.

The recommendation of WHO advising travelers not to go to Toronto was rapidly cancelled following a sharp response from the Canadian authorities concerned with the economic repercussions. In the month of May, Russia closed passages through 31 of its 52 border-crossings with China and Mongolia to prevent the propagation of SARS. The propagation of the illness in developing countries, where the health systems were precarious or deficient, was catastrophic. On Wednesday May 2, 2003, WHO declared that Africa '*could not be allowed*' to be infected by the epidemic of atypical pneumonia, because '*the consequences would be devastating*' for the continent and for the rest of the world.

Specific measures at hospitals

The contamination of hospitals was a crucial factor for the extension of the epidemic. Two of the principal establishments in Beijing closed their doors and were placed in quarantine, with their patients and nursing staff inside, after numerous cases of contamination were noted outside the isolation perimeter for ill patients. The Ditan Hospital, specialized in infectious diseases, was also closed. The People's Hospital of the University of Beijing, with 1,000 beds and 2,300 employees, was placed in quarantine when 50 members of the medical staff were contaminated. Some panicked patients attempted to sneak away in the dark of night to escape the quarantine. The medical personnel paid a very heavy loss to SARS. At the beginning of the epidemic, the Canton hospitals admitted the majority of fatal and non-fatal cases of SARS in China. Many dozens of physicians and nurses died, as well as some patients admitted for various other pathological conditions. In this manner, a patient hospitalized for a leg fracture and another for appendicitis died after contracting SARS.

In Toronto, where 50 to 60% of cases of SARS were members of the health care personnel, some draconian procedures were taken to limit the risks of contamination in hospitals: prohibition of external visits, obligatory wearing of personal protective equipment, placing health care workers potentially exposed to a contagious ill patient in quarantine for 10 days, closure of certain hospital centers where the epidemic was not under control, such as the hospitals in Scarborough or in Sunnybrook. The Saint Michael Hospital, which had a traumatology center, decided to treat all pathological conditions with the exception of SARS for fear of not having the ability to provide care for victims of even minor traffic accidents. According to Dr. Fabrice Brunet, half of the capacity of the health care system of Toronto was paralyzed by the SARS epidemic and the costs to the hospitals of this city could exceed 62 million Euros.

The safety of the hospitals brought about an overall strategy, which included above all, always regularly washing hands before and after any contact with an ill patient, as well as personnel protection by means of adapted personal protective equipment (mask, surgical cap, glasses, gown, shoe covers). 'Surgical' masks and the N95 protective masks were the best means of protection from SARS in case of close contact with a hospitalized ill patient. The 'surgical' masks were covered with an impermeable film, to prevent the wearer from spreading droplets while talking, coughing, or sneezing. On the other hand, paper masks offered uncertain protection and constituted an insufficient barrier against respiratory secretions from the fact of humidification by the saliva. An investigation published in the British weekly journal, *The Lancet*, confirmed these data. In this article, the group of Dr. W.H. Seto, from *Queen Mary Hospital* in Hong Kong, reviewed the manner in which members of the health care staff were protected while treating the first ill patients afflicted with SARS from March 15th to 24th, 2003. It appeared that 13 members of the staff were contaminated, of whom 6 were nurses, 2 were physicians, 4 were care-giving aides, and 1 was another staff person. No member of the staff having formally respected the four prescribed precautions (wearing a mask, wearing gloves, wearing a smock, regular hand washing) was infected. On the other hand, the 13 contaminated persons had omitted at least one of these measures. Only two of them had worn a protective mask, but these were paper masks. Dr. Seto stated:

> The wearing of a mask on the condition that it is a surgical mask or of the N 95 type combined with hand washing seems absolutely essential to the safety of the caregivers.

On the other hand, the other associated measures did not seem to carry supplementary protection.

Some Chinese nurses complained of being out of stock of masks or the absence of masks of sufficient quality in their hospitals. The masks offering good safety were frequently reserved for personnel directly treating patients with SARS, while the rest of the staff had only the right to paper masks. In Hong Kong, a campaign called 'Project Shield' was launched to offer protective equipment to medical personnel.

The admission of ill patients to specialized units for infectious pathology, anticipated from the arrival of a suspected case, contributed to limiting the transfer of contamination in the hospitals. Direct hospitalization, by the intermediary of the pre-hospital care system, in suspected cases detected in airports, allowed bypassing generally over-crowded emergency services. The pre-hospital care system groups were equipped with protective equipment and ambulances specially dedicated to the transport of contaminated patients. The vehicles were decontaminated after each mission. In Toronto, the Canadian Health authorities urgently adopted this type of procedure, as was indicated to the daily newspaper, *Le Monde*, by Dr Fabrice Brunet:

> In France, the mechanism is based on the 15 centers, the pre-hospital care service (SAMU), and several hospitals for accommodating the SARS cases. All the hospitals in Toronto have applied the same rules, as in a scenario of bacteriological warfare.

Within the hospital, the diagnosis should be made as rapidly as possible. In France, nasopharyngeal samples were initially sent to the Institute Pasteur in Paris. The initial delay of response of several days was reduced to several hours with the utilization of rapid detection tests. The quality of epidemiological studies done within the hospital allowed finding the precise context of the contamination in nearly all the cases of patients hospitalized, and of putting together the chain of contamination. From the hospital admission of a suspected patient, the physicians very precisely analyzed the history and his recent contacts and put together the trail, contact by contact, sometimes in collaboration with other countries. The health questionnaire, established in the airports, permitted finding subjects suspected of infection. In Toronto, one nurse from the Mount Sinai Hospital who was afflicted with SARS had traveled on board two trains. The Health authorities disseminated the following message:

> If you have taken the train at 16:30 leaving the Toronto Union Station to that of Appleby in Burlington on April 14th, or that at 7:32 in the opposite direction the following day, stay home and also contact your health service.

Although no cases of transmission of the illness by blood transfusion had been reported, on May 15, 2003, WHO transmitted some recommendations concerning blood donations. Persons having been in contact with a patient suspected of having SARS were excluded from donating blood for 3 weeks. Persons suspected of having SARS must wait to donate. In cases of SARS considered as probable, any blood donation was proscribed for three months which followed the conclusion of treatment. All blood donors developing symptoms of the illness in a delay of one month after donating blood were required to notify the public health authorities, in order to ensure the recall of the involved blood products. France had anticipated these measures for excluding the donation of blood from the month of April from the following groups: persons presenting with suspected symptoms, persons having traveled recently to countries affected by the epidemic, and persons having been in contact with travelers returned from an area at risk for less than 2 weeks. WHO added that 'these recommendations can also serve as a basis for defining the precautions to take for transplantation of organs and tissue and cell grafts.'

Political, economic, and social consequences

After 5 months of a wait-and-see policy, contradictory declarations, and shilly-shallying; the Chinese authorities took exceptional measures to attempt to alleviate the populace's anxiety and to stop the epidemic. The government pronounced some political sanctions against the Minister of Health, Zhang Wenkang, and the mayor of Beijing, Meng Xuenong, who were dismissed for their 'bad' management of the crisis and for having attempted to suppress information on the severity of the epidemic. Ms. Wu Yi, the 'Chinese iron lady,' was nominated as 'commander in chief' in the 'war' against the virus. The celebrated Chinese actress, Gong Li, chose to portray a courageous nurse who devoted her life and soul to SARS victims on the screen.

However, the disastrous management of the onset of the crisis and the disinformation from the authorities resulted in a complete loss of confidence in official announcements. The sudden rapid increase in cases placed under quarantine, the thousands of persons confined to their residences or confined in hospitals, resulted in panic reactions and fed the psychoses in certain places. Students were precipitously returned to their provincial families despite official prohibitions against travel. In the same manner, seasonal travelers and the 'Floating Population' of Beijing (4 million persons) were sent from the Capital to their residence villages. Some patients afflicted with SARS slipped out of designated hospitals for fear of being abandoned in their death throes. The total absence of transparency from the beginning of the crisis only increased the most maddening rumors: the SARS virus was a biological weapon released by George Bush's administration against China and the deceased were piled up by the hundreds in a secret hospital in the city, Martial Law had been declared and the capital had been quarantined. These rumors were amplified by tens of millions of text messages disseminated by cell phones, illustrating the key role of information technology in this type of crisis. For example, 7 million new SMS's (*Short message systems*) were exchanged in China in a country which already had 221 million cell phones. Here is an example of the SMSs which were circulated in the province of Guangdong in the month of April:

> Communiqué from the Ministry of Health: the ceiling of 10,000 cases announced for the epidemic of atypical pneumonia has been exceeded. If you send this message to ten other

persons, your telephone bill will be credited with 188 yuans [20 Euros]. Why don't you try it? It works! Follow-up quickly.

This type of message undeniably spread discord throughout the society. Numerous e-mails avoided censure and disseminated even more fantastic disinformation; China enumerated 60 million postings. The fear of SARS in the countryside provoked some movements of revolt against certain quarantine measures. In this fashion, several thousands of villagers ransacked a high school that the authorities had decided to transform into a quarantine center for suspected cases. Some hospitals were attacked by a hostile mob fearing the presence of SARS patients in these establishments. The police were attacked by the mob. Some entire towns were enclosed in barbed wire barriers to prevent access by citizens suspected of propagating the infection. All these population panic measures were thus susceptible to be transformed in angry reactions with difficult to control political consequences, particularly during a change in government, which was the case in China. The political reliability of the Chinese regime was placed in doubt by numerous governments during the SARS epidemic. According to political analysts, the catastrophe of Chernobyl in 1986, shortly after Gorbatchev's attainment of power, precipitated Pereströika and lead to the downfall of the USSR.

The economic consequences of the epidemic were disastrous. For the countries of South East Asia (with the exception of Japan), the bill for the first 3 months was 15 million dollars; each additional month of the epidemic cost a minimum of 5 million dollars. By the month of May 2003, the Asian Development Bank evaluated the losses for Asia at 28 million dollars if the epidemic continued until September. The Chinese Investment Bank already knew in 2003

the worse case of economic performance since the decline of activity which followed the events of Tiananmen in 1999.

The first sectors affected were tourism: transportation, restaurants, and hotels. The loss for air transportation was twice that which occurred during the First Gulf War. No cases of SARS transmission during airline transportation were ever reported. The Thai Airways company proposed to insure up to the sum of 100,000 dollars any person who contracted the illness on board one of its aircraft. A public health crisis prolonged disorganization of industrial production and international commerce. According to *Time* magazine, the global cost of the epidemic for the month of May was 30 million dollars.

By the month of June 2003, the epidemic seemed to be on the way to extinction after having caused 8,464 illnesses and 799 deaths in thirty countries, mostly in Asia. Only Canada was still confronted with some new cases in the hospital milieu. SARS afflicted, in most cases, persons aged 65 years and older with an overall mortality rate of about 15%. Certain studies, looking for the animal reservoir of the virus, pointed to the rabbit, a small animal whose meat is well liked by the Chinese. The researchers have shown that in the rabbit cells and saliva, a coronavirus quite genetically similar to that retrieved from humans afflicted with SARS can be found. An expert from the WHO announced in the month of June 2003:

We hope to achieve replacing the SARS virus into its bottle, but it falls on us to acquire the certainty that it cannot get back out even if it takes months, or even years.

The first epidemic of the 21st century was therefore rich in lessons on how to combat an unknown virus, whatever its origin. It is still too early to reach definitive conclusions, but the propagation of the coronavirus has allowed us to pinpoint certain deficiencies in our public health protection [1]. The director of the Department of Infectious Diseases at WHO, David Heymann, asked about the principal lessons of the epidemic, responded:

> They are multiple. We learned that unknown infections are the frontier, but that information and advice to travelers can contain international propagation. Likewise, epidemics can be contained with classical measures, such as isolation of ill patients, and quarantine of persons who have been in contact with them, but also through instituting international collaboration between laboratories, health care givers, and epidemiologists. We have also seen the negative impact of emerging illness on the economy, especially in countries where the public health care infrastructure is weak. At the same time when information is furnished by the afflicted country, this epidemic has also shown the importance of international surveillance networks. Finally, the necessary role of WHO to disseminate information and contribute to the worldwide effort against this new disease has been demonstrated.

The establishment, in Europe, of an organization equivalent to the CDC in Atlanta has been proposed in order to improve the public health competency of the continent in the area of emerging infectious diseases.

References

1. Benkimoun P. Malgré le recul de l'épidémie de SRAS, l'OMS invite à rester vigilant. *Le Monde*, vendredi 20 juin 2003, p. 27.
2. Evans A, Finkelstein S, Singh J *et al*. Pandemic influenza: A note on international planning to reduce the risk from air transport. Aviat Space Environ Med 2006, 77: 974–976.
3. Nowak M. Pneumopathie, les lendemains d'une épidémie. La Recherche, juin 2003, **365**: 38–45.
4. Vildé JL. Une pneumonie atypique. Pour la science, édition française de *Scientific American*, mai 2003, **307**: 28–29.
5. Webster R, Walker E. La grippe. Pour la *science*, édition française de *Scientific American*, mai 2003, **307**: 30–33.

15

Anthrax

Patrick Barriot

Bacillus anthracis is one of the pathogenic agents always referred to in cases of biological threats [2,14]. The formation of extremely resistant spores, in particular to mechanical forces, makes it an agent of choice that could be dispersed by numerous means. During the 20th Century, *Bacillus anthracis* led to numerous programs of offensive research with the aim of increasing its virulence and its resistance to antibiotics or vaccines [8]. In the month of October 2001, a bioterrorist attack utilizing booby-trapped letters revealed numerous flaws in civil defense operations [9]. In France, the last reported case was found in 1996. The French government, under the auspices of the Biotox plan, declared that patients with this disease must be cremated rather than buried.

Pathophysiology

Bacillus anthracis is a bacterium that normally develops in the soil and generally affects ruminants (cattle, goats, and sheep). The spores are in an encapsulated form, highly resistant to germination, and can penetrate into the human body through the dermal, pulmonary, or gastrointestinal routes. The spores can penetrate the epidermal barrier through small scrapes and scratches. The cutaneous form of anthrax is expressed by a pustule with a black center, excoriated, and evolving into an edematous or necrotic ulcer. When inhaled, the spores can attack the pulmonary alveoli and suddenly set off a lethal form of the illness. Pulmonary anthrax is expressed in the form of a febrile bronchopneumonia, not contagious, causing a major alteration of health status. In the 2 to 5 days which follow the inhalation of the spores, a dry cough develops which rapidly develops into respiratory distress. In the absence of initiation of early antibiotic treatment, the mortality rate is very high, on the order of 80%. In a few rare cases, ingested spores can cause injury to the gastrointestinal mucosa and result in ulcerations. Gastrointestinal anthrax is expressed as bloody diarrhea. Person-to-person transmission of anthrax has only rarely been described in the setting of contamination in laboratories.

Treating Victims of Mass Destsuction   Edited by Patrick Barriot and Chantal Bismuth
© 2008 John Wiley & Sons, Ltd

Whatever its mode of penetration into the body, *Bacillus anthracis* is capable of being transported by the cells of the immune system and injuring the lymphatic ganglions where they multiply. The illness of anthrax or 'black fever' results from the production of toxins that are dispersed into the lymphatic system and into the circulatory system. These toxins are responsible for the tissue lesions, in particular to the lungs. The infectious agent of anthrax illness secretes three different proteins: antigen protector (AP), edematous factor (EF), and lethal factor (LF). The AP protein combines with the LF protein to form the lethal toxin, responsible as its name indicates, for the patient's death. The AP protein combines with the EF protein to form the edematogenic toxin that causes edema formation. It is important to emphasize that antibiotic treatment is only efficacious early, before *Bacillus anthracis* has secreted its toxins.

Militarization of anthrax

At least three facts have been made public, stating that offensive research programs have been conducted on *Bacillus anthracis*. In July 1942, a bomb containing anthrax was tested by the British armed forces on the small Scottish island of Gruinard, engendering the death of all the sheep as well as long-lasting contamination of the soil. On Friday March 30, 1979, a negligent act resulted in the release of 50 grams of militarized anthrax spores from the Sverdlovsk biological weapons production facility (Ekaterinburg, Urals). These spores, which were dispersed into the atmosphere of Sverdlovsk resulted in the deaths of one hundred persons [11,15,16]. Finally, it has recently been confirmed that anthrax spores were used in booby-trapped letters on the east coast of the United States, coming from the Ames strain cultivated in the Fort Detrick USAMRIID American military laboratory and tested at *Dugway Proving Grounds* (Utah). The technique of militarization of anthrax, developed in the Fort Detrick laboratory, revealed a perfect mastery of the virulence of this agent and of the physical state of aerosols. The very high concentration of spores (thousands of millions of spores per gram) and their very high volatility allows them to disperse through the structure of closed paper envelopes. The spores have an optimal size and weight for penetrating the pulmonary alveoli (1.5 to 3 microns) having also been exposed to a chemical treatment improving their capacity for diffusion in the air. The problem of static electricity, which causes the spores to aggregate, is in effect one of the principal obstacles which must be overcome to militarize anthrax. However, the spores found in the booby-trapped letters were mixed with a product dried over a base of silicon oxide (silica), a procedure specially developed in the American military facilities of *Dugway Proving Ground* (Utah).

Anthrax booby-trapped letters

On October 4th, 2001, the American authorities announced that a man had deliberately been contaminated with anthrax contained in an envelope. On the East coast of the United States, a series of postal workers were contaminated with anthrax spores, causing the deaths of 5 persons amongst the 24 persons who contracted the illness [3,4,10]. The initial cases were diagnosed late because the early symptoms suggested a benign respiratory pathology of the bronchitis type. Later, hospitals were inundated by persons wanting rapid diagnostic tests that were not available. In Washington, D.C., more than 3000 persons were examined in less than 48 hours.

Ciprofloxacin, an antibiotic recommended for treating anthrax, was widely prescribed on a large scale as a preventive security measure. This medication is commercialized by the German firm, Bayer, who received an emergent order for a total of 95 million dollars. Faced with the high cost of antibiotics, the American authorities threatened to no longer respect the patent's need for ciprofloxacin and to produce a less costly generic formulation. This practice was violently condemned by the Bush Administration when some third world countries wanted to manufacture generic medications to treat AIDS. To prevent the fight against anthrax becoming an economic war, the public health authorities of the United States recommended another antibiotic, doxycycline produced by an American firm them, Pfizer. Altogether, more than 30000 Americans received antibiotic treatment, amongst 5000 whose treatment lasted for 60 days.

The contamination first involved postal sorting centers and was propagated to post offices and to the Secretarial staffs of public buildings. Postal workers were therefore the first persons to be exposed. It was nevertheless necessary to wait many days before gloves and masks began to be distributed to postal workers, as well as the establishment of procedures for detection and identification of the pathogenic agent. Two postal workers from Brentwood died after having inhaled anthrax spores. A union delegate declared on a television network: '*We have been told, this last week, that there is no risk and we have no reason to be tested. Sampling has been delayed and two of us have died.*' Two complainants accused the US Postal Service of having exposed postal workers to the anthrax bacillus and of having delayed furnishing them with antibiotics had their depositions taken. These litigants testified that the reception of contaminated letters by members of Congress had lead to a general and immediate distribution of antibiotics to the Congress. The CDC in Atlanta had probably underestimated the severity of the situation at the onset of the crisis, thinking that the spores could not escape from closed envelopes. During a media interview, a representative of the CDC clumsily confessed that '*it was not thought that there was such a risk.*' The Director of the CDC, Jeffrey Koplan, was forced to resign 3 months later for this bad evaluation.

Overall, the attacks with anthrax bacillus caused 5 deaths in the United States. Thirty other persons contracted the illness between October 5th and November 21, 2001. In France, numerous false alarms of contaminated letters were reported. Recalling the events of 2001, Christian Sommade stated in the month of February 2003:

The crisis of envelopes with anthrax as understood in France during the autumn of 2001 was, with more than 5,000 false alarms, a formidable exercise on a large scale which permitted us to assess our reaction capacity. However, at the time of review, we are forced to state that we were poorly prepared or unprepared for such an eventuality. [...] The procedures followed in 2001 were perfected in a crisis where a real danger was not confirmed. And as nothing was, all is well over! On the contrary, I believe that the conclusions were quite different.

Detection, identification and decontamination

The bioterrorist attack with booby-trapped letters revealed the absence of a rapid screening test for anthrax, while hospitals were besieged by a population that wanted to be reassured. This probably contributed to the excessive prescription of prophylactic antibiotics. A short time thereafter, the Mayo Clinic announced the development of a screening test for anthrax illness in humans giving a response of less than one hour. On its part, the group from the Pathogenesis and Bacterial Immunology Laboratory at the Rockefeller University in New York discovered a viral bacteriophage specific for the anthrax bacillus of which an enzyme (Ply G Lysine) allowed the destruction and rapid detection of the bacillus with a luminescent reaction. The destruction of the bacillus causes liberation of ATP, utilized by the enzyme luciferase to degrade luciferin, thus producing an easily detectible luminescent reaction. Laboratories of molecular genetics studied the genome of the anthrax strain disseminated by letter. Timothy Read's group who conducted research on the anthrax bacillus at TIGR (*The Institute for Genome Research*) and the group of Paul Keim from the University of Arizona compared this strain to the Ames strain, cultivated by civilian and military laboratories in view of basic research. The comparison of genomic markers confirmed that the strain of *Bacillus anthracis* utilized for terrorist purposes was derived from the Ames strain.

Numerous systems, whose efficacy has not always been demonstrated, have been commercialized with the aim of destroying anthrax spores. The postal sorting centers, particularly exposed, were equipped with equipment allowing irradiation of letters and thus destroying the pathogenic bacteria. The total cost of these disinfection operations was more than 14 million dollars.

Treatment

Antibiotic treatment, to be efficacious, must be administered early, before the bacillus has secreted its toxins. In the absence of this early treatment, the mortality rate of pulmonary anthrax can reach 80–100%. Two antibiotics are efficacious against *Bacillus anthracis*: ciprofloxacin and doxycycline. In cases of the pulmonary form of the illness, it is recommended to administer emergent treatment by the intravenous route. Otherwise treatment is done by the oral route for a duration of 60 days by the following dosing schedules:

- Ciprofloxacin intravenous (400 mg i.v. every 12 hours) followed by ciprofloxacin by the oral route (50 mg 2 or 3 times/day for 60 days);

- Doxycycline intravenous (100 mg i.v. every 12 hours) followed by doxycycline by the oral route (100 mg twice daily) for 60 days.

The first animal vaccinations against the anthrax illness were conducted in 1881 by Louis Pasteur, who noted that sheep that were placed into pastures where animals that died from anthrax had been buried became resistant to the illness. The vaccine, developed from an attenuated live culture of anthrax bacillus, was revealed to be perfectly efficacious for protecting various sorts of animals, but the immunity is of short duration and it is necessary to repeat the vaccine each year. Since that date, no satisfactory vaccine has been developed for humans [6,17]. During the 1991 Gulf War, the Americans addressed the Soviet Union to buy the vaccine produced by the Institute of Scientific Research for Microbiology of the Ministry of Defense. In 1985, this institute had available nearly 10 million doses of anthrax vaccine available. However, the first Gulf War was already over before the Soviet authorities had decided not to authorize the sale of their vaccine. From 1998, the American company Bioport has commercialized an 'anti-anthrax' vaccine of dubious efficacy. In June 2002, a lack of sufficient material lead to an interruption of vaccinations for the thousands of military personnel susceptible of being exposed to anthrax, particularly in Iraq. The Bioport firm then restarted its production of vaccines in the anticipation of a second generation vaccine, resulting from genetic engineering. Meryl Nass, a physician specialist on anthrax illness, declared to the media in the month of October 2001:

> I have seen so many persons devastated by this vaccine that I think it should be avoided. If the situation becomes such that it is the only solution, I would be led to accept it. But we are not there.

Moreover, the Soviet Biopreparat biological program, revealed by Ken Alibek, had permitted development of a *Bacillus anthracis* strain insensitive to known vaccines.

Researchers in genetic engineering have attempted to develop synthesis inhibitors capable of neutralizing the *Bacillus anthracis* toxins. The principle is the production of traps which divert the toxin from its target and prevent penetration of the cellular membrane. Some researchers from Harvard have discovered a peptide capable of binding to the antigen protector (AP), in this fashion blocking the action of the anthrax bacillus toxin. This peptide has been named 'PVI' for polyvalent inhibitor which prevents the appearance of the symptoms of the illness in rats. The development of specific antibodies capable, like peptides, of binding to the toxins is also being studied.

Bacillus anthracis is thus a pathogenic agent cultivated by numerous military research centers for the resistance of its spores and its capacity for penetrating by the respiratory route [1,5,7,12,13]. These military laboratories carry a real danger for the civilian population and the environment. We have seen as proof that the British Porton Down center was responsible for the contamination of Gruinard Island which lasted several decades, that the Soviet center for the production of biological weapons at Sverdlovsk was the cause of a wave of contaminations within the civilian population, and that the American laboratory at Fort Detrick cultivated the strain utilized for the bioterrorist attacks of October 2001.

References

1. Barakat L, Quentzel H, Jernigan J *et al*. Fatal inhalational anthrax in a 94-year-old Connecticut woman. *J Am Med Assoc*, 2002, 287: 863–868

2. Binder P, Lepick O. Les armes biologiques. Paris, Presses Universitaires de France, 'Que-sais-je?', 2001.
3. Borio L, Frank D, Mani V et al. Death due to bioterrorism-related inhalational anthrax: report of two patients. *J Am Med Assoc*, 2001, 286: 2554–2559.
4. Bush L, Abrams B, Beall A, Johnson C. Index case of fatal inhalational anthrax due to bioterrorism in the United States. N Engl J Med, 2001, 345: 1607–1610.
5. Friedlander A. Microbiology: tackling Anthrax. Nature, 2001, 414: 160–161.
6. Hannoun C. La vaccination. Paris, Presses Universitaires de France. 'Que sais-je?', 1999.
7. Hansen W, Freney J. Le charbon: maladie d'hier, arme biologique d'aujourd'hui. Pour la science (édition française de *Scientific American*), 2001, 290: 8–15.
8. Inglesby T, O'toole T, Henderson D *et al*. Anthrax as a biological weapon: 2002 updated recommendations for management. *J Am Med Assoc*, 2002, 287: 2236–2252.
9. Lepick O. Armes biologiques: le jeu trouble des États-Unis. Libération, jeudi 7 février 2002, p. 4.
10. Mayer T, Bersoff-Matcha S, Murphy C *et al*. Clinical presentation of inhalational anthrax following bioterrorism exposure: report of 2 surviving patients. *J Am Med Assoc*, 2001, 286: 2549–2553.
11. Meselson M, Guillemin J, Hugh-Jones M *et al*. The Sverdlovsk anthrax outbreak of 1979. Science, 1994, 266: 1202–1208.
12. Mina B, Dym J, Kuepper F *et al*. Fatal inhalational anthrax with unknown source of exposure in a 61-year-old woman in New York City. *J Am Med Assoc*, 2002, 287: 858–862.
13. Mock M. Les secrets du charbon. Pour la science (édition française de *Scientific American*), 2001, 290: 18–21.
14. Postel-Vinay O. Le dossier du bioterrorisme. Le Recherche, décembre 2003: 70–77.
15. Rich V. Russia: anthrax in the Urals. Lancet, 1992, 339: 419–420.
16. Wachtel C. Armes biologiques: le problème russe. La Recherche, juin 1998: 37–41.
17. Wiesen A, Littell C. Relationship between prepregnancy anthrax vaccination and pregnancy and birth outcomes among US Army women. *J Am Med Assoc*, 2002, 287: 1556–1560.

16

Biotechnologies: protection or threat?

Patrick Barriot

Genetic engineering, or 'recombinant DNA' technology, was first developed at the beginning of the 1970s, which marked a true turning point for biology. It gathers together all the tools and methods employed for conferring new properties on living cells by modifying their genetic material. The discovery of restriction enzymes, true molecular scalpels, opened the pathway to 'genetic surgery' with which one can fabricate hybridized molecules and manipulate genomes. These enzymes possess the property of invariably recognizing the same DNA sequence and of cutting the molecule at this precise location. At the beginning of the 1970s, for the first time, Hamilton Smith's group in the United States purified one such enzyme and identified its restriction site. Since this time, some hundreds of restriction enzymes have been isolated, but other enzymes, such as ligases and polymerases, are also necessary for genetic manipulations. These molecular tools allow cloning a foreign gene in a bacterium, after which it produces numerous copies of this DNA and assures synthesis of the coded protein. Biotechnologies also open up high performance techniques, such as methods of sequencing that decrypt the base chains of a DNA molecule or the technique of chain amplification, known under the name of 'PCR' (*polymerase chain reaction*), that allows reproduction of millions of copies of a DNA fragment. PCR allows making infinitesimal quantities of DNA *in vitro*. Automation of these techniques and computerization constitute the strongest driving forces for the evolution of genetic engineering, as has been witnessed by the number of genomes sequenced in the last few years. The international consortium of the '*human genome project*' (HUGO) has sequenced the 3.12 million base pairs which make up the 25 000 genes distributed on the 23 pairs of human chromosomes. Knowing the genome sequences of microorganisms may allow '*in vitro*' synthesis of certain of these agents from their chemical formula.

While the pharmacopoeia currently rests on only about 500 protein targets, it is now a matter of identifying the hundreds of thousands of proteins in cells and of analyzing the processes, normal or pathological, in which they participate. Scientists in this era

Treating Victims of Mass Destsuction   Edited by Patrick Barriot and Chantal Bismuth
© 2008 John Wiley & Sons, Ltd

of 'genomics' and 'proteomics' have an arsenal of techniques with which to character-
ize proteins, visualize them, and even follow their activities within the cell. Functional
genetics also addresses the mechanisms of the methylation of genes and epigenetic
phenomena which modify gene expression. The structure and function of chromatin,
histones, and different RNAs are the objects of intense study. Certain 'RNA disruptors'
are capable of silencing specific genes; others can block the entry of viruses, such as
poliomyelitis virus, into cultured human cells. Knowledge of molecular mechanisms
of gene expression allows the study of cerebral functions, particularly the storage and
utilization of information in the brain or the relationships between genes and behavior,
with the possibility of developing new molecules for behavior modification.

A step currently being attempted is the creation of new genomes and new forms of life.
Craig Venter, who deciphered the complete genome of the variola [smallpox] virus, has
undertaken to create *in vitro* a microorganism carrying the minimum number of genes
necessary for its survival. In collaboration with Claire Fraser, Director of The Institute
for Genome Research, he has sequenced the genome of *Mycoplasma genitalium*, a small
bacterium possessing only about 500 genes. In order to understand the genes truly indispensable for life, they inactivated the genes of this bacterium one by one. According to
them, 170 of the 500 genes (about 36%) are superfluous. They thus intend to reduce the
genome of the bacterium by inactivating all of the genes which are not strictly necessary
for life. As a second step, they want to assemble these indispensable genes in an artificial
chromosome that they will insert in place of the natural chromosome of *Mycoplasma
genitalium*. It is a matter of recreating a living system and of modeling it in order to furnish a powerful mathematical tool to biologists. Craig Venter is associated in this project
with Hamilton Smith, winner of the Nobel Prize for Physiology and Medicine. The US
Department of Energy has financed this project to the extent of 3 million Euros. Craig
Venter emphasized that an American bioethics committee had given the green light to
research on synthetic bacteria in 1999. This model could furnish formidable industrial
applications, but it could also open up development of unsuspected biological weapons.
The creation of unknown forms of life could lead, sooner or later, to the creation of unknown pathogenic agents. In fact, Venter stated that he has kept part of his results secret
because he understands the repercussions for terrorist purposes.

On their part, some Japanese researchers have undertaken to enlarge the genetic code
and to create artificial proteins by incorporating modified amino acids. A group directed
by Shigeyuki Yokohama from the University of Tokyo has modified the structure of
DNA and some different molecules which assure gene expression. Their technique, entirely acellular, allows manipulation of the entire fabrication chain, from the DNA up to
the protein, passing through messenger RNA. This technique calls upon a pair of complementary modified bases which direct the insertion of an artificial amino acid into a
synthetic protein. The first base is inserted into a strand of chemically synthesized DNA.
During the transcription of this strand, the second base is inserted into the corresponding
position in the messenger RNA, and can dictate the insertion of an artificial amino acid
into the protein which is then synthesized. The authors hope to generalize their method to
all sorts of artificial amino acids. Some studies on synthetic bacteria have also been performed by the American group of Peter G. Schultz from the Scripps Research Institute

in La Jolla, and the Franco-American group of Phillipe Marlière, founder and scientific director of the Evologic Company. These studies have lead to the creation of new strains of *Escherichia coli* of which the genome contains some artificial elements coding for a modified amino acid. The principal objective is to obtain novel proteins that do not exist in nature that could have multiple industrial or medical applications. Phillipe Marlière intends to enlarge the range of biological molecules by liberating the fundamental rules inscribed in the genetic code. A proponent of 'directed evolution,' he has declared:

> *'Naturalism is the yoke of biological science. It is not in scrutinizing, angstrom after angstrom, the existing that we progress, but by fabricating artificial and alternative biodiversities.'*

All these technologies thus allow modification of existing pathogenic agents, but also the *in vitro* synthesis of all parts of a microorganism.

Industrial and pharmaceutical applications

The bacterium *E.coli*, called 'good for all genetic works,' is the material of choice for the creation of transgenic bacteria carrying a foreign gene that is expressed in the form of a protein. This non-pathogenic bacterium is normally found in the digestive tract and nasal cavities in humans, as well as in the digestive tracts of numerous animals. The first stage of genetic recombination is hybridization: the study gene or 'gene of interest' is hybridized with a DNA vector, so called because it introduces the genetic construct into the bacterium. Specific vectors for *E. coli* are represented by its plasmids and bacteriophages that are well known. The second stage consists of introducing the recombinant DNA into the recipient bacteria. A chemical or electrical treatment (electrocoporation) of the bacterial envelope is necessary for penetration of the vector. Once inside the bacterium, the genetic construct is reproduced to millions of examples and the recombinant bacterium expresses the protein encoded by the foreign gene. Some bacteria called 'bioreactors' already produce antibiotics, human hormones such as insulin, erythropoietin, and human growth hormone, vaccine antigens (hepatitis B vaccine) or interferon. Initially, it was only possible to synthesize molecules encoded by a single gene, but this has now been extended to complex molecules. Recently, hydrocortisone was synthesized by genetic manipulation of a unicellular yeast: *Saccharomyces cerevisae* or 'baker's yeast.' The thirteen genes controlling the different steps of the synthesis of hydrocortisone were inserted into the genome of the yeast, allowing industrial production of this corticosteroid. This is the first time that so complex a character has been conferred upon a microorganism.

Biotechnologies are also applicable to plants and animals. Some transgenic plants are utilized as bioreactors to produce peptides or proteins for pharmaceutical usage. Contrary to bacteria, often utilized for the production of proteins, plant cells have the enzymes necessary for the maturation of proteins after their synthesis. In the eukaryotes, i.e. plants and animals, proteins can undergo numerous modifications before becoming biologically active, including the addition of hydrated carbon molecules, such as sugars, polysaccharides, and glucosides. Several firms are working on fruits and

vegetables that produce bacterial or viral antigens for vaccine development, e.g. a vaccine against hepatitis B in potatoes and one against cholera in bananas. Some American
biologists have developed a transgenic potato capable of making a vaccine against the
Norwalk virus, a food-borne virus which infects more than 23 million persons in the
United States each year. This genetically modified potato produces viral antigens capable
of immunizing persons who consume it. The Novartis firm has developed a transgenic
potato which has resulted in production of antibodies against a strain of *Escherichia
coli* responsible for gastroenteritis in 11 persons who ate it. Claude Leclerc, head of the
Biology Unit for Immune Regulation at the Institute Pasteur, has, however, stated:

> *'Obtaining an immune response does not strongly signify that the individuals are pro-
> tected against the disease. This work is still very preliminary. To measure the efficacy of
> a vaccine, it is necessary to test it on hundreds to thousands of persons and measure its
> impact on the disease.'*

The market for recombinant proteins should reach 60 million dollars in 2004–2005. In
the next few years, 10% of American corn production will be dedicated to pharmaceutical
cultures; true plant pharmacies capable of furnishing edible medications or vaccines. About
20 enterprises such as ProdiGene, Monsanto, or Dow Chemical, as well as several universities are carrying out experiments in open field locations.Other transgenic plants, carrying
bacterial genes which direct the synthesis of enzymes responsible for the hyper-accumula-
tion of nickel, arsenic, zinc, cadmium, or copper, may decontaminate contaminated soils by
concentrating toxic substances or heavy metals in their stems or leaves (phytoremediation).

The insertion of a gene coding for a human protein into the genome of an animal
capable thereafter of excreting this protein in its milk or its eggs presents a considerable
therapeutic and above all an economic opportunity. These genetically modified animals
can serve as bioreactors, otherwise called living assembly lines, for the production of
advantageous human proteins (monoclonal antibodies, antithrombin III, factor IX, serum
albumin, alpha-glucosidase, hemoglobin). The PPL Therapeutics Company announced,
in the June 29, 2000 edition of the scientific journal *Nature*, that they had successfully
cloned some transgenic ewes that produced human alpha-1-antitrypsin in their milk, in
view of a treatment for cystic fibrosis. In the future, human proteins of medical interest
will be produced in the egg whites of poultry. Transgenic silkworms can also synthesize some proteins of therapeutic interest which are harvested from their cocoons. Some
Canadian scientists have created transgenic mice capable of producing human growth
hormone in their sperm. These researchers wrote in November 1999 in *Nature Biotechnology*: *'Sperm is a body fluid which can easily be collected on a continual basis.'* The
end objective is to produce proteins for therapeutic usage in the sperm of bulls or boars.

The shortage of human organs for transplantation has stimulated the creation of
'humanized' transgenic pigs, which have been modified such that their organs carry
fewer antigens to stimulate an immune response after transplantation. This type of
manipulation exposes the recipient to the risk of transmission of porcine pathogenic
agents, especially as the grafted patient is in an immune suppressed state: in particular,
it increases the risk of emergence of a new human virus from a porcine virus. A British
oncologist has discovered a porcine virus capable of infecting human renal cells. An

American group directed by Daniel R. Solomon (Scripps Institute, La Jolla, California) has confirmed this risk experimentally by demonstrating that it is possible to infect human cell lines cultivated in the laboratory with endogenous retroviruses present in all pigs (PERV). The latter can break the species barrier and infect rats which have been grafted with porcine pancreatic cells. *A priori*, such a risk of infection is thus not excluded in humans. Furthermore, the possibility of monitoring and curbing PERV in transplanted tissues, evoked in passing, seems today totally illusory. The group of André Jestin, from the French Agency for the Health Safety of Foods, has noted not less than 11 PERVs, of which 4 can present some risk of infection. Jon Allan virologist from the Southwest Foundation for Biomedical Research (San Antonio, Texas) affirmed on his part that the results of the latest research concerning porcine retroviruses

> *'Should compel those responsible for public health, in the United States as well as elsewhere, to consider organ grafts between animals and humans as a breeding ground for retroviruses susceptible to produce recombinant viruses for affectations of a new type.'*

Evoking the risks for contamination of the human species with an unknown virus, Frank Grosveld, Professor of cellular biology at the Erasmus University in Rotterdam stated: *'Actually, a person cannot measure these risks.'* Professor Robert Ducluzeau, Director of Research at the INRA and member of the French Ethics Committee, has indicated that for him *'the appearance of new illnesses breaking the species barrier is not a myth and one must not underestimate this danger.'*

Many researchers are studying the genomes of insects that intervene in the transmission of infectious diseases. The complete sequence of the mosquito *Anopheles gambiae*, vector of malaria, was published in the journal *Science* on October 4, 2002. A group from the CNRS of Montpellier, France, has placed in evidence, in the genomes of the mosquitoes *Anopheles gambiae* and *Culex pipiens*, a mutation which confers resistance to organophosphate and carbamate insecticides. The manipulation of the genetic heritage of these insects aims to prevent them from reproducing or from transmitting illnesses such as malaria, dengue fever, or Chagas' disease. Some even envision vaccination campaigns by means of the bites of genetically modified mosquitoes. However, Marjorie Hoy, an entomologist from the University of Florida, *'We should be very prudent, because our ignorance in the matter of genetic transmission is great.'* Procedures for monitoring genetically modified insects have not been established: a biologist who wished to transport some eggs of transgenic mosquitoes recently asked the advice of the Center for Disease Control in Atlanta, because it was a species capable of transmitting Yellow Fever. However, as these eggs were not effectively carriers of the disease, the Center indicated that this was not within its remit. The Director of the Department of Health and Safety at the time acknowledged that he had not considered the question of genetically modified insects.

Fundamental research on pathogenic agents

Fundamental research on the genomes of pathogenic organisms advances at a rapid pace. The genomes of viruses such as that of the variola virus and the poliomyelitis virus are today already entirely sequenced, as well as the genomes of numerous bacteria:

Chlamydia pneumoniae, Escherichia coli, Haemophilis influenzae, Helicobacter pylori, Listeria monocytogenes, Mycobacterium leprae, Mycobacterium tuberculosis, Neisseria meningitides, Pseudomonas aeruginosa, Treponema pallidum, Vibrio cholerae, Yersinia pestis. In 1998, researchers at TIGR (Rockville, Maryland) succeeded in sequencing the genome of the Ames strain of the anthrax bacillus.Sequencing of the genome of pathogenic agents allows the study of metabolic pathways utilized by the pathogenic agents and the different factors which determine their virulence. The group directed by Craig Venter has established the sequencing of the genome of Vibrio cholerae, the bacteria responsible for cholera, which is present in the form of two circular chromosomes. The first chromosome contains the genes which direct the replication of DNA, cellular division, and synthesis of membrane elements. It also carries the principal genes for virulence, that of the cholera toxin. The genes implicated in metabolism are situated on the second chromosome of which a part, called intergon, confers resistance to many antibiotics on the bacterium. This work was published in the August 3, 2000 edition of the scientific journal *Nature.* Dr. Jean-Michel Fournier, Director of the Cholera Unit of the Institute Pasteur in Paris, has stated:

> 'This decryption offers us some powerful tools for progressing in the understanding of Vibrio, its physiology, its metabolism, its survival in the environment, the phenomena of regulation between its two chromosomes, or the transfer of genes between the bacteria.'

The complete sequencing of the leprosy bacterium (or the bacterium of Hansen's disease), Mycobacterium leprae, was published in *Nature* on February 21, 2001 by a group of researchers from the Bacterial Molecular Genetics Unit from the Institute Pasteur in Paris, directed by Professor Stewart Cole. He compared the Hansen's bacillus to another pathogenic mycobacterium:

> 'We have compared it to Mycobacterium tuberculosis, its cousin. It inhabits the same cells and comes into contact with the same immune response. However, we have perceived that, unlike M. tuberculosis, M. leprae has lost many genes in the course of evolution. Certain of these genes, such as those which allow it to produce energy, have been submitted to so many mutations in M. leprae that they can no longer function. [...] We have not discovered an evident system which allows it to incorporate iron in M. leprae. However, all organisms have need of iron for their growth; M. tuberculosis, itself, has shown a very efficacious system for finding the little iron available.'

M. leprae has in this manner lost nearly 2 500 genes, which always exist in the genetic heritage of *M. tuberculosis.* In *M. leprae,* only those genes persist which are implicated in the activities essential to the life of the bacterium. For this reason, the Hansen bacillus only develops with difficulty in different surroundings, but it nevertheless possesses the capacity of causing a formidable disease with a difficult diagnosis. As Professor Cole emphasized: 'In *multiplying very slowly,* M. leprae has the advantage of not killing its host and thus has the ability to live as long as it does.' Decrypting of the genome of the 0157 strain of *E. coli,* responsible for formidable gastrointestinal poisonings, sometimes fatal, has allowed comparison with the genome of the non-pathogenic strain of *E. coli.* In this manner, researchers have placed in evidence the genes responsible for the acquisition of virulence. Certain of these pathogenic agents arouse the interest of military personnel. As Olivier Postel-Vinay remarked, two of the authors of the study on sequencing the plague agent, published in *Nature* on October 4, 2001, came from a British military laboratory, and acknowledgements were addressed to a biologist from an American military laboratory. The precise knowledge of the nucleotide chains within the genome allows establishing a true plan for assembly of pathogenic agents which could lead to their synthesis *in vitro*. In this manner, Eckard Wimmer from the Stony Brook University of Medicine (United States) and his group have fabricated the poliomyelitis virus *in vitro*, which is one of the smallest existing viruses (a chain of 7,500 chemical groups). Eckard Wimmer has stated:

> '*Our results show that it is thus possible to synthesize an infectious agent in vitro, in following only the information given by its written sequence.*'

This version of synthesis possesses the same properties as its homologues present in nature and it has proven its efficacy in killing rats into which it has been inoculated. The sequence of the genome of the poliomyelitis virus is freely available in databases on the Internet and there are a good hundred laboratories in the world capable of performing this synthesis. The variola virus contains some 185 000 nucleotides, but its in vitro synthesis is envisioned in about 2 years from now.

Moreover, the decryption of the human genome goes, amongst other things, to allow precise definition of the genetic differences existing between different human populations, notably resistance to certain illnesses. As an example, a gene for predisposition to leprosy situated on chromosome 6 has recently been identified within a Vietnamese population. The identification of such genes could permit elaboration of new therapeutic strategies and early detection of individuals 'at risk' in order to afford them better protection. In the case of leprosy, 90% of subjects exposed to the bacillus do not develop any form of the disease. In practice, with some genetic tests, it is thus possible to select persons who should be treated with antibiotics. However, identification of predisposing genes could also open the route to development and utilization of genetic weapons taking specific ethnic groups for their targets. In this manner, it would be possible for terrorists, belonging to a given ethnic group, to develop biological vectors (viruses, bacilli) inoffensive to them, but fatal to their neighbors. The risks of these 'genetic weapons' or 'bacterio-ethnic weapons' have been denounced by numerous scientific and humanitarian associations.

Biotechnologies and militarization of pathogenic agents

Because of genetic engineering, it is possible to amplify the virulence of natural infectious agents and to develop biological weapons called 'third generation' [12–14]. This exacerbation of virulence can be obtained in different manners:

- In conferring on the micro-organism resistance to vaccines or antibiotics.
- In equipping it with new pathogenic properties.
- In making possible its spread.

- In creating new modes of transmission, in particular transmission by the respiratory route.

- In permitting to escape the usual methods of detection.

The techniques of hybridization permit combining on the same plasmid the genes conferring resistance to several antibiotics. These plasmids can be easily transferred not only from one bacterium to another but also from one bacterial species to another. The hybridized molecules can in this manner spread into very numerous bacterial species and resistance to several antibiotics can be transferred to pathogenic species. From 1973, during the decline of the USSR, the Soviets had conferred resistance to antibiotics onto several bacterial agents (anthrax, plague, tularemia, melloidiosis). The Soviet biological program, BIOPREPARAT, revealed by Ken Alibek, former Director of the Soviet program for biological weapons, had also allowed development of a strain of *Bacillus anthracis* insensitive to known vaccines [1,11,16]. Moreover, some foreign genes intruded into a bacterium such as *E. coli* can confer on it some new pathogenic properties and can prove to be extremely dangerous for humans or animals. Some American researchers have isolated the gene coding for the lethal factor of *Bacillus anthracis* and have introduced it into the genome of *E. coli*. The protein secreted by *E. coli* exerts the same lethal factor as that produced by *B. anthracis*. The genes coding for the cholera toxin have also been inserted into the genetic heritage of coliform bacteria [3,8]. It would thus be very difficult, approaching impossible, to rapidly detect them by means of biological analysis – such coliforms secreting in situ, in the human gastrointestinal tract and nasal passages in humans could be a formidable method of propagation of illnesses. In the same manner, a strain of Yersinia pestis has been genetically modified in a fashion to produce a peptide capable of destroying the myelin sheaths which protect the nerve fibers. Following the example of bacteria, researchers have successfully incorporated into a commonplace virus responsible for rhinopharyngitis, a scorpion gene and a snake gene coding for a lethal toxin. Ken Alibek affirmed that the USSR attempted in the past to produce a modified variola virus by genetic engineering against which vaccines would be inefficacious. The techniques of recombinant genetics also allows the creation of viruses which do not exist in nature and of which we are ignorant of their mechanisms of action. One could thus fear the appearance of a 'super virus' combining, because of hybridization, the pathogenic properties of several viruses. Some techniques such as directed mutagenesis, which provoke point mutations in the genome of the virus, also serve to activate augmentation of the virulence. Some genetic engineering companies are developing 'methods of hyper-mutability' with the aim of provoking a large number of mutations within the genomes of different micro-organisms in the hope of discovering mutant strains susceptible of presenting a commercial or military interest. These genetic engineering tools conceived for producing therapeutic molecules can also direct the synthesis of toxic molecules.

Biological weapons of the fourth generation could be made up of 'phantom' viruses which would be introduced secretly within a given population and remain silent until a signal activates their pathogenic activity. Likewise are studies of the synthesis of completely new pathogenic agents, the stimulation of mechanisms of apotosis (cell death), or activation of natural mechanisms capable of stopping the expression, it doesn't matter of which gene, in the organism by means of RNA inhibitor molecules.

Biotechnologies and development of new treatments

Biotechnology methods allow the study of the mode of entry of toxins into the cells and the development of synthesis inhibitors responsible for neutralizing them. Toxins bind to membrane receptors before penetrating into the interior of the cell. The cellular receptor for a *Bacillus anthracis* toxin has been recently isolated and cloned. These studies lead to the production of traps responsible for diverting the toxin from its cellular target and in this manner blocking the mechanism of access to the cytoplasm. The agent of the anthrax illness secretes three different proteins: antigen protector AP, edematous factor EF, and lethal factor LF. Innocuous when separated from each other, these proteins form some formidable toxins once they are assembled two by two. The protein AP combines with the LF protein to form the lethal toxin, responsible as its name indicates for the patient's death. The AP protein combined with the EF protein corresponds to the edema toxin which causes edema formation. The liaison of the AP protein with a second protein requires that it first be bound to the substance of a cell, and that it has been cleared by a particular enzyme. The Harvard researchers have discovered a peptide capable of binding to the truncated AP molecule and neutralizing it. This peptide, named PVI for polyvalent inhibitor prevents, in rats, the appearance of the symptoms of the illness. This strategy could be applied to the neutralization of other circulating toxins, such as those of *Clostridium botulinum* or *Staphylococcus aureus*. It is also possible to neutralize some toxins by means of antibodies, according to Michèle Mock, Director of the Toxins and Pathogenic Bacteria Unit of the Institute Pasteur, '*The utilization of inhibitors of synthesis is not the only route of research. Serotherapy is another. This is based on the utilization of antibodies which can, like the peptides, bind to toxins and neutralize them.*'

Genetic engineering currently attempts to develop a vaccine against the anthrax illness. Since the first animal vaccinations conducted by Louis Pasteur in 1881, no satisfactory vaccine has been developed for humans. The vaccines for veterinary usage are fabricated from attenuated strains, but the utilization of live vaccines is contraindicated in humans because of the risks. In the United States, the only existing vaccine against anthrax leads to adverse effects and does not confer long-duration immunity. Since 1998, it is no longer produced. Some vaccines coming from genetic engineering and directed against the toxins of the bacteria are currently being studied. The toxins are in effect a privileged target for vaccine research, especially as they are insensitive to antibiotics. An experimental vaccine against the anthrax illness has been successfully tested by Professor Michèle Mock from the Institute Pasture in rodents contaminated with the bacillus. This new vaccine is elaborated in part from a protein which enters into the composition of the toxins and components of the spore. In the United States, the Batelle Foundation, based in Columbus, Ohio, is researching a genetically modified variant of anthrax bacillus in order to test the quality of the vaccines which are available to the armed forces ('Project Jefferson'). Other American scientists have attempted to develop a prototype of a vaccine against a particularly deadly form of meningitis caused by meningococcus type B (*Neisseria meningitidis*). After having sequenced the genome of the bacterium, they identified some membrane proteins capable of stimulating the production of antibodies which can destroy the bacterium.

Biotechnologies and genetic therapy

Genetic therapy consists of replacing a deficient gene with a functional gene. This latter, also called 'gene medication', is generally inserted into a virus responsible for penetrating into the diseased cells. Different types of viruses can be used as vectors. An international group of American, French, and Swiss researchers has performed some studies of gene therapy in monkeys with experimental Parkinson's disease. These scientists utilizing the brains of ill monkeys that had an inactivated AIDS virus into which they have inserted a gene which stimulates the production of dopamine which is impaired in Parkinson's disease. Inactivated AIDS virus was chosen as the vector of the gene because of its ability to specifically and durably infect the neurons. The results published on Friday October 27, 2000 in the American journal *Science* were spectacular, with a significant reduction of incapacitation of dopamine in the brain. One of the authors of this study, Phillipe Hantraye (CRA - CNRS) declared: '*Our idea was to demonstrate that genetic therapy can work in Parkinson's disease. For this we have utilized the AIDS virus, stripped of all power of replication and all pathogenic effects, into which we have inserted the genetic coding for a growth factor for neurons, GDNF (glial-derived neurotrophic factor).*' Numerous genetically modified viruses, most of them adenoviruses, serve as vectors in experiments of genetic or anti-cancer therapy. An adenovirus vector for genetic therapy can be utilized to introduce a gene endowed with a lethal or incapacitating action into the human body. Recently, a group of American researchers announced having developed an 'intelligent viral bomb' capable in mice of destroying brain tumors of the glioblastoma type. The genetically modified virus, injected directly into the brains of mice, is incapable of proliferating in normal cerebral cells, although it can multiply in tumor cells and destroy them.

Biotechnologies and development of identification and detection systems

Contrary to chemical agents, methods to rapidly detect the presence of pathogenic micro-organisms, either in the patient or in the environment, have been lacking. The classical techniques of culturing impose a delay of several days. New techniques detect components of the genome of the pathogenic agent or of proteins which it produces (surface antigens or toxins). The method of molecular hybridization, developed in 1975 by Edwin Southern, is based on the complementarity of the two long filaments in the double helix of DNA. Today, this has led to the production of DNA 'chips' or 'microarrays', capable of rapidly detecting the presence of fragments of bacterial or viral genomes in a sample. Because of the contribution of fabrication techniques for electronic circuits, this technology allows analysis of thousands of genetic fragments with a minimum of operations. It however imposes two prior conditions. The first is the knowledge of the sequence of the genomes of the organisms that one wishes to detect; the sequence which allows fabrication of a synthetic DNA probe. The second is the extraction of the DNA from the cells collected from the patient or in the contaminated site in order to amplify them by PCR before reacting them with the 'biochip' probe. This latter is made up of a substrate of some square centimeters, in glass or in silicon, on which are fixed the sequences previously synthetized of the genome researched. If the complementary fragment is present in the analyzed sample, it will appear with the molecular probe placed in the substrate, according to the property of hybridization of the DNA. A fluorescent marker can be activated during hybridization; the presence of the microbiological genome is confirmed by an optical reading system. The first 'biochip' was fabricated in 1991 by researchers from the California firm Affymetrix who developed a chip permitting analysis of mutations of the AIDS virus (HIV-1) and of locating in them, in particular, the mutations responsible for resistance to certain medications. The most sophisticated chips allow immediate and simultaneous detection of hundreds of thousands of DNA sequences. In the United States, the *Massachusetts Institute of Technology* (MIT) is working on the development of DNA chips capable of detecting a biological attack. In France, the Institute Pasteur and the Institute Mérieux are working on similar projects. For the detection of pathogenic agents in the environment, the principle consists of aspirating several cubic meters of air with a 'sniffer' and then to place the contents of the sample in solution, to filter it, and to analyze it before reacting it with the probes of DNA chips. All these operations can be carried out in situ in the space of several hour if a 'biochip' can conduct several analyses in parallel.

The utilization of monoclonal antibodies, detecting very small concentrations of specific microbial antigen, also allows development of rapid tests for diagnosing viral or bacterial illnesses. A French-Madagascan group has developed a rapid diagnostic test (in 15 minutes) for plague. Previously, the delay of laboratory response was 3 or 4 days.

Biotechnologies also allow envisioning the establishment of a detailed databank of the genomes of pathogenic agents susceptible of being militarized. This databank would allow rapid identification of the strains involved and their origin. Following the bioterrorist attack of October 2001 in Florida, the group of Timothy Read who directs research on the anthrax bacillus at TIGR and that of Paul Keim at the University of Arizona had the idea to compare the strain spread by letters to the Ames strain. Isolated for the first time from a Texas cow that died of anthrax illness in 1981, the Ames Strain had been sent at that time to civilian and military laboratories for basic research and testing of the efficacy of potential vaccines to control the anthrax illness. In comparing the genomic signatures of the two strains, Timothy Read and Paul Keim confirmed that the strain of *Bacillus anthracis* spread in Florida was derived from the Ames strain. The knowledge of the sequence of the genome of this bacterium will allow future investigators to recognize and identify its variants if a new anthrax attack should be perpetrated.

Risks due to this research

The laboratories where manipulations of micro-organisms or genetic manipulations such as the construction of plasmids conferring resistance to antibiotics, the development of viral vectors for genetic therapy, hybridization of animal viruses, or the transfer of DNA from higher cells take place, represents a permanent danger to the heart of large urban areas. The risk of an accident or terrorist attack liberating contagious germs must not be underestimated. A biotechnology laboratory can create voluntarily or involuntarily a pathogenic agent with unkno wn powers [2,5–7,9,10]. In 1972, Paul Berg (Stanford University, United States) successfully hybridized a bacteriophage and a carcinogenic monkey virus (SV 40) but he refused to introduce the hybrid into *E. coli*: because he feared the consequences. He announced then: '*I have decided to give up my experiments because I have not managed to persuade myself that there is no risk.*' Rewarded with the Nobel Prize in Chemistry in 1980 for his work, Paul Berg was questioned on the dangers of such constructions and on the risks of making the appearance of new bacteria virulent to humans. He proposed an international moratorium with the aim of temporarily halting genetic manipulations in order to provide '*an evaluation of the potential dangers.*' A conference chaired by Paul Berg was organized at Asilomar in 1975 in order to define the rules for security in the matter of genetic engineering and the methods of surveillance for biotechnology laboratories classified P1 to P4. The initial 'P' is the abbreviation for 'pathogen.' The level which follows, from 1 to 4, designates the level of required confinement, according to the more or less significant danger of the microorganisms studied. Level 1 concerns biological agents that do not cause illness in persons in good health and which, from this fact, can be manipulated without special protection. Level 2 concerns pathogenic agents of little danger such as the agents of listeriosis or rubeola. Access to P2 is limited and manipulations are done with smock, gloves and mask. Level 3 concerns micro-organisms which cause severe illness but which are not transmitted by simple contact, such as prions or HIV. In a P3 laboratory, the access and airflow are controlled while the wastes and work clothes are decontaminated. Level 4 concerns very dangerous viruses which are easily transmitted person-to-person and which cause incurable illnesses. At this time, only viruses such as Ebola, Marburg, Lassa or simian herpes are classified as P4. The safety regulations are draconian: seismic standards, bullet-proof glass and structures resistant to rocket/ missile attack, strains of viruses preserved in liquid nitrogen, work in level 3 PPE, artificial depressurization of the laboratory [negative pressure], air filtration, surveillance by a central computer, surveillance of animal vivariums with video cameras, airlock decontamination with showers, sterilization of all wastes. In France, the high-security P4 laboratory Jean Mérieux of the Mérieux Foundation and the Institute Pasteur are located in the Gerland quarter, on the left bank of the Rhone, in the center of the Lyon metropolitan area. This institution, classified as a 'National Sensitive Point', shows that the study of these viruses is more dangerous.

A manipulated bacterium, escaped from a laboratory, could be rapidly disseminated and launch an epidemic difficult to control and treat. On September 11, 1978, Janet Parker, a photographer, died of smallpox in a hospital in East Birmingham where she had been admitted on August 25th, thought to have contracted a 'severe influenza.' Her mother, also contaminated, died several days later. The investigation first established that Janet Parker, attached to the Anatomy Department of the University of Birmingham, had contracted the Abid strain of the virus (major variety), from a little Pakistani boy from whom samples had been sent to Kew in 1970. However, some cultures of this strain were stored on the floor above her workplace, in the laboratory of Henry Bedson, a defective laboratory in which safety conditions did not exist. Professor Henry Bedson, who committed suicide 5 days after the death of Janet Parker, carried out research on the identification of animal variola viruses (monkey pox, cow pox, rabbit pox, etc.) and on hybrid human-animal viruses. The variola viruses are distinguished by their extreme genetic instability and the spontaneously exchange genetic material between themselves, forming natural hybrids. At the time when Janet Parker was contaminated, Henry Bedson was studying virus hybrids of cow pox and human variola, which had been created by Professor Dumbell from the Department of Virology at St. Mary's Hospital Medical School (London). Several specialists have suggested that Janet Parker died as a victim of a hybrid virus coming from genetic manipulation.

At the end of the 1980s, a series of genetic engineering experiments performed in the United States by the *National Institute of Allergy and Infectious Disease* envisioned developing an animal model allowing the study of AIDS. To this purpose, researchers introduced the genome of AIDS into mouse embryos. The adult mice expressed the human AIDS virus in their cells. Critics of these experiments reported the existence of a risk, small but real, that the mice could accidentally escape from the laboratory and breed with wild mice, in this manner favoring the propagation of AIDS in the animal world. In February 1997, in an article published in the journal *Science*, Dr. Robert Gallo was questioned about the opportunity to utilize such an animal model. He made note that the AIDS virus carried by the mice could combine with other murine viruses and result in the creation of an even more virulent form of AIDS. A new strain would have in effect acquired some new biological characteristics, among them: *'The capacity to reproduce more rapidly and to infect new types of cells.'* The major risk was that it could be transmitted by new routes, which could include the respiratory route. Recently, some Australian researchers from the University of Canberra accidentally created a dangerous virus while studying how to prevent rodents from reproducing and proliferating. The group of Ronald Jackson and Ian Ramshaw introduced the gene coding for interleukin-4 into the mouse variola virus (mouse pox), because this protein has the property of sterilizing female rats and mice by hindering early embryonic development. In nature, the virus is transmitted by oral-nasal contact, in other words, when the mice meet they rub noses. But interleukin-4 also has the property of inhibiting the immune system. They found that the modified virus killed all the strains of mice infected in several days, including those with natural resistance to the variola virus. Moreover, the vaccine against rodent variola was inefficacious against this new virus. Bob Sea-mark, Director of the Center for the control of risks in Canberra declared:

> *'Our studies envisioned only limiting the proliferation of rodents who destroy the grain harvests throughout the world and particularly in developing countries.'*

If it were to have escaped from the laboratory, this new virus could have contaminated species of animals other than mice, in particular rabbits and kangaroos. Phillipe Horellou (Antoine-Béclère Hospital/INSERM) has emphasized this danger:

> *'This is what is very worrisome in this experiment; it is that the virus could pass from mice to rabbits. The evaluation of risk then becomes much more difficult to do.'*

This work was published in the February edition of the *Journal of Virology*. The risk of utilization of such a virus by bioterrorists has been evoked and Ron Jackson has recognized:

> *'One can only imagine that if an insane act placed human interleukin-4 into a human smallpox virus, a virus similar to the mouse pox virus, it would acquire lethality in a very significant manner. When one sees the consequences that can occur in mice, I do not wish to be the one who makes the experiment.'*

Some researchers from the University of Tokyo (Japan) have manipulated human and simian AIDS viruses to create a hybrid carrying the human interleukin genes and capable of neutralizing the defensive immune reaction. In a general fashion, the insertion of foreign genes into a viral genome could set in motion some unforeseen interactions, which could encompass activations or inhibitions.

Military research laboratories also represent a risk of dissemination of pathogenic agents. In 1988, a serious accident occurred in the Russian Vektor Center for Virology and Biotechnology. During the inoculation with the agent of Marburg hemorrhagic fever into a laboratory animal, two employees were infected and one of them died. The USAMRIID (US Army Medical Research Institute of Infectious Disease), located at Fort Detrick in Maryland, has shown several failures concerning safety over the course of the last few years. In April 2002, the USAMRIID revealed that active spores of the anthrax bacillus had been discovered outside the confined rooms where they were studied. Three samples collected in a changing room, an office, and a hallway were found to be positive. On June 17, 2002, during cleaning operations, a biologist from Fort Detrick discovered a phial containing a pathogenic agent developed in the 1960s and abandoned there for decades. The Ames strain of anthrax bacillus, contained in the letter bombs which were circulated in the fall of 2001, were cultivated at the USAMIID.

In 2001, the *Imperial College of London* was condemned for having taken ill-considered risks in manipulating some extremely dangerous viruses (a viral hybrid of dengue and hepatitis C, as well as the AIDS virus).

Genetic engineering in the future will allow *in vitro* synthesis of pathogenic agents eradicated by long vaccination campaigns such as the poliomyelitis or smallpox viruses. At the same time, when the WHO promised the eradication or poliomyelitis by the end of the year 2002, because of massive vaccination campaigns carried out since the 1950s, a group of researchers announced the *in vitro* synthesis of this viral pathogen. There thus exists a real danger of re-introducing a viral agent believed to be eradicated and which could be revived, in a few hours, from the sequence written in its DNA. In the end, some other infectious agents, such as that of variola, could be assembled without natural strains. While humanity believes itself to be definitively free of a natural scourge, biotechnological progress could reintroduce it at any time.

The dangers due to this type of research are beginning to be taken into account. In France, the law of July 12, 1992 on experimentation in genetic engineering placing in work some pathogens for humans or the environment is a first response to this concern about control. In the United States, since 1997, the National Institutes of Health (NIH) no longer finance studies of recombinant DNA permitting rendering of bacteria resistant to a medication. The CDC in Atlanta has established a list of pathogenic agents on which all research is submitted to close surveillance. The '*Patriot Act*' of October 26, 2001 punishes the possession of 36 pathogenic agents. A new regulation, the '*Biopreparedness*' Act reinforces this mechanism. About one hundred pathogenic agents (for humans, but also for animals and plants) are from now on subject to several rules and all researchers who wish to work with these microbes must be accredited by the Department of Justice. Finally, the citizens of seven countries, of which Iraq is one, are no longer authorized to stay in the American laboratories concerned.

Biotechnologies and open societies

In January 2001, the group of Australian researchers discussed above provoked turmoil by publishing their disturbing results in the *Journal of Virology*. The elaboration of a contraceptive for rodents, from a mouse variola virus, had accidentally produced a formidable pathogenic agent possessing all the characteristics of a biological weapon, even if the mouse variola had no impact on human health. At the end of this experiment, the Australian researchers launched a call for a revision of the Convention for the Prohibition of Biological Weapons signed in 1975 by 140 countries in Geneva. Anabelle Duncan, Director of the sector for the Division of Molecular Biology for the CSIRO, declared:

> '*Discoveries of this type can be made at anytime. It is indispensable for the authorities, to assure that they are not destined for destructive purposes.*'

The publication of techniques allowing amplification of the virulence of infectious agents could benefit terrorist organizations. For this reason, the Bush administration exercised, across the Atlantic, some intense pressure on the scientific community in order that they not disseminate certain results. In January 2002, more than 6500 scientific documents in this manner disappeared from public databases. During the annual conference of the American Association for the Advancement of Sciences in Denver, Colorado in February 2003, the editors of principal scientific journals and medical scholars launched an appeal to not publish certain sensitive studies, susceptible to inspire bioterrorists. This appeal, which advocates self-censorship and recommends to editorial boards to withdraw those elements judged to be dangerous, was published in

Proc Natl Acad Sci USA (Tuesday February, 18, 2003), *Nature* (Thursday February 20, 2003), and *Science* (Friday February 21, 2003):

> 'On certain occasions, a publisher can conclude that the potential danger of a publication exceeds its beneficial potential for society.... There are some data, which, although not yet on a list or with a precise definition, represent a sufficiently significant risk to be utilized by terrorists and which should not be published.'

Donald Kennedy, Editor-in Chief of *Science,* raised the issue in his editorial of February 21, 2003: '*the establishment of bridges between the research and security communities.*' Shortly after the publication of the appeal launched by the journals, the *Public Library of Science* (PLOS) association, an important organization advocating open access to the scientific literature, published this response:

> 'The benefits and the dangers represented by a discovery are rarely immediately evident and research which would be a source of great benefits for society has often some dangerous direct applications. A process in which the publishers are authorized to withdraw a publication on the strength of their appreciation of its dangers and its potential benefits becomes simply arbitrary censorship.'

And Nicolas Cozzarelli, publisher of *Proc Natl Acad Sci USA*, has added:

> 'All work which has value for terrorists has value for the fight against terrorism.'

Echoing the beliefs of Paul Berg, concerning genetic engineering, several scientists have launched a warning on the extraordinary dangers of biotechnologies, even calling for the immediate cessation of certain studies. In a disturbing article published in the journal *Wired* in the month of April 2000, Bill Joy, Scientific Director and founder of *Sun Microsystems* judged it preferable to '*renounce the exploration and development of technologies so dangerous that it would be better if they were never accessible*' [4]. Not hesitating to compare biotechnologies to weapons of mass destruction, Bill Joy affirmed:

> 'The power of destruction of some new technologies will be greater than that of an atomic bomb [...]. My article is not extremist. I believe I have even underestimated the seriousness of the situation. For example, for the biotechnologies. While the danger of the chemical industries and the like is generally recognized, the dangers, much more serious, that I have denounced, are unknown' [15].

References

1. Alibek K. La guerre des germes. Paris, Presses de la Cité, 2000.
2. Binder P, Lepick O. Les armes biologiques. Paris, Presses Universitaires de France, 'Que sais-je?', 2001.
3. Ho MW, Cummings J. Des OGM thérapeutiques aux armes bactériogiques. L'Écologiste (édition française de *The Ecologist*), 2003, 2: 45–47.
4. Joy B. Why the Future doesn't need us. Wired, San-Francisco, avril 2000.

5. Kohler P. L'ennemi invisible. Paris, Éditions Balland, 2002, 250 pages.
6. Leglu D. Bioterrorisme: la Menace à venir. Paris, Éditions Robert Laffont, 2002, 299 pages.
7. Lepick O, Daguzan JF. La terrorisme non conventionnel. Paris, Presses Universitaires de France, 2003.
8. Mamère N, Massey J. Un OGM peut en cacher un autre. Libération, vendredi 11 juillet 2003, p. 8.
9. Massey J. Bioterrorisme, l'état d'alerte. Paris, Éditions de l'Archipel, 2003, 360 pages.
10. Mollaret HH. L'arme biologique. Paris, Éditions Plon 2002, 214 pages.
11. Postel-Vinay O. Le dossier du bioterrorisme. La Recherche, décembre 2003: 70–77.
12. Rifkin J. Bioterrorisme high-tech et révolution génétique. Le Monde, samedi 6 octobre 2001, p. 16.
13. Rifkin J. Le siècle biotech. Paris, Éditions La Découverte & Syros, 1998.
14. Rifkin J. The biotech century: harnessing the gene and remaking the world. New York, Jeremy P. Tarcher/G.P. Putnam's Sons, 1998.
15. Un génie de l'informatique sonne l'arame (interview de Bill Joy par Zac Goldsmith). L'Écologiste (édition française de *The Ecologist*), 2001, 3: 44–46.
16. Watchel C. Armes biologiques: le problème russe. La Recherche, juin 1998: 37–41.

17

Nuclear and radiological weapons

Patrick Barriot

After frantically seeking to obtain nuclear weapons in the 1950s and 1960s, the United States and the USSR engaged in different processes to limit and reduce their nuclear arsenals. In July 1968, they were the promoters of the Nuclear Non-Proliferation Treaty (NPT), which stipulated that only the five countries having experimented with an explosive device before January 1, 1967, were to be considered as being 'equipped with weapons.' In exchange for the renunciation of nuclear weapons, all States who signed the NPT obtained the guarantee that this type of weapon would never be used against them. The contractual renunciation of atomic weapons is also supported by the agreement of the great powers to 'pursue in good faith negotiations for disarmament.' Currently, more than 180 countries have adhered to the NPT, of which the application was extended in 1995, for an indefinite duration. An additional protocol of the NPT, allowing unannounced inspections by the International Atomic Energy Agency (IAEA), was put in place after the discovery of a clandestine program of armament by Iraq in the 1990s. India and Pakistan, having not adhered to the treaty, have not violated any engagement by developing nuclear weapons. In regard to the NPT, they are not 'legally equipped with' such weapons. At this time, eight States have nuclear weapons. The NPT was completed by the Total Prohibition Treaty on Testing of September 24, 1996. Beginning in 1969, negotiations between the United States and the USSR pursued the limitation and then the reduction of strategic weapons. The SALT (Strategic Arms Limitation Talks) agreements anticipated a quantitative but also qualitative limitation on intercontinental nuclear launches. With the START (Strategic Arms Reduction Talks) accords, the United States and Russia to engaged reducing their stores of offensive nuclear weapons by 30 per cent. In 2000, the five States officially possessing atomic bombs were engaged to progressively reduce their arsenals totally. The ABM (Anti-Ballistic Missile) Treaty of 1972, which prohibited developing an anti-missile system, is also a masterpiece in the process of reduction of armaments.

Treating Victims of Mass Destsuction   Edited by Patrick Barriot and Chantal Bismuth
© 2008 John Wiley & Sons, Ltd

First- and second-generation weapons

Scientific progress opened the route, in the 1940s, to high-technology weapons: the war of physicists. First-generation nuclear weapons first saw the light of day shortly after the discovery of the fission of uranium by neutrons, announced in January 1939 by O. Hahn and V. Strassmann in the German journal *Naturwissenschaften*. An element is said to be 'fissile' when its nucleus can, in certain conditions, split and produce energy. During the same year, physicists from the College of France, H.H. von Halban, F. Joliot and L. Kowarski, demonstrated that during this fission the split nuclei themselves emit neurons, causing new fissions and can set in motion a chain reaction that can generate considerable quantities of energy. They also investigated the notion of 'critical mass', below which the nuclear chain reaction cannot develop. At this time, a weapon capable of liberating an enormous quantity of energy could be conceived of by starting a chain reaction in a critical mass of fissile materials. On May 4, 1939, Frederic Joliot, Lew Kowarski and Hans Heinrich von Halban deposed, under the number 445686, a patent having the title 'Improvement of explosive charges.' The fabrication of a bomb producing an explosion equivalent to 1000 tons of dynamite was envisioned. Albert Einstein wrote to President F.D. Roosevelt on August 2, 1939, in these terms: 'Over the last four months, it has become possible – through the work of Joliot in France as well as that of Fermi and Szilárd in America –to start a chain reaction in a large mass of uranium … This new phenomenon could also lead to the construction of bombs and it is conceivable – although much less certain – that extremely powerful bombs of a new type could be constructed' [1]. In his directive of August 30, 1941, to the Committee of the Heads of Major States, Churchill took a position in favor of focusing on a uranium bomb in the name of progress: 'Although I am for my part satisfied with existing explosives, I think that we must not make obstacles to progress.' The Nazi threat of resorting to 'terrifying secret armies' set off a gigantic allied research effort, called the Manhattan Project, with the view of developing a controlled chain reaction. On December 2, 1942, Professor Enrico Fermi and his group succeeded in creating 'the first autonomous chain reaction, initiating in this fashion the controlled liberation of nuclear energy.' A thousand scientists, working within the Los Alamos laboratory under the direction of the physicist Robert Oppenheimer, developed the first bomb, which was tested at the Alamogordo Bombing Range on July 16, 1945. That day, President Truman, who was attending the Potsdam conference with Stalin and Churchill, received a coded message describing the first atomic experiment in these terms: 'The results have surpassed all our hopes.'

First-generation weapons utilize heavy atoms, Uranium 235 or Plutonium 239, which liberate an enormous quantity of energy as well as particles such as neutrons. Natural uranium essentially contains two isotopes: 99.3 per cent of U-238 and 0.7 per cent of U-235. Only U-235 is fissile. The process of enrichment consists of eliminating a part of the U-238 to obtain a mixture richer in U-235. Several procedures can be used to separate U-235 and U-238. The old technique of gaseous diffusion has been replaced by a technique of centrifugation of uranium hexafluoride. The U-238 eliminated during the enrichment phase is called 'depleted uranium'. It is thus a waste product of the nuclear industry. A mixture containing 97 per cent U-238 and 3 per cent U-235 is used as a fuel in nuclear power plants. To fabricate a nuclear weapon, the process of enrichment must be pursued until the proportion is more than 90 per cent U-235. Plutonium is a byproduct of the fission of uranium in nuclear reactors. This fissile element, which does not exist in nature, can serve in the manufacture of a nuclear bomb in the same way as U-235. Special reactors dedicated to the production of plutonium of military quality have been constructed in the eight States with nuclear weapons at their disposal.

The energy liberated by a fission weapon varies by several kilotons. During an explosion at altitude, the effect of the wind from the shock wave corresponds to 50 per cent of the energy dissipated, the thermal effects to 35 per cent, and the nuclear radiation (initial and delayed) to 15 per cent. The first fission bomb was tested by the United States on July 16, 1945, in New Mexico. The bombs dropped on Hiroshima (August 6, 1945) and Nagasaki (August 9, 1945) were both fission bombs, or 'A bombs'. In the first, it was a matter of the fission of U-235, while the second put into play the fission of P-239, *Little Boy* and *Fat Man* had, respectively, a yield of 15 and 22 kilotons of trinitrotoluene (TNT). The yield of a nuclear weapon is measured by comparing it with the energy which would be developed by a quantity of TNT, a conventional explosive taken as a reference. A 1-kiloton weapon produces energy equivalent to that which would be released by the explosion of 1000 tons of TNT. Pure fission weapons have subsequently been conceived to attain yields of several dozen kilotons. The program of development of an operational nuclear bomb includes the production of fissile materials of military quality, the development of the firing mechanism, and of the detonator, as well as the acquisition of vectors. The quantity of fissile materials necessary for the fabrication of a rudimentary weapon is estimated to be 25 kg of highly enriched uranium or 8 Kg of plutonium. It is accepted that a moderately industrialized country without a nuclear infrastructure must dedicate nearly 10 years of effort to develop an explosive device.

Thermonuclear weapons (hydrogen bombs, or H bombs) represent second-generation, or fusion, weapons. They utilize the fusion of two light nuclei: tritium (H3) and deuterium (H2). This fusion necessitates a prior reaction of fission to initiate the thermonuclear reaction. Plutonium, called 'military quality', is generally preferred to U-235. The energy liberated by this type of reaction is immense. While the yield of fission weapons is measured in kilotons, that of fusion devices is measured in megatons. A 1-megaton weapon emits as much energy as the explosion of a million tons of TNT. The first thermonuclear H bomb, with a yield of 15 megatons (1 000 times the yield of *Little Boy*) was tested on Bikini atoll in 1954. The highest-yield nuclear bomb, tested by the USSR at the beginning of the 1960s, had a yield of between 50 and 100 megatons. The effects of thermonuclear bombs are three-fold: the production of heat, blast effects (shock waves), and the release of ionizing radiation. It must be added that the explosion of an H bomb in the stratosphere produces a powerful electromagnetic implosion capable of destroying electronic materials. Constant efforts at miniaturization have been made to render the bomb lighter and transportable by all sorts of delivery mechanisms, in particular by intercontinental missiles [2,3]. The declared nuclear powers have probably reached the limit of possible improvements. Thus, the end of nuclear testing does not penalize them, while it galvanizes other countries to frantically develop their nuclear weapons.

Third-generation weapons

The third-generation groups together weapons derived mostly from the preceding technologies, but in which certain effects are accentuated or reduced according to the tactics adopted for the terrain. The modified bombs therefore constitute a bending of the doctrine of deterrence, because they are conceived to be used on the battlefield. Such weapons required numerous technological developments, and the stopping of nuclear testing hindered their development. In 1999, the American Senate refused to ratify the Treaty for the total prohibition of nuclear testing, expressing the willingness of the United States to resume the tests interrupted in 1992. At the end of December 2001, the Pentagon's Nuclear Posture Review addressed the American Congress and stipulated that the United States could not maintain the position which consisted of 'developing their nuclear arsenal without new testing'.

Neutron bombs

The neutron bomb, or 'weapons of reinforced radiation', is a thermonuclear bomb of low yield which provokes the emission of a flux of very high-energy neutrons. The neutron radiation emitted from the fireball is responsible for the majority of deaths. On the other hand, the blast effect and the thermal effect are reduced, and the radioactive fallout and the residual radioactivity are nearly nonexistent. In amplifying the emission of neuron radiation, it is possible to extend the zone of destruction of living beings beyond the perimeter of the mechanical destruction of materials. For this reason, the neutron bomb is qualified by certain people as a 'weapon of reduced collateral effects'! The neutronic flux is provoked by the fusion of deuterium, or triatoms, of very high temperatures, the initiation of the reaction is obtained by laser beams. A one-kiloton device has a destructive radius of 400 meters, while the zone corresponding to 100 per cent mortality is extended up to 1000 meters from the point of the explosion. The neutron flux still provokes 50 per cent mortality at 1500 meters and is attenuated at about 3000 meters. The neutrons traverse the thickest arm, or plating, and cause the deaths of a tank's crew without causing much damage to the environment or to buildings. Neutrons have a penetrating power much greater than charged particles. Their biological effects, disseminated in the body, are principally due to the ionization provoked by protons when they are placed in motion. Neutrons and gamma radiation also destroy the electronic components of targeting devices. The first studies on neutron bombs were carried out in 1960. President Regan planned to make and stockpile neutron bombs in 1981. Several countries equipped with a nuclear arsenal, France among others, are also in a position to produce them.

Bombs with an increased penetration effect

Numerous munitions (artillery shells, missiles, bombs), designed to 'kill tanks' or to 'break bunkers,' are now equipped with depleted uranium, which is, as we have seen, a waste product of the nuclear industry. In the United States, the factories that manufacture these munitions are called 'dirty plants'. The U-238, or depleted uranium, is an extremely dense and heavy metal, endowed with a strong power of penetration. It has replaced projectiles with tungsten products in recent years. In this manner, the French Leclerc tank is equipped with depleted uranium shells. When the munitions pierce the target, the explosion liberates radioactive particles. Used for the first time during the first Gulf War in 1991 by the United States and the United Kingdom, these munitions were employed by NATO in Yugoslavia in the spring of 1999, and then again against Iraq by the American-led coalition in the spring of 2003. In total, many tens of thousands of these shells were fired and tens of tons of depleted uranium have been abandoned on battlefields.

The United States has also developed a new generation of miniaturized nuclear weapons, such as the BL 61-11 ('Robust Nuclear Earth Penetrator' or 'mini-nuke'), designed to deliver energies of less than one kiloton, in the hectoton range. The BL 61-11 was developed by the Los Alamos Scientific Laboratory in 1989, and its existence was officially recognized in 1997, in defiance of the NPT. This tactical weapon, based on plutonium, which measures 3.5 m long and weighs 315 kg, is designed to explode 30 m underground and to destroy subterranean bunkers. It is, in fact, a classic thermonuclear bomb equipped with a penetrator of depleted uranium. Its ability to penetrate the soil is not truly established, and so it has not been shown that the explosion would be deep enough to avoid radiation being emitted into the atmosphere. The American Senator Steve Buyer declared on October 17, 2001: 'Send a small atomic device into the caves of the al-Qaida terrorists and you will destroy them for a thousand years.' Moreover, the conceivers of this nuclear mini-bomb first made a lighter version (equivalent to 0.3 kilotons TNT) but remain silent about the most powerful version (equivalent to 20 times the Hiroshima bomb, 340 kilotons). In this way, it is possible to pass imperceptibly from a sub-kiloton (or hectoton) weapon to a kiloton weapon and then to a megaton weapon. What constitutes the critical legal proscription beyond which a tactical weapon becomes a pre-strategic weapon and then a strategic weapon? This bomb is presented by the Pentagon as inoffensive as defoliants containing dioxins, munitions with depleted uranium, or high-strength microwave weapons.

Radiological, or dirty, bombs

These are devices that are made up of a conventional explosive around which are placed some radioactive products. Victims of radioactive contamination are therefore added to those of the explosion. This type of weapon, based on 'radioactive poisons,' had been envisioned by American researchers during the Second World War. In 1987, Iraq experimented with a radioactive weapon containing some radioactive material from Al-Tuwaitha nuclear center, essentially Zirconium-95. The studies had been interrupted in view of the disappointing results of the experiments. A rudimentary weapon of this type could, however, be used by terrorist groups because it is very much easier to procure some radioactive elements than fissile materials of military quality. During the second quarter of 2003, looters stole some radioactive elements, which could serve for the fabrication of 'dirty bombs,' from the Al-Tuwaitha atomic complex.

Electromagnetic bomb (e bomb)

We have seen that the explosion of an H bomb in the stratosphere produces an electromagnetic pulse (EMP) capable of destroying electronic materials. An electromagnetic energy source, of at least a terawatt, can be produced by a non-nuclear generator, or 'flux compressor,' that is capable of producing an EMP and of directing it onto a target by means of an antenna. The initial studies on the electromagnetic bomb were undertaken by the USSR and the United States during the 1960s. The principle consisted of creating an EMP of tens of millions of watts from a 'flash,' without producing a shock wave, a thermal effect, or ionizing radiation. This electromagnetic 'flash,' which propagates at the speed of light, is devastating for all materials containing electronic equipment. It renders useless all systems that are 'non-hardened' (not integrated into a Faraday cage) against this effect. Hence, it acts on telecommunications control centers, radar detection centers, and guidance control and autopilot systems. It could, among other things, be used from the ground to disorient pilots. The E bomb, conceived to selectively destroy electronic and computer equipment, is thus the opposite of the neutron bomb, which was developed to kill living beings while leaving equipment intact. It is presented as a 'clean weapon which does not kill,' but which returns the enemy to the Stone Age by destroying all his technological equipment. This bomb can be transported by a cruise missile of the Tomahawk or Storm Shadow types, by an attack drone, and it can also be deployed from light ground vehicles. In the opening days of operation Desert Storm in 1991, the American Navy launched against the Iraqi forces some Tomahawks charged with flux compressors producing an EMP of 3 000 megawatts. These weapons were also used in Kosovo in 1999 and again in Iraq in 2003.

The E bomb is an umbrella term for a vast range of weapons using a source of electromagnetic energy that can be created, pulsed, and directed by means of an antenna. They are generally classified as a function of the wavelength of the beams that they emit or according to the type of modulation of the beams. Numerous systems that can generate powerful EMPs with a very large spectrum of frequencies (from several kHz to many hundreds of mHz) have been developed. The 'radar killers' use radio frequencies and hyper frequencies, or microwaves. Their strength of emission can reach many thousands of millions of watts. The usage is present exclusively against equipment. Researchers from British Systems have developed a weapon that emits on a very large wavelength band several impulses of incredible strength obtained by a generator called Vircator (virtual cathode oscillator).

The weapons and their delivery systems

Nuclear weapons exist in the form of artillery shells, bombs, and missiles. The range of the missiles range from medium range, to intermediate range, and intercontinental ballistic missiles with the power to cover more than 10 000 km. The installation of nuclear bombs onto missiles, from the 1950s, considerably extended the range of the threat. Cruise missiles of the Tomahawk and Storm Shadow types are equipped with electronic guidance systems and are capable of flying at low altitudes for nearly 2000 km. They can transport a conventional weapon as well as a nuclear mini-bomb, a neutron bomb, or an electromagnetic bomb. A nuclear weapon is called 'strategic' or 'anti-city' when it is capable of devastating a country and abruptly killing hundreds of thousands of civilians. It is called 'tactical' or 'anti-forces' when it is aimed at enemy troops on a battlefield.

Strategic missiles can be launched from underground silos or from ground vehicles. They can also be launched from nuclear missile launch submarines (HML 5) or from bombers. The United States and Russia have numerous intercontinental missiles with multiple nuclear warheads with the strength of many megatons and a range of 12 000 km at their disposal. During the Cold War, American missiles were destined to hit Soviet territory, and vice versa. The type of weapons carried as well as the number of missiles and their technological performances determined their capacity for destruction. Missiles with multiple warheads MIRV (multiple independently targeted reentry vehicle) were developed by both parties. The Soviet SS20 missiles, deployed in the territory of certain State members of the Warsaw Pact, were opposed to American Pershing II rockets installed in West Germany. Intercontinental ballistic missiles were essential instruments of the politics of detente. For this reason, the ABM Treaty of 1972 prohibited the development of antimissile systems. The French strategic nuclear forces combined a ground component represented by ground-to-ground ballistic missiles such as the S-3 capable of carrying a megaton charge for 3,500 km, a naval component represented by the new generation SNLE equipped with multiple warhead M-45 and an aerial component represented by IV-P Mirages armed with ASMP nuclear missiles (medium range air-to-ground) with a yield of 500 KT.

Tactical weapons are weapons designed for use on the battlefield. Their strength is on the order of one kiloton and their range is some hundreds of kilometers. The French tactical nuclear forces (or pre-strategic) combined mainly an aerial component represented by the Mirage 2000 N armed with AGMR and a naval air component represented by the Rafale, which was also equipped with AGMR. The ground component was equipped with Pluton type nuclear weapons, which were subsequently replaced with Hades type weapons, with a range of 500 km that could be equipped with neutron bombs. This ground component has in part been dismantled for budgetary reasons.

Several countries have looked to equip themselves with intercontinental missiles; in the first rank are North Korea, Iran, and Pakistan. In countries that proliferate, the majority of the missiles are derived from the Soviet Scud. Iraq possessed Al-Hussein missiles, with a range of 850 km, and Al-Samoud ground-to-ground missiles, with a range of 150 km. North Korea developed Nodong ground-to-ground missiles (range 1500 km) and Taepodong 1 and 2 missiles (range between 2000 and 2500 km). The Taepodong 3 missile could reach 6000 km. The United States, which wished to preserve its strategic supremacy by making a 'sanctuary' of its territory, announced the deployment of an 'antimissile shield' responsible for protecting American territory against an eventual salvo of missiles launched by a 'Rogue State'. SM-3 missile interceptors could be fired from ground launchers positioned in California and Alaska or from missile-launch cruisers equipped with the Aegis system. Detection and alert radars were placed, amongst other sites, in Greenland. This shield would be capable of destroying enemy missiles in all flight configurations (in the initial propulsion phase, in midcourse of the trajectories, and on final approach to their objectives) according to the concept called 'multilayered.' It constituted a violation of the ABM Treaty of May 26, 1972, created to manage the process of armament reduction.

Nuclear arsenals in the world

The arsenals of nuclear powers comprise tactical and strategic weapons of the first, second and third generations. Thirty thousand nuclear warheads are currently distributed amongst the five major nuclear powers (China, the United States, France, the United Kingdom, and Russia). In 1990, the United States and Russia each possessed nearly 12 000 nuclear warheads. This number was reduced by half the first time, and by 2010 the United States should have 2500 warheads and Russia 1800 warheads. During the breakup of the USSR in 1991, the new countries which proclaimed their independence retained in their territories some tactical nuclear weapons. Of them, four (Belarus, Kazakhstan, Ukraine, and Russia) also possess strategic weapons, equipped with intercontinental ballistic missiles or bombers. An agreement signed in Minsk on December 30, 1991, concluded that only Russia was authorized to retain nuclear weapons. The transfer to Russia of all tactical and strategic nuclear weapons was to be effective at the end of 1994. The exact number of nuclear warheads in the Russian arsenal at the end of the Cold War cannot be precisely known, nor can the number of warheads dismantled in accordance with the START agreements.

Three countries which currently have nuclear weapons have refused to sign the NPT: India, Pakistan, and Israel. In 1995, Canada furnished India with a natural uranium and 'heavy water' reactor, which could serve for the production of plutonium for military purposes. After the Indian explosion in 1974, the Pakistani government intensified its own offensive nuclear program. The construction of a facility for uranium enrichment in Pakistan began at the end of the 1970s after that country had obtained certain Dutch technology. The United States closed its eyes to this program for the acquisition of nuclear weapons because it needed the alliance with Pakistan in order to oppose the Afghan mujahideen who fought against the Soviets. The Hebrew State possessed between 100 and 172 nuclear warheads, without official recognition. In 1956, France aided Israel to acquire nuclear weapons. They constructed the Dimonu reactor, which served to produce military plutonium as well as a facility where plutonium could be extracted from combustion products. According to Joseph Cirincione, from the

Carnegie Endowment for International Peace: 'It is not currently in the interest of Israel to possess nuclear weapons, and … chemical and biological weapons, because of its pre-eminence in the region in matters of conventional weapons, and let the matter rest. And it is the retention by Israel of weapons of mass destruction which incites the other countries of the region to equip themselves also.'

Three other countries, in recent years, have developed nuclear energy which could be developed into weapon systems. Regarding Iran, France built, at the end of the 1970s, the research reactor of Osiraq (or Tammuz). This latter was destroyed on June 7, 1981, by Israeli aircraft, although it could not produce fissile material for military use. In the 1980s, a German engineer helped Iraq to develop a clandestine program for uranium enrichment by centrifugation. This program was suddenly stopped in 1991. Under pressure from the United States and the United Kingdom, who accused Iraq of having reactivated its program for the acquisition of nuclear weapons in the 1990s, the UN Security Council adopted Resolution 1441 on November 5, 2002, demanding the return of International Atomic Energy Agency (IAEA) inspectors to Iraq to search for nuclear weapons. The American–British accusation was founded on contracts for the acquisition of uranium between Iraq and Niger from 1999 to 2001. The President of the United States, George Bush, evoked this order in a speech in 2002. However, the Director of the IAEA, Mohammed El Baradei, demonstrated that the documents furnished by the British Secret Service in September 2002 detailing the purchase of uranium by Iraq were 'not authenticated' [4]. In other words, they were falsified documents. The inspectors on the ground did not discover any proof of a nuclear program. On the other hand, Iran and North Korea seem to have developed military nuclear programs. In 1993, North Korea launched an initial crisis by announcing its withdrawal from the NPT, although it had been a member since 1985, and in building an enrichment facility close to the Yongbyon reactor. At the end of 2002, it gave notice of its intention to activate its Yongbyon facilities, in violation of the 1994 agreement concluded with the United States, and expelled the IAEA inspectors. North Korea seems to have received significant technical aid from Pakistan to launch its enrichment program. North Korea, which also has a ballistic missile program, publicly gave notice of its intention to equip itself with nuclear weapons on Monday June 9, 2003: 'We have no other option other than nuclear dissuasion because the United States pursues its hostile politics and continues to exert a nuclear threat to the Democratic People's Republic of Korea. Our desire to possess nuclear dissuasion should not been seen as blackmail, but to reduce our conventional arsenal and to place our human resources and our funds in the service of constructive economic activities and for the lives of the people.' The same day, the White House declared that: 'North Korea must completely and immediately dismantle its nuclear weapons program.' The United States claimed that Iran also developed a nuclear weapons program camouflaged as a civilian program, with Chinese and Russian technology. In 1991, Iran imported 1.8 tons of natural uranium of Chinese origin, without a special hearing of the IAEA. A facility for uranium enrichment with 200 centrifuges was built in Natanz. A unit for the production of heavy water in Arak was built in anticipation of the acquisition of Canadian reactors, which would be capable in the future of producing plutonium. A program of development of laser techniques was also begun. Since 1995, Iran constructed, with Russian aid, the nuclear center at Bouchehr, with a power of 1000 megawatts. Moscow may have furnished Tehran with the nuclear fuel, then reprocessed in Russia the used nuclear fuels. Iran, which has been a signatory to the NPT since 1974, refused to sign the additional protocol allowing unannounced inspections by the IAEA. The Russian Minister of Foreign Affairs, Igor Iranov, stated on May 28, 2003, that Russia would not accept pressure from the United States to put a stop to its nuclear cooperation with Iraq. The Pentagon thought there might be a possibility of a 'surgical' aerial assault of the Bouchehr Center, similar to that which had allowed Israel to destroy the Iraqi nuclear reactor in 1981 before it could be activated.

Terrorist projects

The terrorist threat can be defined in four different forms: hijacking a commercial airplane which could be crashed into a nuclear installation (a reactor for the production of electricity or a facility for the reprocessing of spent radioactive fuels), the explosion of a nuclear device, the explosion of a radiological bomb, and the dissemination of radioactive products [5,6].

An airplane crash could damage the concrete confinement shield or the cooling system of a nuclear reactor. A reactor is enclosed in a concrete shield that is supposed to resist crashes by airplanes of middle category (not exceeding six tons of weight and 12 m^2 of impact surface) but not the crash of a commercial Boeing 747. If the cooling system came to be damaged, the elevation of temperature of the fuels would set off a melt-down within the reactor core and a dispersion of radioactive products in the environment. A very large commercial airplane has fuel tanks containing 100 tons of kerosene and would set off a violent fire, which would be particularly difficult to manage. Facilities for fuel reprocessing could also be targeted. These installations, as we have seen, are designed for the extraction of nuclear fuels from residual enriched uranium, plutonium, and radioactive wastes. The most vulnerable part of the facility is represented by the fuel storage ponds. In Europe, two installations are currently in service, one at La Hague (France) and the other at Sellafield (Great Britain). In France, a pilot may not penetrate within a radius of 5 km around a nuclear center and he is prohibited from flying at less than 36000 feet. The French Minister of Defense has placed a radar station and a battery of ground-to-air missiles near the La Hague site. The Air Force has taken steps to be able to launch combat aircraft within a few minutes to protect this installation as well as the nuclear reactors of the French electric board (EDF). A fighter plane can receive the order to shoot down a hijacked commercial aircraft whose hijackers intend to strike a nuclear installation. Nevertheless, despite the Vigipirate plan, two unidentified aircraft (a single-engine airplane and a helicopter) flew over the Civaux (Vienne) nuclear center at low altitudes in June 2003. The organization 'Out with Nuclear' immediately declared in a communiqué: 'The protection of French nuclear installations is not only faulty, but it is sometimes completely nonexistent. We thought that these flights would allow for a demonstration, before a true attack, of the security plans. It must be plainly seen that they are nonexistent.' On this occasion, the Out with Nuclear network emphasized the dangers of transporting nuclear waste by railway, as was the case in Bordeaux on May 19, 2003: 'A commando had only to use plastic explosive on the nuclear railcar.'

Three serious events of accidental origin have occurred at nuclear installations in recent years. The fire in the reprocessing facility of Windscale (United Kingdom) in 1954 and the destruction of the Three Mile Island reactor (United States) in 1979 did not have any health repercussions because the radioactivity remained confined in the interior of these installations. The dramatic accident of Chernobyl in 1986 followed the explosion of a mixed civilian and military reactor, which breached the interior confinement. The fusion of the reactor core caused the dispersal into the atmosphere of a large quantity of radioactive elements (300 million curies). The health and environmental consequences were thus very heavy. As always when it comes to accidents, the resistance to earthquakes of the EDF centers has been the object of lively debate, and there also seems to exist a difference of opinion concerning the risk between the authorities of Nuclear Safety and the EDF.

The manufacture of an explosive nuclear device by a terrorist group is considered improbable because of the classified nature of the technologies involved and the system of international surveillance. Besides the technical and scientific knowledge, numerous other major obstacles would have to be overcome. It would be necessary, in the first place, to obtain fissile materials of 'military quality': Uranium 235 enriched to 93% or plutonium-239 containing less than 7 per cent plutonium-240. The quantity of fissile materials necessary for the construction of a rudimentary weapon is estimated at 25 kg of highly enriched uranium or 8 kg of plutonium. If natural uranium were purchased in an African country, it would be necessary to conduct an enrichment program by centrifugation or by the other procedures (gaseous diffusion, chemical process, or electromagnetic process) available. For plutonium, it could only be produced in a reactor designed for military purposes or in a reprocessing facility allowing from extraction nuclear fuels. It is nevertheless possible to overcome these obstacles by stealing fissile materials stored in those countries equipped with a nuclear arsenal. Russia is frequently cited, owing to its defective security mechanisms. Warheads dismantled by the START agreements represent nearly 1000 tons of plutonium. Russia, however, is not the only place where the theft of fissile materials could occur. Some serious failures in the security of American installations, such as Rocky Flats and Los Alamos, have also been cited. Once fissile materials have been obtained in an adequate quantity, the nuclear weapon is still not built. The system of firing and detonation, by means of electrical devices and conventional explosives compressing the uranium or plutonium for a sufficient time to set off the chain reaction, requires high-level specialists in detonation. For all these reasons, it is improbable that an isolated terrorists group could manage to develop a nuclear device. The Japanese sect Aum Shinrikyo had attempted to acquire fissile materials for this purpose, but failed. The situation would be different if such a group received help from a country possessing a nuclear arsenal. It has been shown, for example, that Bin Laden had discussions with a Pakistani scientist who had occupied high positions in the nuclear program of that country.

The diversion or theft of low-yield nuclear weapons, such as a suitcase bomb, represents a real threat, which, however, is difficult to evaluate. In 1946, Robert J. Oppenheimer declared that two or three persons carrying a bomb in a suitcase could destroy the city of New York. A confidential report on this subject (the Screwdriver Report) was produced by the Atomic Energy Commission. In October 1997, General Lebed confirmed that certain low-yield weapons, which could be transported by a single person, had been constructed for the Russian Secret services and, from this fact, did not appear in the official inventory of the Russian Ministry of Defense. These weapons were destined to equip commandos involved in sabotage operations. Bin Laden had successfully acquired a "portable" nuclear bomb of this type (a so-called 'suitcase bomb'). The American authorities, amongst others, fear that terrorists could transport a nuclear weapon of this type into a United States port via a maritime route.

The construction of a bomb for the dispersion of radioactive materials, called a 'radiological bomb' or 'dirty bomb', is a more concrete threat. It is a matter of a device with a conventional explosive charge around which is placed radioactive waste meant to contaminate an urban site. The radioactive waste cannot in any case set off a chain reaction and is incapable of causing a nuclear explosion. It is much easier for a criminal organization to procure radioactive elements than military-quality fissile materials. In this case, the objective is not to kill a large number of persons but rather to create panic. Amongst the reprocessing wastes, radioactive plutonium would be the most dangerous product, but it is much more difficult to obtain than some radio elements used for medical or industrial applications (isotopes of cobalt, iridium, strontium, cesium, or iodine).

The intentional diffusion or dispersion of radioactive products, in liquid, solid, or gaseous form, should also be considered. Jean-François Lacronique, President of the Administrative Council of the Institute for Radioprotection and Nuclear Safety, recently emphasized: "It is also necessary to take into account as possible some forms of attacks with slow or insidious onset, and not limited to the anticipation of attacks with an explosive manifestation: the contamination of water supply reservoirs, the dispersion of radioactive elements into the environment or into collective living centers would also be acts of which the clinical expression would differ and could affect numerous persons before even being identified.' Such a situation occurred in an accidental fashion in Goiäna, Brazil. During the demolition of a clinic, a cesium-137 source used for medical purposes was abandoned in a dump; more than 1000 persons were contaminated of whom four died. The decontamination of certain neighborhoods required considerable resources. In 1995, a Chechnian group threatened the Russian government with a 'radioactive' weapon by placing some cesium-137 elements in the Izmailovsky Park in Moscow. According to Ken Alibek, the Russian mafia assassinated the chief of the enterprise, Ivan Kivelidi, and his secretary by placing radioactive cadmium in their telephone. The prevention of such acts rests in large part on the control of facilities using radiological elements for medical or industrial purposes, and on the surveillance of those agencies managing reprocessed wastes, even when they have been vitrified. Unfortunately, it must be recognized that numerous radioactive sources, lost or not registered in the countries of the former USSR, could fall into the hands of terrorists.

As an example, some hundreds of radiothermal generators, designed to power naviga-tion beacons, have disappeared. They exist in the form of metal cylinders filled with cesium or strontium. In February 2002, three Georgian forestry workers were seriously contaminated after having discovered a beacon of this type in a forest.

From non-proliferation to counter-proliferation

Numerous treaties and international accords govern the processes for the limitation and reduction of nuclear arsenals: the NPT, the Treaty for Total Prohibition of Nuclear Testing, the SALT and START agreements (treaty between the United States and the USSR on the reduction and limitation of strategic offensive arms) and the ABM Treaty. In 1990, the United States and Russia each possessed about 12 000 nuclear warheads. This number has been reduced to 6000 and should be reduced by a further two-thirds by 2012. The end of the Cold War has opened the way for nuclear disarmament; the Americans and Russians are committed to progressively reducing their arsenals to fewer than 2000 warheads each. In addition, various facilities with the IAEA in the first rank, exercise close international surveillance in the area of non-proliferation. The movement of fissile materials and sensitive materials is rigorously controlled, as are centrifuges for uranium enrichment and systems for missile guidance. Unfortunately, in reality, one cannot look at the situation with any real optimism. It must be recog-nized that the reduction of nuclear weapons is of a purely quantitative nature and that the course to weapons is pursued on the technological level. The reductions effected in the arsenals concern obsolete or unsuitable weapons, while third-generation weapons are developed in utmost secrecy. The dismantling of warheads in Russia also exposes the risk of diversion of stored fissile materials in conditions of doubtful security. We have seen that the warheads retired from missiles concerned in the START agreements represent nearly 1000 tons of highly enriched uranium and 200 tons of plutonium.

The United States has gone through a dangerous step in planning preventive attacks against countries that are at the point of acquiring prohibited weapons or of procuring intercontinental missiles. The Israeli Army has set a precedent by bombing the Iraqi reactor at Osiraq in 1981. The Administration of Bill Clinton had envisioned bombing the North Korean reactor at Yongbyon in the 1990s. In March 2003, an American-led coalition launched a preventive attack against Iraq, wrongly accused of retaining weapons of mass destruction. The *Washington Post*, in its edition of July 30, 2002, raised the possibility of attacking the Iranian nuclear center at Bouchehr before nuclear fuel could be loaded, which Moscow stubbornly persisted in delivering to the Tehran government. The official report *Nuclear Posture Review* indicated that Washington had developed miniature nuclear weapons in order to destroy subterranean installa-tions used to shelter prohibited weapons. The Pentagon estimated that there exist some 10 000 subterranean sites on the planet where weapons of mass destruction are stored. The tactical nuclear weapons developed by the United States for counter-proliferation are essentially targeted against seven countries: Russia, China, Iraq, Iran, North Korea, Libya, and Syria.

The United States put in place the principle of not attacking or threatening signatory countries of the NPT (called 'first strike'). A signatory country to the NPT, which doesn't possess any nuclear weapons, is in future vulnerable to a preventive attack by means of a 'nuclear mini-bomb.' This reduces to nothing the principle of dissuasion, and certain countries are tempted to develop their own weapons of mass destruction in order to retaliate. In developing a range of miniaturized nuclear weapons and launching the recent antiballistic missile defense program, the United States bypassed the Nuclear NPT as well as the ABM Treaty of 1972. The possibility of using a nuclear weapon in a 'first strike', be it sub-kilotonic, removes the border between conventional weapons and weapons of mass destruction. Nuclear weapons are, in reality, integrated into the conventional arsenal in this way. We assist a dangerous slide from a defensive and diplomatic concept, non-proliferation, to an offensive and military concept, counter-proliferation. This risky strategy, without doubt, could restart the course to weapons and nuclear proliferation.

A new American doctrine, which developed the concepts of preventive strikes, counter-proliferation, miniaturized nuclear weapons, and anti-missile shields, is in the process of undermining the foundations of dissuasion. The risk of a nuclear confrontation between the United States and Russia having disappeared, the Americans think that the NPT has lost its *raison d'être* following the end of the Cold War and only preventive strikes can be effective against rogue states capable of suicidal behavior and inaccessible to the logic of dissuasion. We threefore assist, fundamentally, calling into question all the principles which govern, up to today, nuclear disarmament.

References

1. Feld T, Weiss Szilard G (eds). *The Collected Works of Léo Szilard*. Cambridge, MA: The MIT Press, 1972.
2. Gallois PM. *Naissance et Décline de l'Arme Nucléaire*. Lausanne: Éditions L'Âge d'Homme, 2002.
3. Le Guelte G. *Histoire de la Menace Nucléaire*. Paris: Hachette, 1997.
4. Leser E. Les faux sur l'achat d'uranium au Niger provoquent une polémique à Washington. *Le Monde*, 18 juin, 2003: 3.
5. Le Guelte G. *Terrorisme Nucléaire: Risque Majeur, Fantasme ou Épouvantail, Institut de Relations Internationales et Stratégiques*. Paris: Presses Universitaires de France, 2003.
6. Lepick O, Daguzan JF. *Le Terrorisme Non Coventionnel*. Paris: Presses Universaires de France, 2003.

18

The effects of nuclear and radiological weapons on humans

Patrick Barriot

On August 6, 1945, the B-29 Bomber Enola Gay dropped a 15-kiloton A bomb which exploded 600 meters above the center of the city of Hiroshima. According to official estimates, 350 000 people were present in the city that day. About 78 000 people died on the morning of August 6. In December, 1945, the toll had increased to 140 000 deaths. Medical care was overwhelmed because the majority of the nurses and doctors in the city were dead or injured. These numbers are approximations and the total number of victims remains unknown. Three days later, on August 9, 1945, a bomber carrying a larger 22-kiloton plutonium bomb made Nagasaki its objective. At the site of the explosion in the center of the city, *Fat Man* exploded over a city district, causing the deaths of 38 000 persons according to certain sources, or 70 000 according to certain other estimations.

The announcement of the nuclear bombardment of Hiroshima was received with enthusiasm by the Allied countries, and the press reported the good news. In its edition of Wednesday August 8, 1945, the daily newspaper *Le Monde* announced the nuclear bombardment under the title 'A scientific revolution.' Albert Camus was one of the rare people to not share this passion in his editorial dated August 8 in the journal *Combat*: The world is what it is; that is to say it's nothing. Everyone has known this since yesterday, thanks to the massive chorus that radio, the press and information agencies have just sparked off on the subject of the atomic bomb. We learn, in effect, amidst a mass of enthusiastic commentaries that a town of average importance can be totally razed to the ground by a bomb the size of a soccer ball. American, English and French newspapers promulgate elegant essays about the future, the past, the inventors, the cost, the peaceful intention and the military repercussions, the political consequences and even the independent character of the atom bomb ... Meanwhile, it might be thought that there is something obscene in celebrating in this manner an invention whose primary aim is to unleash the most tremendous destructive force that man has demonstrated for centuries.

Treating Victims of Mass Destsuction   Edited by Patrick Barriot and Chantal Bismuth
© 2008 John Wiley & Sons, Ltd

The effects of first- and second-generation weapons

The A bomb sets off three types of devastating effects: the thermal flux, which represents 35 per cent of the energy liberated by nuclear fission, the shock wave, which represents 50 per cent of the energy liberated, and nuclear radiation, which represents 15 per cent of the energy liberated. During the explosion of a bomb of this type, the majority of deaths are due to the thermal effects and the shock wave.

Thermal radiation and shock wave

The explosion of *Little Boy* formed a fireball, more brilliant than the sun, of many millions of degrees in the atmosphere which hung for several seconds over the center of the city of Hiroshima. On the ground, the temperature reached several thousand degrees under the detonation point. Within a 1-km radius, the thermal flux reduced everything to cinders. Up to 4 km from the epicenter, human bodies and buildings spontaneously burst into flames and persons located in an 8 km radius had third-degree burns. The flash of dazzling white light caused definitive blindness by burning retinas up to several kilometers away.

The brutal expansion of hot gasses created an overpressure shock wave; true ramming gasses launched at a speed close to 1000 km/hr and reduced everything to dust within a radius of 2 km. Two-thirds of the buildings in the city were entirely destroyed. The shock wave, constituting a extreme overpressure front was followed by a depression, accompanied with extremely violent winds of which the direction was opposite to the depression phase. The winds swept up everything in their path and transformed them into lethal projectiles. Casualties suffered from a variety of injuries, from severe burns to blast-injury lesions – in particular, pulmonary, multiple-trauma and multiple-penetrating injuries, and crush syndrome.

Irradiation

During the first minute following detonation, the initial nuclear radiation is made up of electromagnetic radiation (X-ray and gamma) and neutrons which can travel several kilometers. Although the energy of this radiation only represents 3 per cent of the fatal energy of the explosion, it causes 'radiation sickness' in numerous victims. The biological risk of X-ray and gamma radiation is due to the power of ionization, that is to say that these types of radiation are capable of displacing an electron from an atom and furnishing an energy at least equal to the electron's bond energy. These radiations which have wavelengths less than 1 nm, have long trajectories and their penetration into the tissues is so much greater because their energy is greater. One might also view them as beams of photons. The photon travels at the speed of light and carries an energy which depends on the frequency of the beam. The neutron is an elementary particle, one of the two constituents of the nucleus, with a mass very close to the proton but without an electrical charge. Neutrons have a significant penetrating power and their biological effects, scattered throughout the body, are mainly due to the ionization caused by protons which they set in motion.

External irradiation results from exposure to ionizing radiation [1]. The absorbed dose is the physical parameter which characterizes an irradiation and measures its significance. Its unit is the gray (Gy). The dose equivalent, proportional to the absorbed dose, takes into account the nature of the radiation involved and its potential level of harm for human tissues. Its unit is the sievert (Sv). Radiation, in passing through living material, effects energy transfers which cause physical-chemical phenomena cause physical and chemical damage at the sites of cellular lesions. The ionization of an atom in the interior of a molecule sets in motion the breakdown of that molecule. The breakdown of a water molecule results in the formation of free radicals cells responsible for molecular lesions. The physical-chemical damage caused by the passage of ionizing radiation into living material damages all biological molecules, in particular DNA molecules, whose role is essential. The majority of the DNA lesions are repaired by enzymatic repair systems. When the DNA is not suitably repaired, the cells autodestruct by apoptosis. The absence of repair has serious genetic consequences. Certain lesions, compatible with cellular reproduction, can cause cancer, if they affect somatic cells, or genetic abnormalities, if they affect germinal cells. The cellular injury is proportional to the mitotic activity. The cell lines with a very active genetic turn-over replacement (gastrointestinal epithelium, hematopoietic cells, male sperm cells) are very sensitive to ionizing radiation.

With irradiation doses less than or equal to 2 Gy, the prognosis is good even without treatment, and hospitalization is not necessary. With doses greater than 2 or 3 Gy, the existence of nausea and vomiting denote serious irradiation. The LD_{50} (lethal dose in 50 per cent of cases) in humans is situated at about 3.5 Gy. The illness has, generally, four phases:

- An initial phase of two or three days of nausea, vomiting, fever, and a rapid decrease in the number of lymphocytes; the clinical examination at this stage is most often normal.

- A latent phase, which is shorter when the dose is higher; it lasts for about two weeks with doses between 3.5 and 4.5 Gy, and eight to 10 days with doses greater than 8 Gy.

- A critical phase, which is manifested by intense asthenia, an elevated fever, chills, buccal ulcerations, leucopenia and thrombocytopenia signaling bone marrow aplasia. The patient is at risk for infectious and hemorrhagic complications. With doses greater than 8 Gy, one can observe gastrointestinal manifestations of the type of bloody diarrhea and a painful erythema, which extends all over the body. The prognosis is extremely poor without bone marrow grafting. Above 15 Gy, there are neurological manifestations such as disorientation, obtundation, and seizures, and death is inevitable whatever treatment is undertaken.

– When the evolution is favorable, a phase of remission and recuperation begins after eight to 10 days of bone marrow aplasia. Its duration is usually short because cellular regeneration is rapid.

The delayed effects of irradiation are represented by teratogenicity (irradiation of an embryo or fetus during pregnancy), carcinogenicity (in particular leukemias and solid tumors), and genetic effects. 'Genetic effects' refer to those lesions caused in viable germ cells (spermatozoids and ova), that may result in biological abnormalities in the children of exposed subjects. The genetic risk seems to be three times less than the risk of cancer. The survivors of Hiroshima and Nagasaki have been monitored for 50 years by a research organization, the RERF (Radiation Effects Research Foundation) in order to evaluate the carcinogenic effects of photons and neutrons. An excess of cancers, in particular leukemia, has been found in this population.

Contamination

Residual radioactivity is made up of the debris from a detonated device and by the reaction of the released neutrons on different elements in the atmosphere. The effects of the radioactive fallout from a nuclear weapon can be felt over a much wider area than any of the other effects of its detonation, and some of these effects will not manifest themselves for months or even years. The fallout contains charged particles (alpha and beta) whose trajectories are relatively short and not very penetrating. The alpha particle is a nucleus of helium composed of two protons and two neutrons whose travel distance in water is measured in microns. Beta radiation is composed of electrons whose travel distance in water or in human tissue is some millimeters.

External contamination is caused by radioactive material coming into contact with the skin. A particle counter detects the presence of these radioactive elements, identifies their location and estimates their significance. The depositing of beta emitters on the skin can cause severe burns and, in this case, external decontamination is a priority. Different levels of severity can be observed: erythema with temporary epilation, dry dermatitis with permanent epilation, exudative dermatitis with excoriations, cutaneous radiation necrosis. The treatment of radiation dermatitis is best carried out in a major burn center because these cutaneous lesions are not dissimilar to thermal burns.

Internal contamination is due to the presence of radioactive particles in the interior of the body [1]. Their absorption can be by the respiratory route (inhalation of particles in the ambient air), the gastrointestinal route (ingestion of radioactive substances contained in food or beverages or present on an object where the hands carry the contaminant(s) to the mouth), or the transcutaneous route (wounds or dermatological illnesses contaminated with radioactive dust). The total amount of gamma ray emitters present in the body can be measured by whole-body gamma scanning. Measuring the concentration of isotopes in excreta (urine and feces) and exhaled air facilitates the detection of alpha or beta radiation emitters, which cannot be detected by external counting.

Very little information is available on the victims of the Hiroshima bombardment, and it is difficult to distinguish, among the causes of early deaths, which were due to traumatic causes and which to the effects of radiation. The chronic effects, such as radiation-induced cancers, can manifest themselves many years after initial exposure to the radiation, and the studies sometimes contradict each other. In the end, the Hiroshima bomb was a low-yield fission bomb (15 kilotons), as compared to modern fusion bombs developing yields of many dozens of megatons. It is difficult to imagine the ravages of an H bomb on a large metropolitan area.

The effects of third-generation weapons

We have already discussed the effects of the neutron bomb on the human body; it has the stated objective of eliminating living beings. The contaminant effects of depleted uranium munitions on exposed populations, who might inhale or ingest radioactive particles, are the subject of lively debate. They are flatly denied by the authorities, who point out that Uranium-238 is effectively radioactive but that its radioactive period is between 4 and 5 million years [2,3]. The amount of radiation emitted is proportionate to the amount of time that has passed since the initial explosion and is thus very small; it would require very long periods of exposure and large quantities of particles before any deleterious effects are seen . This raises several questions. The first concerns the effective exposure of certain populations to large amounts of U-238. Some tens of thousands of depleted uranium shells were fired during recent conflicts and some tens of tons of depleted uranium were abandoned on certain battlefields, in particular in the Iraqi desert. The second concerns the non-radiological, but rather chemical, toxicology of heavy metals such as plutonium or uranium. The renal toxicity of uranium, for example, is well established. A third question concerns the eventual association of depleted uranium with another radioactive product coming from enrichment operations. In the absence of international clinical, toxicological, and epidemiological studies of the Iraqi and Yugoslavian, civilian populations, no satisfactory answer can be reached.

Microwave weapons produce a large quantity of electrical energy transformed into microwaves that are released in the form of tightly focused wave beams, or pulses, of variable duration. The wave beams can be directed onto the target by means of an antenna. The HPM (High Power Microwaves) generators, produced by the Soviets from 1983, produce formidable hyperfrequencies, directed against electronic systems but also against human beings. It can be a matter of a non-lethal weapon emitting microwaves designed to produce a burning sensation in the skin. During civil disturbances, such a weapon could disperse crowds within at least a 500-metre radius [4]. If the strength of the microwave beam is significantly increased, exposed living organisms can literally be cooked by the elevation of bodily temperature caused by the agitation of water molecules in the interior of the body. The thermal effects of microwaves on human beings are thus equivalent to those of a microwave oven.

Raytheon, the American armaments giant, is the conceiver of microwave ovens and HPM generators.

Some weapons of low and very low frequencies can produce waves intended to disrupt certain biological processes. The modulation of the signal can interfere with cerebral processes to bring about debilitation or submission. The applications are military, but also civilian, in the context of the maintenance of order. It is equally possible with such weapons to disturb a person's cardiac rhythm from a distance, resulting in death.

It would be salutary to emphasize once again the indirect effects of so-called 'non-lethal' weapons [2,3]. We have mentioned the disastrous effects of graphite bombs when they deprive emergency services of electricity. In this way, an electromagnetic bomb can cut the electricity supply to a hospital and render all of the medical equipment that has electronic or computer circuits useless [7]. A pilot disoriented by an 'E bomb' can crash and cause the deaths of a large number of passengers. Yet, this is how this bomb is described in the highly reputable weekly journal *Le Point:* 'The damage created is such - power surges, the erasing of magnetic memory, the paralysis of components - that the civilian and military installations – radio and television networks … telecommunication centers and radars – are found to be instantaneously "struck down" from within. And this, without that which one has to deplore, the slightest collateral damage. In microseconds, alert systems, command posts, and anti-missile defenses are paralyzed. Regarding airplanes and helicopters in flight, their fate is no more enviable than that of a swarm of flies that encounters a cloud of insecticide.' [5]

The notion of 'non-lethal' weapons is, in fact, only theoretical and does not tally with the realities on the ground.

The consequences of a terrorist act

With regard to terrorist attacks, we can learn much from two recent accidents. The incident at Chernobyl (Ukraine) gives an idea of what would happen were a commercial aircraft to crash into a nuclear reactor (Table 18.1). The accident at Goiänia (Brazil) demonstrates what might happen were radioactive products to be criminally dispersed in an urban setting.

On April 26, 1986, the No. 4 reactor of the Chernobyl nuclear center (Ukraine) exploded. As a consequence, a considerable quantity of radionuclides was discharged into the atmosphere over a 10-day period. The heaviest particles were deposited at least 100 km from the epicenter, while the more volatile elements such as cesium and iodine were transported over very long distances. The displacement of the radioactive cloud over Europe contaminated millions of persons, most often with low doses. Several human groups have been followed for health effects: the initial intervention groups, the "liquidators" charged with decontamination of the site, persons evacuated from the 30 Km zone, and the populations living in the contaminated zone.

Table 18.1 Emergency measures in the event of an accident in a nuclear installation

Initiation of the particular plan of intervention (PPI) and the ORSEC radiological plan (ORSECRAD)

Declaring the alert by siren or loudspeaker

Broadcast of instructions by radio

Decision to evacuate the population or shelter in place, according to the circumstances

Distribution of stable iodine compounds

If the decision to shelter in place is made, remain indoors and in shelter, if possible in a basement or, when there is none, block all openings; do not go outside during the first few days unless absolutely necessary

If one is caught outside by surprise, breathe through a filter (wet handkerchief) and cover exposed skin areas; return home, shower, and change clothes

Restriction of consumption of well water and of foodstuffs produced in the exposed region (fruits and vegetables, milk, etc.); canned and packaged foods should be consumed as well as mineral water

The initial response groups present at the site in the immediate aftermath of the accident suffered external beta and gamma irradiation, receiving doses of up to 15 Gy. Two hundred and thirty-seven persons engaged in firefighting received between 1 and 3 Sv in a few hours and presented acute irradiation syndrome, which accounted for 28 deaths. The majority of them developed radiation burns, caused by depositing of redioactive particles on the skin. Three other deaths were caused by trauma or thermal burns, making the number of initial deaths rise to 31.

A considerable increase in the frequency thyroid cancer in the inhabitants of the regions near Chernobyl was detected. The incidence of thyroid cancer in children and adolescents was multiplied by 100 in the most contaminated regions of the Ukraine and Belarus. In the case of a nuclear reactor accident, the chemical family of the iodines constitutes an important part in the released substances. In the absence of preventive treatment with stable iodine to saturate the thyroid, radioactive iodines preferentially bind to this latter. For the evacuated populations and the liquidators, the development of excess leukemias or solid tumors was likely but not demonstrated. The consequences of the Chernobyl accident on the mental health of the exposed populations represented a major public health problem. Pregnant women and the mothers of young children con-stituted a group at risk. Numerous pregnant women decided to have elective abortions, sometimes on the advice of their doctors. The authoritarian management of protective measures and the opacity of official information aggravated the distress of the various groups affected, and in particular those that were displaced. Moreover, the persistence of anxiety and depressive disorders was associated with the absence of good-quality social support.

The accident at Goiänia, a city of about one million inhabitants located 200 km from Brazilia, occurred in September 1987. Two junk scavengers discovered a metallic capsule abandoned by a private radiation therapy clinic, which contained Cesium-137 in the form of a powder. The persons in direct contact with the radioactive material presented with nausea, vomiting, headaches, and diarrhea, symptoms which were thought to be explained as gastroenteritis. During the actual diagnostic evaluation that was done, more than 100 000 persons were submitted for screening with detectors. Two hundred and forty-nine persons presented with detectable external or internal contamination and 49 persons needed to be hospitalized, of whom 21 were treated in intensive-care units. Five persons directly exposed to cesium-137 died and one person required an amputation. It took a considerable effort to decontaminate the surrounding area.

Therapeutic management

Classic emergency medical/surgical treatment is most important in radiation biology management (Tables 18.2 and 18.3). If there are associated injuries, in particular traumatic lesions or burns, requiring urgent care, their treatment takes priority over the care necessary for irradiation or contamination.

An irradiated patient (irradiation only, without external or internal contamination) does not represent a risk to others: he/she cannot irradiate or contaminate them. If possible, such patients should be admitted to a special service equipped with reverse isolation chambers. In the case of bone marrow aplasia, treatment is based on symptomatic resuscitation, blood and platelet transfusions, and the prescription of antibiotics and antimycotics. A bone marrow graft can be necessary. A blood sample should be done in the first few hours for lymphocyte and granulocyte counts, HLA (Human Leukocyte Antigen) typing and karyotype.

Table 18.2   Actions to take in the event of whole-body external irradiation

1. External irradiation is secondary to an exposure to X-rays or gamma rays, or even a flux of neutrons. Simple irradiation is not dangerous for persons who come near the victims.

2. The intensity and precocity of the symptoms have great diagnostic and prognostic value. The early appearance of nausea and vomiting is a good indicator of the dose received.

3. For associated injuries, emergency medical/surgical treatment takes precedence over the treatment of irradiation.

4. Where exposure to a flux of neutrons is suspected, remove and isolate metallic objects carried by the victims whenever possible.

5. Symptomatic treatment combines:
   - treatment of associated injuries
   - treatment of nausea and vomiting
   - early rehydration in the event of severe vomiting and diarrhea
   - sedation in the event of anxiety or agitation.

6. In the event of severe irradiation, rapid hospitalization in reverse sterile isolation with early HLA typing.

Table 18.3 Actions to take in the event of contamination

1. A subject who is a victim of external contamination might transfer his/her contamination by simple contact. The risk to response groups, and in particular health care personnel, however, is moderate if the instructions for precautions are followed.

2. Where external contamination is suspected, response groups should don NBC protective clothing or, when this is not available, masks, surgical caps, protective eyewear, gowns, and shoe covers.

3. External decontamination should be done whenever possible to avoid internal contamination of the injured person and that of his/her family. Complete disrobing is followed by prolonged rinsing with a mild soap solution, while protecting natural orifices and injured areas.

4. For associated injuries, emergency medical/surgical treatment takes precedence over treatment of the contamination. When the patient is in an unstable condition, external decontamination should only be done once the patient is stabilized.

5. For internal contamination:
   – Early administration of potassium iodide in the event of exposure to radioactive iodine:
      o adults: 130 mg/day
      o children 3 to 12 years old: 50 mg/day
      o children less than 3 years old: 25 mg/day
   – Early administration of chelators for heavy metals:*
      o four injections of Prussian Blue if exposed to radioactive cesium
      o DTPA (wound irrigation, nebulization, or perfusion) if exposed to plutonium or transuranics
      o intramuscular injections of BAL (dimercaprol) if exposed to radioactive polonium
   – Symptomatic measures
      o protection and irrigation of the eyes and skin
      o significant hydration to induce diuresis (collect the urine)
      o medications to diminish gastrointestinal absorption (collect the feces)

*For emergency recommendations, availability, and dosing schedules, in the US contact REACTS, Oak Ridge, TN 1-865-576-1005

In summary, a contaminated patient can be responsible for the transfer to others of radioactive particles deposited on their clothing or skin. Such patients should be decontaminated before admission to the health care building, at least when their clinical condition does not necessitate emergency care [6].

Decontamination

Heath care personnel in charge of decontamination should wear surgical-type garb with cap, mask, protective eyewear, gown, gloves, and shoe covers. After use, these should be placed in plastic sacks. Response personnel should be monitored with a particle counter. Several rules regulate the process of radiological decontamination:

– undress and wash with tap water and soap (repeat two or three times);

– prevent transformation of external contamination into internal contamination;

– avoid the creation of a cutaneous injury by aggressive scrubbing;

– protect the eyes, nose, mouth, and auditory canals during decontamination of the face or hair;

– avoid placing the hands in the mouth and smoking;

– dry carefully and re-dress with clean clothing;

– monitor residual radioactivity by means of detectors;

– store contaminated clothing in plastic sacks;

– do not spread the lavage water.

Anti-radiation and anticontamination treatments

In an irradiated subject, the treatment of bone marrow aplasia is based on transplantation of stem cells from the bone marrow removed by biopsy of the least irradiated areas and stimulated by injection of growth factors. These factors, such as Neupogen® commercialized by the Angen laboratory, are sometimes poorly tolerated and can cause adverse effects, such as fever and vomiting. The injection of growth factors costs 2500 euros (3000 dollars) and the graft technology costs 10 000 euros (11 500 dollars). This type of treatment would be difficult to carry out on a large scale if it became necessary to treat a large number of irradiated persons.

The Hollis–Eden private company based in San Diego, California, under contract with the Armed Forces Radiobiology Research Institute (AFRRI), has developed a medication (molecule HE-2100) capable of neutralizing the effects of nuclear irradiation. This medication, based on DHEA (dehydroepiandrosterone) metabolites (in particular androstenediol), triggers the production of growth factors in the irradiated organism which stimulate the bone marrow cells. The molecule developed by this laboratory might have been commercialized under the name of Neumune in 2007, under the restrictions of an agreement with the FDA; however, its commercial development has been curtailed in early 2008. Hollis-Eden has received eight million dollars of subsidies to develop this molecule, which has been successfully tested in primates irradiated with a dose of 4 Gy. The administration of HE-2100 reduced the severity of the aplasia. Studies in humans should begin next. This product is interesting for two reasons. On the one hand, it does not seem to have any toxicity and one can hope that it would be well tolerated in clinical use. On the other hand, its cost is limited, which constitutes a major advantage were there a large number of irradiated patients needing treatment. Treatment of one patient costs between 50 euros (60 dollars) and 100 euros (125 dollars), at a dose rate of one dose per day for about five days. The experiments in primates were, however, carried out by means of low-intensity irradiation (4 Gy). In human pathology, the ideal treatment should work with irradiation of more than 6 Gy.

In the case of internal contamination, the treatment should aim either to reduce absorption or to increase the elimination of radionuclides. The efficacy of the treatment decreases rapidly with time. These must therefore be instituted on simple presumption of internal contamination. The risk depends on the radionuclides involved and their metabolism in the body. In certain cases, chemical toxicity unique to the involved element can be added to the emission of ionizing radiation. Anthropogammametric examination (whole-body counting) can detect the existence of internal contamination and chart its elimination. The treatment of internal contamination aims to reduce the absorption of contaminant products or of accelerating their elimination.

The risk of developing thyroid cancer, due to exposure to radioactive iodine, should be managed by the early administration of stable iodine capable of saturating the thyroid and preventing binding of radioactive iodine by this gland. The dosing schedule in adults is 100 mg of iodine in the form of potassium iodide (or 130 mg of potassium iodide) administered orally. In children, the recommended dosing schedule is 50 mg for those between 3 and 12 years of age, and 25 mg for children less than 3 years old. The efficacy of this treatment is maximal between 6 hours before and 3 hours following exposure. The French government recently requested that pharmacies in its territory set up stockpiles of potassium iodide tablets. Since 1997, this measure only concerned populations living in close proximity to nuclear centers (within a 10 km radius). This has subsequently been extended to throughout the county. The tablets, stockpiled by pharmacists, facilitate a response when faced with the health consequences of a radioactive cloud. After the Chernobyl accident, the administration of stable iodine in the Ukraine seems to have been very limited and often done too late to be efficacious. Only 25 per cent of persons questioned who resided in the most contaminated areas received potassium iodine. The mean duration of prophylaxis for these persons was 6.2 days. In Poland, more than 20 million tablets were distributed following the Chernobyl accident.

The administration of heavy metal chelators should be envisioned according to the type of radioactive agents. DTPA (diethylene-triamine-penta-acetate) is utilized in cases where internal contamination with plutonium or transuranic elements that are alpha emitters is suspected. It is available in the form of injectable ampoules and in capsules of micronized powder. It can be prescribed as a perfusion (one ampoule four times a day, about 1 g for an adult) or by nebulization (micronized powder). In cases of skin contamination or burns, it is recommended to break an ampoule of DTPA on the skin or the burn and then to cover the area with sterile compresses. This treatment is contraindicated in renal insufficiency and in pregnant women, as well as in cases of uranium contamination (risk of acute toxic nephritis). DTPA is not commercially available, but is available through the Army Medical Service (France) or REACTS (Radiation Emergency Assistance Center/Training Site; USA). BAL (British Anti-Lewisite; dimercaprol) is used in cases of internal contamination with polonium, at a dosing schedule of one ampoule intramuscularly every 4 hours. Prussian Blue is used in cases of internal contamination with cesium, at a dosing schedule of 1 g three times daily.

Some non-specific treatments are generally added: gentle laxatives to facilitate gastrointestinal elimination, bronchial lavage and significant hydration (at least two liters per day). Stools and urine should be collected and handled with extreme caution.

On the occasion of the fiftieth anniversary of the use of nuclear weapons against Japan, a Gallup poll revealed that Americans more than 50 years of age approved of this decision in an overwhelming majority (80 per cent). The results were similar to those of a survey of August 26, 1945, revealing that 85 per cent of Americans were in favor of the atomic bombings, 10 per cent were opposed, and 5 per cent had no opinion. On April 21, 2003, Mr. T. Akiba, Mayor of Hiroshima, addressed the following letter to the President of the United States: 'I have received a report that your government has submitted to Congress a request for funds for the development of small nuclear weapons with a yield of five kilotons or less whose manufacture has been prohibited since 1993, and which contradict the Furse–Spratt prohibition of weapons of this type. This clear indication that the United States intends to manufacture small nuclear weapons evokes the horrible possibility that such nuclear weapons will be used. As Mayor of the City of Hiroshima, victim of an atomic bomb, I am indignant at the barbarity with which you have behaved, not only in attacking Iraq, killing or mutilating thousands of innocent Iraqis, but also in developing nuclear weapons. You trample on the hopes of a vast majority of the peoples of the world who search for peace, and, in the name of the residents of Hiroshima, I protest most vehemently. This announcement, accompanied with declarations concerning the necessity of resuming underground testing and of rapidly developing new tactical nuclear devices is an extremely regrettable, head-on denunciation of nuclear disarmament.'

References

1. Tubiana M, Lallemand J. *Radiobiologie et Radioprotection.* Paris, Presses Universitaires de France/Que sais-je?, 2002.
2. Abdelkrim-Delanne C. Ces armes si peu conventionnelles. *Le Monde Diplomatique,* juin 1999: 11.
3. Wright S. Hypocrisie des armes non létales. *Le Monde Diplomatique,* décembre 1999: 24.
4. Dao J, Pentagon unveils plans for a new crowd-dispersal weapon. *The New York Times,* mars 2, 2001.
5. Brosselin S. Bombe 'E', l'arme qui foudroie. *Le Point,* novembre 1, 2002: 68–69.
6. Mavrakis D. Accidents nucléaires et radiologiques: prise en charge précoce. *Urgence Pratique,* 2002; **55:** 11–17.
7. Poupée K. Un test pour les armes électrométiques. *Le Monde Diplomatique,* avril 2003: 15.

19

Chinks in the armor

Patrick Barriot and Chantal, Bismuth

In a country where internal security is a national priority, the political will is expressed before all in the allocated budgets. Before the attacks of September 11, 2001, the annual budget for the struggle against biological and chemical terrorism in the United States was 1.5 million dollars. The American Defense budget for 2004 proposed by the Bush administration was 380 million dollars, or about 18 million more than in 2003. The Department of Homeland Security, equipped with an annual budget of 38 million dollars and anticipating integrating some 170 000 employees, has been created following the September 11, 2001 attacks. It is charged with developing an overall strategy in matters of civil defense: networks, education of health and emergency response personnel, constitution of stockpiles (vaccines, antidotes, antibiotics), improvement of health surveillance, animal-breeding facilities and agriculture, fundamental and applied research studies, etc. It thus becomes a matter of bold political moves expressing the will of the people in the light of these new threats [1, 2, 3]. A note from the Secretary General for National Defense (SGDN), sent to Lionel Jospin on December 12, 1998, revealed the pitiful level of civil defense in France. The budget for civil defense, managed by SGDN, was on the order of some millions of francs. In January 2003, the *White Book of the French High Committee for Civil Defense* was presented to the Minister of the Interior. It emphasized, in 10 reports and propositions, the principal gaps of the French action plans for civil defense as well as the means of remedying them. Stress was placed on, among other things, the necessity of a law for setting up a program of civil defense, for the creation of a Secretary of State for the protection of populations and for a true training academy for civil defense, to carry out research and development of civil defense strategies for the long term, on the development of a better partnership between the public and private sectors and to subsidize those private firms involved with the public sector. For the first time, an actual plan of action was articulated. Christian Sommade, Secretary General of the French High Council for Civil Defense (HCFDC) emphasized: 'Contrary to the United States, were are not in overall middle-term thinking. One tackles the problems blow by blow. We still ask ourselves how we will react in case of an attack, such as that perpetrated with sarin gas

Treating Victims of Mass Destsuction   Edited by Patrick Barriot and Chantal Bismuth
© 2008 John Wiley & Sons, Ltd

in the Tokyo subway. Anticipation is still the master word.' In Great Britain, experts doubt the effectiveness of intervention when faced with bioterrorist aggression on a large scale. Éric Alley, Professor Emeritus at the Institute for Civil Defense and Studies of Catastrophes, stated: 'The government has not made a real effort to be ready in the event of a terrorist attack.'

Plans

Deputy Pierre Lellouche, Member of the Commission for Defense of the French National Assembly and co-author of the report *France and the Bombs*: *The Challenge of the Proliferation of Weapons of Mass Destruction* declared in 2001: 'The Biotox plan, I don't know what it is. I add that I don't know anyone who knows what this plan is. Before, we had Piratox. Now we have Biotox. If one doesn't want this to be from intox, we should tell the French people what it is. Last year, France spent four million francs on civil defense. That is to say for nothing. Are we prepared? The answer is "no." The physicians are not trained. Not for recognition of smallpox. Because it has been eradicated, most people do not learn to discern the symptoms. Nor for noting the difference between anthrax and bronchitis.' In February 2003, Christian Sommade, Secretary General of the HCFDC was also pessimistic: 'It is unfortunately a very French tendency to think that, when a plan exists, the problem is solved ... It is true that the Biotox plan lists the means and determines the responsibilities of each one facing the crisis. Still, it is necessary that those who are to intervene must be trained and equipped with the technical means necessary for their missions, which is – as always – far from being the case.'

The first-aid plans in practice envision situations which involve some dozens of victims, rarely some hundreds and never several thousands. They have proven their efficacy in response to relatively well-circumscribed and controlled events, and it is dangerous to transpose a proven action plan to non-comparable situations. The Euratox exercise which simulated chemical contamination of 2000 persons in a stadium revealed the limits of the management of a flood of victims passing through a decontamination line. The occurrence of an epidemic of smallpox or the explosion of a thermonuclear bomb would create an unforeseen and radically different situation, with a considerable number of victims. One should ask whether our response plans would allow us to function when faced, for example, with a chemical catastrophe such as that of Bhopal. It is therefore urgent to reconsider the response plans, pre-hospital and hospital, as a function of the emergence of new threats and to reflect on the long-term nuclear, radiological, biological and chemical (CBRN) risks. The great flood of contaminated or contagious victims should be considered in a very concrete fashion. The recent SARS epidemic revealed, amongst other things, that modern hospitals are not adapted for the management of numerous contagious patients before they are placed in isolation chambers. The response plans should also consider algorithms for the triage of victims and for temporary morgues, while respecting the dignity of the dead. Above all, it is necessary to retain only the thinking which informs a plan when the application of a plan becomes ineffective when confronted with the realities on the ground, and to be able to coordinate, on a nationwide scale, trained personnel, training programs and preparations. They should be perfectly understood by all of the response personnel, and validated by simulations and exercises on the ground. That is to say that confidentiality, the blanket ban of 'defense secrets', seriously harms the effectiveness of civil defense.

Professor Henri Mollaret, bacteriologist, has criticized a form of administrative inertia that could lead to inaction: 'I have been invited, in France, to sit on a certain number of commissions, and I must note that they have always been to me a constant source of distress. In this fashion, in 1980, the Secretary General for National Defense assembled a crisis team to deal with a hypothetical bioterrorist attack on French soil. One time each month, we would meet, between experts and the responsible persons, at Les Invalides to decide this or that agent should appear on this or that list. Everyone was in agreement on smallpox, plague, anthrax, or botulinum toxin, but it was imperative that we ended up with an overall idea of [how to deal with] the entire group of [biological] agents. But we had nothing. Or, more precisely, we had an empty administrative straitjacket [both that and 'straightjacket' in US English] totally incapable of enabling the types of action we in power needed to take, actions of which we became the victims because the notes on what actions to take in the event of biological attack were restricted to the central management of the Army health service. It was, I believe, the most miserable operation, those responsible generally having the conviction that no one would ever use biological weapons. The necessary measures have, as far as I am concerned, never been taken. But nothing would be easier for terrorists than to procure and to disseminate the most fatal strains of pathogens. I also know some biologists who, still more recently, commercialized all sorts of strains, including that of the plague.' [4]

Warning and chemical detection

Numerous systems exist that are capable of rapidly detecting the presence of chemical agents on persons or in the environment. Units of the French Army are equipped with systems for the detection and identification of vesicants and organophosphates. The AP2C apparatus for detection of contamination, based on the principle of flame photometry, rapidly and sensitively detects these agents in the vapor state. It can be equipped with a warning system that has a detection radius of some meters. Detection vehicles can be equipped with either a transportable mass spectrometer coupled to a gas chromatography device or with an infrared photo acoustic spectroscope. The mobile means can refer to a database, which will enable the automatic identification of toxicants within a matter of minutes.

Studies in the field of detection and identification of chemical agents are being conducted to develop new receptor systems with enhanced performance. The group of receptor systems consists of semiconductor probes, electrochemical probes, sound wave probes, and fiber optic probes. The group of bioprobes consists essentially of immunological probes made up of specific immunoreactants for certain toxicants.

The identification of the principal chemical agents can be performed very rapidly by examination of a sample of air. In the United States, the Laurence Livermore National Laboratory has created a system (BIDS) which tests the air quality every 30 minutes and sets off an alarm in the presence of chemical agents. This system, which has been set up in a Metro station in Washington, can be linked to a device for checking the dispersion of chemical agents in a tunnel or in an air-conditioning system. The deployment of chemical agent detectors on a large scale, however, involves a considerable cost.

Warning and biological detection

Unlike those for chemical agents, there are currently few high-performance systems for the rapid detection of the presence of pathogenic microorganisms, either in the patient or in the environment.

Two types of techniques have been developed for the detection, in the patient, of biological agents. The first group is based on the detection of the genome of the pathogenic agent by means of genetic probes. The method of molecular hybridization, which is based on complementing of the two long strands in the double helix of DNA, enables the development of 'DNA chips', or 'biochips', capable of rapidly detecting the presence of fragments of bacterial or viral genomes in a sample. In the United States, the Massachusetts Institute of Technology (MIT) has worked on the development of DNA chips capable of detecting a biological attack. In France, the Pasteur Institute and the Mérieux Institute are working on identical projects. These biotechnologies also facilitate the development of a detailed database of the genomes of pathogenic agents capable of being militarized. This database would permit the rapid identification of involved strains and of their origin. The second group is based on immunological techniques which detect, by means of specific antibodies, the toxins or membrane proteins of microorganisms. The utilization of monoclonal antibodies, which detect very small concentrations of specific microbial antigens, facilitates the development of rapid tests for diagnosing viral or bacterial illnesses.

The detection of pathogenic agents in the environment can also benefit from the techniques of molecular genetics. The principle consists of aspirating a few cubic meters of air with a 'sniffer' and then placing the contents of samples collected on a filter in solution and analyzing them before reacting them with DNA chip probes. All these operations can be carried out in situ over the course of a few hours; a biochip can manage several simultaneous analyses. Some systems for the identification of biological particles in the environment by size analysis and with fluorescence have also been developed.

In the case of biological risk, all warning systems used to rely on old national and international public health networks. The international network of the WHO is equipped with informatics software (GPHIN), developed in Canada, which daily analyzes the websites of a thousand research journals for public health events. This software revealed on November 27, 2002, in a Chinese daily newspaper, the explosion of pneumonia affecting the Foshan region, but no one paid any attention. The international network of the WHO, however, presents two drawbacks: on the one hand, it is dependent on an alliance with the CDC (Centers for Disease Control and Prevention) in Atlanta and, on the other hand, it depends too much on the goodwill of the public health authorities of member countries to report useful information.

The Chinese authorities had in this manner concealed the SARS epidemic for several months. The ProMED network (Program for Monitoring Emerging Diseases) founded in 1994 by the Foundation of American Scientists is capable of rapid reaction owing to Internet support (automatic search engines). It allows for the establishment of connections between apparently independent events. The delay of dissemination of verified information in seven languages does not exceed 48 hours. The institution, in Europe, of an organization equivalent to the CDC in Atlanta has been evoked as a means of improving the effectiveness of public health on the Continent in the battle against emerging infectious diseases.

At the same time, it is essential to establish a national warning plan of action worthy of the name. Ill humans or animals are not the best means of detecting an outbreak, in the sense that they alone would not guarantee that the entire public health network would be able to make a rapid diagnosis and then instantly warn a central information center. At the present time, the idea of a network of physicians, pharmacists and veterinarians standing sentinel is still in its infancy. In all likelihood, many days would pass between the initiation of an epidemic and its detection.

Warning and radiological detection

The activity of radiation, expressed in disintegrations per second, or becquerels (Bq), is estimated by particle counters such as Geiger counters graduated in counts/minute (CPM). External contamination, which results from radioelements depositing on bodily surfaces, is detected with a particle counter which localizes the contamination and estimates its extent. The total amount of radioactive agents emitting gamma rays present in the body can be measured by whole-body counting. Measurement of the concentrations of isotopes in the excreta (urine and feces) and exhaled air enables the detection of those emitting alpha or beta radiation which cannot be detected by external counting.

Certain laboratories are equipped with apparatuses capable of detecting and analyzing radioactive gases emitted many hundreds of kilometers away. In 1986, the Chernobyl accident was detected by a Swedish laboratory, from atmospheric samples, although the Soviet authorities attempted to conceal it. In the same manner, it is possible to detect the emissions of xenon or Krypton-85 at a great distance, revealing a radioactive waste re-processing facility.

Group protection

The protection of 'sensitive' sites involves airports, Metro stations, railroad stations, offices and commercial sites, theaters and auditoriums, stadiums, and religious sites, as well as nuclear centers. In France, a pilot must not fly within 5 km of a nuclear center and is prohibited from flying at an altitude less than 36 000 feet above one. The

Minister of Defense has placed a radar station and a battery of ground-to-air missiles close to the La Hague site. The Air Force is in a position to scramble combat aircraft within a few minutes to protect this institution as well as the nuclear reactors of the EDF. And yet, despite the Vigipirate plan, two unidentified aircraft (a single-engine airplane and a helicopter) flew over the nuclear center at Civaux (Vienne, France) at low altitude in June 2003. The protection of the ventilation systems of administrative office buildings and large commercial groups, in particular air intakes, should be enhanced. Detectors for chemical agents could be coupled with devices to check the diffusion of a toxicant in a tunnel or an air-conditioning system.

The protection of sites for supplying potable water should be made a part of all plans to combat terrorism. It is always acknowledged that the dispersion of botulinum toxin in a food supply network or in potable water is not the sum total of the terrorist risk and that the chlorination of water does not eliminate all the dangers.

Public health surveillance of breeding farms and agricultural enterprises is a crucial element of a protection action plan. Since the economy contributes to Western strength, it is incomprehensible that private enterprises have been miraculously spared this new form of warfare, terrorism. We simply recall that on September 11, 2001, Al-Quida not only attacked the Pentagon but also the World Trade Center. Large international enterprises were thus potential targets. And one can only conclude that they will one day be the object of biological or chemical attacks with the view of destabilizing entire sectors of the economy. Contamination by ingestion concerns groups which distribute potable water, but also all those who participate in the food chain, from producers to distributors. The agricultural industry is in the frontline in the fight against bioterrorism, as it is a means of attacking the population via its foodstuffs, and because these industries produce their wealth from the exploitation and transportation of species of animals and vegetables, which could also be struck by viruses or bacteria. The dramatic economic consequences of epidemics of aphthous fever ('hoof and mouth disease') and spongiform encephalopathy ('mad cow disease') demonstrate how this sector is vulnerable to such an attack.

Individual protection

The penetration of toxic agents into the body by respiratory and cutaneous routes implies that individual equipment should combine respiratory and cutaneous protection [5, 6].

Respiratory protection

The first gas mask improvised during World War I was a cotton pad soaked in sodium thiosulfate, glycerin, and calcium, covering the nose and mouth. Currently, surgical masks and N-95 protective masks are the best means for guarding against infectious agents when in close contact with a hospitalized ill patient. 'Surgical masks' are covered with an impermeable film that prevents the wearer from spreading droplets when speaking, coughing or sneezing. The N-95 protective devices are also equipped with a filter and protect the wearer from particles suspended in the ambient air. In summary, paper masks offer an uncertain protection and constitute an insufficient barrier against respiratory secretions because of humidification by the saliva. During the SARS epidemic in China, nurses complained of the lack of masks or the absence of masks of sufficient quality in their hospitals. In Hong Kong, a campaign called 'Project Shield' was launched to offer effective protective equipment to medical personnel.

'Gas masks' are equipped with filtering cartridges combining a gas filter and a particulate filter (Table 19.1):

Filters against gases and vapor are made up of activated charcoal (coconut charcoal) impregnated with metal salts. The filling of the absorbent canister must be adapted to the toxic products to be trapped. The activated charcoal filter can absorb gases and vapors by a purely physical mechanism or neutralize them chemically by action of the metal salts with which it is impregnated. For example, hydrogen cyanide, because of its volatility and low molecular weight, is only weakly absorbed by activated charcoal alone, but certain metal salts react with the cyanide to form a complex which is retained in the canister. Filters against gases are classified into types and classes as a function of their utilization and their protective capacity (see Table 19.1).

Anti-particle or anti-aerosol filters are made up of very fine cellulose or glass fibers. They are folded into pleats in such a manner as to increase the filtration surface. There are three classes of particulate filters, designated by their effectiveness: P1, P2, and P3. The P3 filter stops nearly all aerosols and particulates whose size is greater than 0.15 microns.

Table 19.1 Filter cartridges

The designations (A, B, E, and K) concern activated charcoal filters and specify the toxicants in the gas or vapor states which are adsorbed and retained by their filters.

Designation A: protection against gases and organic vapors having a boiling point greater than 65 °C and specified by the manufacturer.

Designation B: protection against certain gases (excluding CO) and inorganic vapors specified by the manufacturer.

Designation E: protection against sulfur dioxide and gases or vapors specified by the manufacturer.
Designation K: protection against ammonia and amine derivatives specified by the manufacturer.

The designation P designates an 'anti-particulate' filter which stops aerosols and particles of which the size is greater than 0.15 microns.

The indication attached to each designation corresponds to the class of protection:

Class 1: low-capacity filter
Class 2: medium-capacity filter
Class 3: high-capacity filter

NBC type cartridges or A2B2E2K2P3 are wide spectrum

The protection offered by filtration cartridges is, however, limited. Above all, the cartridge must be adapted to the toxicant to be retained and it is necessary to know that the duration of its effectiveness depends on the concentration of the toxicant in the atmosphere. When the concentration of the toxicant increases, the effectiveness of the filtration cartridge can decrease in a dramatic fashion. On the other hand, their use is dangerous in the presence of a simple asphyxiant gas: filtration cartridges can only be utilized in an atmosphere whose concentration of oxygen is greater than 17% (by volume). Certain gases, such as perfluoroisobutene (PFIB), are not stopped by the cartridges of conventional marks. Some mixed gases combine a lethal agent, stopped by the cartridge, and a very irritating and volatile agent, which is not stopped by the cartridge and which obliges the wearer to remove their protective mask.

Special ventilation bags are made up of a bag which covers the head and relies on a bottle of compressed air which at once over pressurizes the interior of the bag preventing penetration of the toxic gas and furnishing breathable fresh air. A collar placed at the bottom of the bag assures a seat at the wearer's neck. This type of ventilation bag is particularly useful for children for whom gas masks adapted to their size are not provided and for persons with beards which limit the sealing of the masks. This type of device is also very useful for first aid to poisoning victims at the incident scene due to the ease and rapidity of use even in cases of wounds involving the face, vomiting, or profuse secretions.

The only absolute respiratory protection is represented by stand-alone isolating respirators of the intervention services, which can be either self-contained breathing apparatus (SCBA) or supplied-air respirators.

Skin protection

The levels of protection can be divided into three principal groups. The highest level is represented by fully encapsulated suits for chemical intervention made of butyl rubber (Level A). They are generally combined with SCBA which can be worn on the inside or with an air-supplied respirator with the air-supply exterior to the suit. The limitation of movements is such that a physician is incapable of working with this type of equipment. The lower levels, with hoods and boots incorporated, are made with lightweight synthetic materials which offer short-duration protection, levels B and C. They are generally worn with a gas mask (filter respirator). These intermediate levels realize a compromise between protection and freedom of movement. They are essentially a matter of filtering levels with layers of activated charcoal (S3P, T3P and TOM), as the Armed Forces are equipped with, conceived to confront chemical warfare agents in the form of liquids or vapors. Their use is only effective when in combination with a protective mask respirator equipped with its filtration cartridges. In October 2002, the American Congress warned that 250 000 CBRN levels of protection delivered to the American Army by the manufacturer, Istratex, were defective. One does not know, moreover, if these levels of protection are impermeable to very small-sized viruses.

The choice of respiratory and skin protection depends, on the one hand, on the degree of exposure to the toxicant and, on the other hand, on the necessary compromise between protection and operational capacity and freedom of movement. It is possible to distinguish schematically two types of protection: protection for intervention and protection for escape. Personnel belonging to groups for intervention and first aid should be equipped with high-level skin protection and with respiratory protection by SCBA or supplied-air respirators. For populations who have to rapidly get to a shelter or to evacuate a contaminated area, escape protection is sufficient: low level with a filtration cartridge mask or a hood for respiratory protection.

Decontamination

Three types of decontamination exist: radiological decontamination, chemical decontamination, and biological decontamination. They also concern persons, equipment, locations, and the environment. Although the decontamination of persons is generally well established and relatively simple, the decontamination of sensitive equipment, locations, and the environment comes up against some major technical and financial problems. The cost of these operations can run into the tens of even hundreds of millions of dollars.

Chemical decontamination

Chemical decontamination is based on the mechanical displacement of toxicants present on the skin or clothing in the form of droplets. It can combine several techniques: mechanical elimination by means of powder absorbents, undressing, lavage with a decontaminant solution, and showering. Utilization, at the beginning and the end of the decontamination line, of the AP2C monitoring apparatus type allows detection of vesicant or organophosphate toxic vapors. Basic decontamination of all suspected droplets on skin or clothes must be begun rapidly with the use of absorbent powders. The Armed Forces are equipped with powdered cloths with one side for dispersing an absorbent powder and the other side for wiping it off. This powder is finely pulverized Fuller's Earth, which acts as a blotter absorbent for toxicants without destroying them. Talc and flour possess approximately the same properties. Initially, it is suitable to sprinkle the toxic droplets with talc or flour and then remove them with paper towels. Absorbent powders have an advantage over water lavage in not increasing the contaminated surface by spreading the toxicant and by limiting the penetration of the toxicant into healthy or injured skin.

Undressing is intended to reduce the duration and intensity of the contamination, whether it is a matter of products with percutaneous absorption or an exclusively local action. It should be done rapidly, taking into account possibly combined traumatic lesions. In the course of undressing, all precautions should be taken to avoid contamination of the healthy skin from droplets present on the clothes. Cutting the clothing off is the most rapid technique and the least contaminating for proximate lesions or healthy skin. Contaminated clothing should be placed in watertight garbage bags. In the event of exposure to a chemical warfare agent, undressing is imperative. Moreover, the action of certain toxicants is particularly insidious as cutaneous penetration of the toxicant is not painful and because the symptoms appear after an asymptomatic interval of a few hours. It thus happens that the victims do not recognize that they have been exposed and do not remove their clothing. For this reason, in the event of a chemical threat, all irritation of the eyes and upper airways, even fleeting, should prompt undressing and, if possible, showering.

Lavage with a decontamination solution is intended to promote the chemical inactivation of the involved product. It is, above all, used for toxicants with percutaneous penetration, but to be effective, it must be applied quickly. To inactivate sulfur mustard, an aqueous solution of 2 g/L of potassium permanganate is recommended. To inactivate the neurotoxic agents, an aqueous solution of sodium hypochlorite at 8 g of active chlorine/L is advocated. When the toxicant is unidentified, it is possible to use an aqueous solution containing both potassium permanganate and sodium hypochlorite.

Showering is above all a means of radiological decontamination (see below under 'Radiological decontamination'). In the context of chemical contamination, showering allows mechanical decontamination of the toxicant, but exposes the victim to the risk of spreading the toxicant on the skin, setting in motion an increased skin surface area for cutaneous penetration. For this reason, decontamination, by means of absorbent powders, of all suspected droplets should precede showering. Furthermore, water is not always available in sufficient quantities and the disposal of contaminated water poses logistical problems. Water lavage must be done with copious volumes of water for at least 20 minutes, following undressing. Ocular lavage should be done systemically, bilaterally, abundantly and for a prolonged time in all victims presenting with ocular irritation. Wounds should also be lavaged with copious amounts of water and then protected with hydrophilic gauze bandages.

Current studies are being carried out on new procedures for the elimination of chemical agents. Biological procedures use enzymes which hydrolyze certain toxic molecules. Chemical procedures use various oxidant compounds, such as perborate ions or chloride agents, which attack oxidizable bonds. In this manner, an enzyme extracted from the common squid, *Loligo vulgaris*, di-isopropyl fluoro-phosphatase, or DFPase, is capable of destroying nerve agents by hydrolysis. On their side, highly reactive oximate ions are capable of binding with nerve agents and degrading them. The time for the degradation half-life is on the order of 15 seconds for Soman, of 5 seconds for sarin, and of 2 minutes for VX. At the same time, American scientists from the Sandia National Laboratories have developed a non-corrosive form which neutralizes chemical agents and possesses a bactericidal component. The organization of a medical center can only be conceived of in an uncontaminated area. It must be made up of two distinct parts. The first part is the decontamination center where, at the reception site, there is triage and decontamination of victims. The second part is the treatment center. These two parts are separated by a barrier and no personnel are authorized to pass from one part to the other, in order to prevent the transfer of contamination.

The decontamination of sites polluted with chemical warfare agents is extremely costly. As an example, the United States abandoned some large stockpiles of chemical weapons on the Panamanian Island of San José after WWII. Currently, Panama cannot carry the financial burden for the dismantling of these weapons and decontamination of the site. One can estimate that the clean-up of these 4000 contaminated hectares alone would cost more than 600 million dollars.

Biological decontamination

In the fall of 2001, numerous systems, of which the efficacy has not always been demonstrated, were commercialized with the view of destroying anthrax spores. According to Meryl Nass, a physician specializing in anthrax illness, the decontamination strategy is not clearly established: 'The decontamination is … a major problem: up to now, I have not met a person who has clearly mastered the technique.' Postal-sorting officers, who are particularly vulnerable, were equipped with devices allowing irradiation of the mail to destroy bacterial pathogens. The overall cost of these operations exceeded 14 million dollars.

In 1986, the British government decided to decontaminate the Island of Gruinard, polluted by anthrax spores since the experiments of July 1942. Over a 4-year period, the island was irrigated with 280 tons of formaldehyde diluted in 2000 tons of sea water. Such an operation was possible because of the small size of the island. For a larger surface area, the operation would be very expensive and much more difficult. On the battlefield, thermobaric weapons would be capable of destroying, by their thermal effects, the pathogenic agents and preventing their dispersal in the air.

Radiological decontamination

If radiological decontamination of persons by showering is a simple and not costly thing, decontamination of urban sites or vast areas has rarely been undertaken. In Goiänia, 25 houses were contaminated with Cesium-137. The decontamination of the different polluted sites in the city involved the treatment of 5000 cubic meters of contaminated rubbish. When it is a matter of vast areas, the problem is nearly insoluble. In the south of Belarus, which received 70% of the radioactive fallout from the Chernobyl accident, 1.5 million persons lived in contaminated areas where the soils had a radioactivity greater than 37 000 Bq per square meter. The Director of the Gomel Hospital, Vlacheslav Ijakovski, deplored the contamination by radioactive cesium of ingested foodstuffs: 'in the villages where the people eat only potatoes from their gardens, fish which they catch, berries from the forest.' In 17 years, the catastrophe cost 295 million dollars in Belarus and the management of its consequences absorbed almost 8% of its budget. Their agriculture cannot develop certain products, such as milk, because they remain contaminated. Fallout from the Chernobyl accident in France has still more long-term controversies. The contamination map for Cesium-137 presented by the IRNS (Institute for Radioprotection and Nuclear Safety) in April 2003 contradicted the official view. The information about the total radioactivity of the soil could vary from 740 Bq per meter squared to more 20 000 Bq per meter squared according to the area.

Treatment

In the eventuality of a CBRN attack, the necessity of starting early specific or non-specific treatment dictates the need for four types of national stockpiles (Table 19.2). According to the type of treatment and the delay of prescription, stockpiles should be managed by hospitals, pre-hospital responders, pharmacies, or military organizations. For example, artificial ventilation of 100 victims requires for 1 hour only:

- more than 60 000 liters of oxygen, or about 100 3.5 L portable bottles filled to - 200 millibars and equipped with hand controls (one ton of supplies);
- 100 ventilators (volume or pressure controlled for transport).

One can easily conceive the quantities of oxygen necessary for several days of treatment.

It is pointless to attempt to put together stockpiles of antidotes against all known toxicants, as was emphasized by Jean-François Lacronique, President of the Administrative Counsel of the Institute for Radioprotection and Nuclear Safety: 'How can we anticipate the makeup of stockpiles of antidotes when one cannot anticipate the extent and the efficacy of these means? Owing to budgetary constraints and simple logistics, it is impossible to accumulate stockpiles of all the imaginable products,

Table 19.2 Component which could be part of stockpiles

I.   Treatment for biological agent attacks:
     Antibiotics: Ciprofloxacin, doxycycline
     Antivirals: Zanarnivir, oseltamivir
     Smallpox vaccine

II. Treatment for chemical agent attacks:
     Antidotes for organophosphates: atropine, oxime, valium
     Cyanide antidote: hydroxocobalamin

III. Treatment for nuclear or radiological attacks
     Potassium iodine pills
     DTPA (Diethylene-triamine-penta-acetate)
     Prussian Blue
     BAL (British Anti-Lewisite; dimercaprol)

IV. Protective measures against CBRN agents
     surgical masks
     filtration cartridge masks
     low-level skin protection
     decontaminating measures

---

throughout the country, and, paradoxically, to give up trying to understand as might be said, "ready for all eventualities"' [7]. It is, however, prudent to stockpile antidotes against organophosphate nerve agents and cyanide compounds [8, 9].

Concerning antibiotics, the public powers in France will be prepared for a bioterrorist attack by anthrax spores and stockpiles of antibiotics that are efficacious against the bacteria are kept in France, in confidential and protected sites. Ciprofloxacin and doxycycline, to treat the majority of bacterial infections most likely to be internationally propagated, must be stockpiled. The treatment, as we have seen, is much more efficacious when it is begun early. Some months ago, the town of Perreux-sur-Marne (Val-de-Marne), confronted with a case of meningitis in a nursery school, had a sad experience with the failure of the antibiotic stockpile. The families, went to the Saint-Camille Hospital in Bry-sur-Marne in order to receive prophylactic antibiotic treatment, could not obtain the medication, neither from the hospital nor from the stockpile pharmacy. The father of one child described the situation to a journalist in the following manner: 'We received a phone call from the Prefecture a little before 11 p.m. My wife and I were very anxious. We went to the hospital with our two children and waited for a long time. At about 2 a.m., the staff on duty presented us with a prescription because all the available doses had been used. And no one could tell us where to find this product.' It was necessary to wait until the following morning before the Saint-Camille Hospital was supplied by the Central Pharmacy of the Paris Public Assistance Hospitals in Paris. At the end of June 2003, several cases of meningococcal-B meningitis were reported in the Metz-Borny district. In July, 3000 homes involving 10 000 inhabitants benefited from short-duration antibiotic prophylaxis without any problems.

Since the bioterrorist threat has become clear, France has built up a stockpile of 72 million doses of smallpox vaccine, 55 million doses of Pourquier vaccine, which are held by the military health authorities, and 17 million doses produced by the French multinational pharmaceutical firm Aventis-Pasteur. The vaccines, as well as the equipment for injection adapted for mass vaccination, are stored in two secure military sites in the north and south of France. In the United States, vaccination of military personnel against anthrax was stopped in 2000 because the American company, Bioport, which commercialized the anti-anthrax vaccine ran out of stock.

Antivirals are practically never cited in the makeup of stockpiles. However, Robert Webster and Elizabeth Walker recently stated, in regard to the fight against influenza epidemics: 'Today, faced with a pandemic, hospitals would be overwhelmed, vaccine stocks rapidly exhausted, the production of new vaccine would be too slow, and the majority of persons would remain vulnerable. Throughout the world, countries devote a tiny part of their budgets to stockpiling medications against influenza. It is the responsibility of biologists to convince governments to promote the production of vaccines and stockpiling of antivirals. For the developed countries, the cost of such programs would be tiny compared to the social and economic disaster which would occur during a pandemic on a worldwide scale.' [10]

Treatment allowing response to the health consequences of a radioactive cloud are also part of the list. The efficacy of treatment with potassium iodide tablets is maximal between 6 hours before and 3 hours following exposure. It must therefore be instituted as early as possible. The French government recently asked pharmacies in its territory to make up stockpiles of potassium iodide. In Poland, nearly 20 million tablets were distributed following the Chernobyl accident. Chelators for treatment (DTPA, BAL, Prussian Blue) should also be stockpiled.

Training response teams

In years gone by, the strategy adopted in numerous countries was based on the creation of units specializing in chemical, biological, or radiological risks. These units were generally reported in the media and placed in advance on the scene during exercises. However, this strategy was hazardous, as emphasized by Christian Sommade: 'I do not totally believe in the concept of specialized units. No matter what their role is, they respond before all to a concern of media display. In the event of a chemical incident, it will take them several hours to arrive on the scene. Given the time it takes for the specialized unit to arrive, it would always arrive too late. It is therefore necessary to train local units. In the case of a biological threat, it is the quantitative aspect and distribution over a very vast area (as a function of the incubation time and mode of attack) which necessitates the mobilization of all first aid and health personnel. Above all, training the rescuers is not sufficient. It is necessary to train the entire intervention chain, all the public and private players, both nationally and locally, who will be appealed to at times of crisis. This can seem a gigantic task, but in an operational network, it is necessary that all the links function in a mode of common understanding. If not, it will be a failure.'

In this chain of operation, Jean-François Lacronique insists, quite rightly, on medical training: 'A weakness has been clearly demonstrated which is important to correct as rapidly as possible: it is a matter of the training of physicians to recognize the illnesses generated by terrorist acts. In effect, the health system will be ... the first victim of a bioterrorist attack, and so it must be ready to raise the ... alarm, organize the medical care, and, above all, to know how to limit the consequences to a minimum, by early and precise interventions' [11].

Exercises and simulations

In the 1950s, the American Army demonstrated the feasibility of a bacteriological attack by dispersing aerosols containing *Bacillus subtilis*, a non-pathogenic bacteria, into various parts of the New York City subway and into underground passages in Washington DC. In a group of comparable studies carried out during the same time period, minesweepers of the American Navy simulated an attack on San Francisco by spraying *Bacillus globigii* and *Serratia marcescens*.

A simulation exercise of an attack with smallpox, called 'Dark Winter', was organized in June 2001 by Johns Hopkins University and the American ANSER Institute for the Department of Homeland Security. The simulated action unfolded during the winter of 2002. At the beginning of December, the clouds of aerosols spread from fake planters.

Each contaminated 1000 persons in office buildings in three large American cities. Nine days later, the US Public Health Service made the diagnosis of smallpox. The illness, disseminated by airline passengers, was found in other countries. At the beginning of February, according to the worst-case scenario, three million persons would have been infected, of whom one million died.

The 'Top Off would have' exercise, conceived in May 1999 by SAIC (Science Applications International Corporation) on behalf of the American government, studied the consequences of the dispersion of pulmonary plague (*Yersinia pestis*) in the ventilation system of the Arts Center in Denver: 950 to 2000 potential victims, would have developed the septicemic form, there would have been some thousands of ill patients, and disorganization of the local government. The Top Off 2 exercise simulated bioterrorist aggression at several points on American territory; the cost of this exercise was more than 3.5 million dollars.

A program for computerized simulation of large-scale terrorist attacks has been developed by a research group from Sadia National Laboratories. This program, called 'Weapons of Mass Destruction: Decision Analysis Center' (WMD-DAC), was conceived to simulate a bioterrorist attack, for example spraying anthrax spores above a large city. Howard Hirano, the director of the project, specified that: 'this program is interactive. That is to say that it allows one to immediately see the consequences of a decision, and one can then go back and take another option.' It is utilized in a 'war room', of which the walls have giant screens dealing with various specialties, each giving specific information to the different person responsible for public health. The responders who make the best decisions can be appointed to command posts in the event of a bioterrorist attack.

The European exercise 'Euratox', which took place in the Canjuers military camp in October 2002, envisioned two types of terrorist action: the explosion of a 'dirty bomb' in a movie theater causing 200 casualties and the dispersion of a toxic cloud by a microlight aircraft flying over a stadium involving the contamination of 2000 persons. This first European exercise, of which the cost was estimated to be 1.2 million euros, brought together 850 first responders from France and five other countries from the European Union. It demonstrated the organizational deficiencies of the response when faced with an attack involving not dozens but hundreds or thousands of persons. Christian Sommade made this analysis: 'This lack of training has notably been highlighted during the Euratox operation, the simulation of a radiological and chemical attack, which was conducted quite recently in Canjuers in the Var: the response of the medical teams, the triage of casualties etc. was universally recognized in France as highly professional. In summary, the intervention at the attack site, the management of the injured, and their decontamination have revealed some shortcomings.' Taking into account the difficulties of financing, it is unlikely that such exercises will be repeated.

Offensive and defensive research

Programs of offensive research conducted with equipment for CBRN weapons have caused numerous accidents and serious environmental contamination. Following experimentation in July 1942, the island of Gruinard was contaminated with anthrax for a half-century. It remained contaminated until a vast decontamination operation was undertaken in 1986. The release of anthrax spores from the Sverdlovsk military laboratory certainly caused deaths, as well as spores disseminated by letter in the United States (spores which might have from a military research center!). Up until 1992, the Soviets tested all their militarized infectious agents on the Island of Vosrozhdenje in the Aral Sea. Numerous cases of plague and anthrax were reported in the region. In 1972, a fishing boat was found run aground, with all its crew dead from plague. For 30 years, some inexplicable epidemics decimated the sheep and the wildlife in the region. The Aral Sea dried up and retreated, the island of Vosrozhdenje was transformed into a peninsula and should soon rejoin the mainland. The animals were then at risk for dispersing in the neighboring regions, transporting with them pathogenic, virulent, resistant, and contagious agents. It is the same with material from chemical weapons. A short time before the end of the Second World War, Panama authorized the United States to carry out studies of chemical warfare agent at three firing ranges on the island of San José, located in the Pacific Ocean. When leaving these sites, the American Army abandoned large stockpiles of chemical weapons (more than 100 000 munitions which had not been used) which have caused severe ecological degradation and will cause pollution of ground water. M. Lindsay-Poland denounced this dangerous situation for the inhabitants of the island: 'The fact that the Americans have neither dismantled these weapons which they have left on the Panamanian island of San José, in spite of declarations formulated by the local government, by the Organization for the Prohibition of Chemical Weapons (OPCW) in 2001 and 2002, constitutes on their part a violation of the International Convention on Chemical Weapons.' Panama is incapable of ensuring the financial obligation for the dismantling of the weapons and the decontamination of the site. It is estimated that just the clean-up of the 4000 contaminated hectares would cost more than 600 million dollars. All the nuclear experimentation sites in the former USSR are seriously contaminated and will be uninhabitable for many years, as well as regions of Australia which served as testing grounds for last-generation nuclear bombs during the Cold War. Numerous establishments performing CBRN offensive research have had significant failures in their safety systems. We have mentioned failures of several military biotechnology laboratories, both Russian and American, with the ability to release and spread extremely virulent pathogens. The theft of fissile materials had certainly occurred in Russia, but serious failures have also been reported in the safety system of American nuclear installations such as Rocky Flats and Los Alamos.

If offensive research constitutes a real threat to civilian populations, defensive research should be strongly encouraged, in particular to develop new treatments (medications, antidotes, vaccines) and new diagnostic tests. Once again, the determination of a country's research efforts can be determined by the amounts invested. The American authorities have decided to double the budget dedicated to basic research via the NIH (National Institutes of Health), which finances numerous university projects, over 5 years. The budgetary envelope has been increased to 27 million dollars, a sum three times greater than that of the total of public national budgets for research and development in Europe. This sum corresponds more or less to the increasing total investments of private American laboratories. Among the priorities of the NIH appear: development of a vaccine against SARS and new treatments against the bioterrorist threat. In France, the funds for functioning and investment for public research were frozen in 2003, see above [12]. Public research is suffocated and the private sector totally lacks motivation. The development of a range of medications requires considerable means which are therefore only committed by the private sector when it is assured a return on its investment. The market for the fight against bioterrorism is hypothetical. That for masculine impotence or for antidepressants is clearly real. Christian Sommade explains the reticence of the industrial firms in this manner: 'Why should the large pharmaceutical groups invest massively in medications of which the usage would only be hypothetical? Why should they spend millions in research for civil defense when, up to now, the French government itself does not make this question a priority, contrary to the United States?' Only the intervention of the government can clear up the situation because, before constituting a market, these research studies constitute a stake for national security. And as far as proof to the contrary, this question is taken over by the government. Moreover, if tomorrow a major incident should occur, there is no doubt that the population will first hold the government accountable. One can very well imagine that the professions of the exposed sectors will join together with national funds intended to finance the research. But, there again, the initiative for its creation devolves upon the government.

Information management

The National Academy of Engineering stated: 'In reality, the journalists are the first responders. Not only are they sometimes the first to arrive on the scene, but also they are the only ones to concentrate their attention on the level of risk and to be able to describe it to the public. They can save lives by the effective dissemination of pertinent information.' If it is correct that the dissemination of pertinent information can save lives, it must be strongly stated that the media often spread unconfirmed or doubtful hypotheses, coming from fake 'experts.' In the United States, the media coverage during the warnings about the anthrax illness showed that no authorization or certification was required to be qualified as an 'expert.' In the *Journalist's Guide to Covering Bioterrorism*, one can read that 'routes to sources lead to a surprising range of persons of which one can hear or read words, without concern for their experience or their education ... Incorrect information or even precise information transmitted in an exaggerated manner can weaken the best of reactions and cause unnecessary deaths, chaos, panic, and instability.' The vague description of symptoms likely to appear following a biological attack or of exaggerated stories can lead a panicked public to overwhelm the hospitals or to demand onerous and useless screening tests. All disinformation, which credits rumors propagated by instant message service and emails, is likely to set in motion a 'mass sociogenic illness', as Peter Van D. Emerson has emphasized: 'The media must not become a tool of terrorism by inadvertently disseminating incorrect information and provoking increased panic.' In an article in the *British Medical*

Journal entitled 'Worse than anthrax: the fear of anthrax', Simon Wessely, Kenneth Craig Hyams and Robert Bartholomew insist on the decisive role of public perception in such circumstances: 'These examples of mass sociogenic pathology remind us at which point it is dangerous to inadvertently exaggerate the psychological reactions to the risk of bacteriological and chemical attacks. This is notably the case when the police send, for the slightest warning, specialized groups garbed in protective suits. Or when the American government announced that it envisioned placing detectors for the identification of chemical warfare agents in the Metro tunnels in Washington.'

We have mentioned in the chapter the risks of biotechnology owing to the dissemination of scientific information which could be utilized by terrorists 'enemies of the open society.' For example, the publication of information on genetic construction could allow for the amplification of the virulence of certain pathogenic agents and the publication of the results of sequencing of a dangerous virus could lead to its synthesis in vitro. Professor Patrick Berche, Chief of the Microbiology Service of the Necker Hospital, made a declaration on this subject to the Academy of Sciences in December 2001: 'Must we not curb the dissemination of our data on the Internet, to prevent, for example, giving ideas on complex genetic constructions? I think especially about the dissemination of studies conducted on the genome of smallpox and works on the sequencing of this virus.'

The manipulation of information regarding weapons of mass destruction has recently allowed justification of a preemptive war. According to a public opinion poll conducted on June 4, 2003, by a center for opinion studies in Washington (the Program on International Policy Attitudes), four out of 10 Americans were not even aware that weapons of mass destruction had not been found. The proportion of those who approved entry into the war reached 52 per cent. The director of the Center said that 'the desire which leads a number of Americans to support the war can lead them to ignore information on the absence of weapons.' One-fifth of those polled even had the 'impression' that Iraq had used its chemical and biological weapons during the conflict! Moreover, the threat of CBRN weapons being aimed at the West aided the military-industrial complex and its desire to produce GNR (genetic engineering, nanotechnologies, robotics) technologies. This, as well as the political maneuverings to encourage and legitimize massive investments into this sector, has served the military-industrial complex's aim to achieve military and economic superiority [13, 14]. In March 2002, at the Massachusetts Institute of Technology, the American Army created an Institute for Military Nanotechnology in association with the weapons manufacturer Raytheon. In April 2000, the cofounder and Director of Development of Sun Microsystems, Bill Joy, published in the American trade journal *Wired* an article entitled 'Why the future doesn't need us' [15]. In this article, dedicated to the dangers of new technologies, Bill Joy repeated in his account certain arguments of Théodore Kaczynski [16] as an appeal to stop the development of GNR technologies.

During an interview with Zac Goldsmith, Bill Joy confirmed the reality of this threat: 'the destructive power of these new technologies will easily be greater than that of an atomic bomb. ... The most irresistible technologies of the 21st century carry the awesome threat of a nature basically different from that of previous technologies. ... [R]obots, genetically modified organisms, and nanorobots are united by a common fearsome … factor: they have the capacity to reproduce themselves. A bomb can only explode once; a robot, on the other hand, can multiply itself and rapidly escape all control' [17].

In France, Jean-Pierre Dupuy, Professor at Stanford University and at the École Polytechnique, member of the General Council for Mines and a specialist in nuclear deterrence, has asked for the creation of a mission charged with the evaluation of the impact of nanotechnologies [9], and gave this warning: 'The continent to explore, here, is immense and of great complexity: it is the disruptions that the development of nano-technologies carries in the conception of weapons …. In does not require hiding that gigantic sums are today swallowed up in research already constituting a new chapter in the course of weapons. This course has already begun very strongly, and no one can see how it can be regulated, much less stopped. … [W]eapons based on nanotechnologies will be weapons of mass destruction on a scale that nuclear, chemical, and biological weapons could never pretend to attain. … Contrary to NBC weapons, weapons based on nanotechnologies will be very easily accessible to small powers or terrorist groups when the techniques are widespread, present in all sectors of economic and social life. … The dissemination therefore will be the internet database. Weapons based on nano-technologies render inoperative the logic of deterrence, and the 'equilibrium of terror' will simply be totally unthinkable' [18].

References

1. Khan AS, Morse S, Lillibridge S. Public-health preparedness for biological terrorism in the USA. *The Lancet*, 2000; **356**: 1179–1182.
2. Simon J. Biological terrorism: preparing to meet the threat. *Journal of the American Medical Association*, 1997; **278**: 428–430.
3. Tucker J. National health and medical services response to incidents of chemical and biological terrorism. *Journal of the American Medical Association*, 1997; **278**: 362–368.
4. Propos du professeur Henri Mollaret, recueillis par Jean-Yves Nau. *Le Monde*, octobre 16, 2001: 20.
5. Barriot P, Chevalier P. Protection des populations civiles contre les gaz de combat. *Journal Europén des Urgences*, 1991; **4**: 5–19.
6. Barriot P, Chevalier P, Pitti R. Intoxications aiguës collectives par inhalation de toxiques indus-triels et de gaz de combat. In: V Danel, P Barriot (eds), *Intoxications Aiguës en Reanimation*, Paris, Arnette, 1993: 203–220.
7. Saviuc P, Danel V. Les antidotes. In: V Danel, P Barriot. Intoxications aiguës en réanimation, 2ᵉ édition, Paris éditions Arnette, 1999: 89–96.
8. Baud FJ, Barriot P, Riou B. *Les Antidotes*. Paris, Masson, 1991.
9. Dupuy JP. Le risqué inouï des nanotechnologies: l'écophagie. *L'Écologiste* (édition française de *The Ecologist*), 2003; **2**: 70–72.
10. Webster R, Walker E. La grippe. Pour la science (édition française de *Scientific American*), 2003; **307**: 30–33.
11. Lacronique JF. Sous la menace bioterroriste. *Libération*, mars 28, 2003: 16.
12. Papon P. 2003, l'année terrible… *Pour la Science* (édition française de *Scientific American*) 2003; **307**: 34–37.
13. L'Amérique a fait de la recherche une machine de guerre. *Le Monde*, mars 19, 2003: 26.

14. L'offensive sans précédent de l'industrie de l'armement américaine. *Le Monde* mars 19, 2003: 21.

15. Joy B. Why the future doesn't need us. *Wired,* San Francisco, avril 2000.

16. Kaczynski T. *La Société Industrielle et Son Avenir*. Paris, Éditions de l'Éncyclopédie des Nuisances, 1998.

17. Un génie de l'informatique sonne l'alarme (interview de Bill Joy par Zac Goldsmith), *L'Écologiste* (édition française de *The Ecologist*), 2001; **3**: 44–46.

18. Dupuy JP. *Pour un Catastrophisme Éclairé*. Paris, Éditions de Seuil, 2002.

Postscript

According to Heraclites, "conflict is the father of all things". The Bible recounts how Cain, who murdered his brother, built the first city and how his descendents invented the forge and music. Since the beginning of time, in all parts of the world, the most respected man in the city has always been the victorious warrior: "*Ritorna vincitor*" (return victorious) sings Amneris in Aïda, during the *Vae Victis* (misfortune to the defeated) of Brennus who threw his Gaulish sword into the Roman balance; it is David and not Goliath who writes history. The Noble Savage conceived in the imagination of Jean-Jacques Rousseau never existed: *homo hominis lupus*, man is a carnivorous animal that has war in his blood. And, if he comes to exorcise his warlike instincts in placing them at the service of a Prince, a cause, or a religion, in the end the question remains the same: I kill my neighbor because he displeases me, or because I covet his fields, his sheep, his wife, but above all because it is in my nature to kill. The condemnation of war, a priori, is one of taking a modern, sentimental, utopian position, and it is not ours to judge if it is the fruit of an excessive outgrowth of Christianity or the outcome of a civilization entering into decline. For whatever reason, war, approved or disapproved, seems inseparable from the human condition.

Public crowds, who believe themselves to be peaceful, that attend military parades seem even to indicate that approval gets the better of disapproval; likewise, the ever-present popularity of Napoleon who left France impoverished, diminished, bled-to-death, who enslaved the French for his purposes, who destroyed the French economy by abolishing the birthright, did however created a flattering warrior myth for the French.

Here, a paradox: although war would seemingly be the least moral of human activities – I am stronger than you, therefore I will devour you – it has, on the contrary, been governed by more or less scrupulously enforced rules; sometimes arising from the forces face-to-face, sometimes imposed by an external authority. The Truce of God, the code of chivalry, respect for prisoners, the Geneva Convention, the International Court of Justice (World Court) in the Hague, it is all one: the desire to curb that which by definition is the negation of curbs.

However, in the 21st century, we have come into a world where the existence of God is doubted, the Church ridiculed, the aristocracies destroyed, the codes ignored, the charters violated, and the international conventions exploited solely when they can serve the strongest of the belligerents. Here is one of the highest benefits (and the most certain) of "Democracy", but it finds in itself a moral nihilism – that the pseudo-Rights of Man are proven to be powerless to limit in the slightest, when accompanied by scientific progress that places within the reach of man not only the elimination of his rival in love, or the purging of his neighbor who owns more cattle,

Treating Victims of Mass Destruction   by Patrick Barriot and Chantal Bismuth
© 2008 John Wiley & Sons, Ltd

or the conquest of a neighboring province, or domination exercised over such-and-such a portion of territory, but a worldwide hegemony, an absolute colonialism and the destruction of anyone who dares oppose the designs of those who possess weapons of mass destruction.

This is the scientific and medical problem addressed by Doctors Bismuth and Barriot. It is true that, as they have shown, the proportion of non-participating parties who are nevertheless victims has always been increasing, whether temporary superiority is found in the hands of dominant forces, bombing Belgrade or Baghdad, or whether it is found in the hands of terrorist forces, destroying the World Trade Center.

It is true that an attack, from a flint weapon, to a knife, to a sword, to a bow, to a musket, to a canon, to an atom bomb, to a thermonuclear device, to a variola virus, duly allows the forces of good or evil to destroy retreats to make progress, and that the virtues of true warriors – courage, camaraderie, sacrifice, responsibility, transcending oneself – no longer seem to have any connection with warfare that is possible with modern methods: bombing done from an altitude of 10,000 meters with an ideal of 0 deaths on one side and 100% deaths on the other.

It is also true, and it here where I have devoted my studies into the techniques of disinformation that may throw the light-of-day onto weapons of mass destruction – that these weapons, whether they are nuclear, biological, or chemical, or even traditional, have no true interest for being employed in future "fall-outs" – I do not wish to speak of radioactive materials, but "informational", if one will allow me this neologism. Dresden: it was not 35,000 German civilians burned alive; it was bringing Germany to it knees. Hiroshima: it was not 157,071 Japanese irradiated; it was putting Japan on the carpet. From the explosion of the bomb(s) to the capitulation of the adversary, there was a shifting effect which can only be explained by media coverage, more and more manipulating, more and more able to be manipulated, and thus the development of such tactics seems to be without limits. There is, in our times, a peculiarly apocalyptic convergence of the means that science delivers to Man to kill men and the means that it delivers to the killer for informing the world how many he has already killed and how many he can still kill – all that, of course, in the service of humanity. Gilgamesh and Joshua only had some heroes on one side and some heralds on the other: we have CBRN weapons and the internet.

Here, moreover, a new theme enters into play: that of "dirty weapons". The dagger in the time of the sword; gunpowder in the time of the saber; the explosive artillery shell in the time of the cannonball; war gases in the time of the machine gun... And, in this perspective, the usage of a repugnant weapon can backfire. In modern conflicts, the first who says to the other "you utilize dirty weapons" is already winning in public opinion, even if he himself is employing them on a daily basis and when the other does not have the means to dream of their possession.

Being neither a scientist nor a politician, I ignore whatever conclusions they can bring to the work presented here. I have, for my part, the temptation of yearning for the era of the blacksmith who forged as he was able, the shaman who treated as he was able, and of the nobleman who ruled as he was able; the techniques of the one, the science of the other, and the authority of the third were closely limited by the methods of cottage-industry craftsmanship. However, in these early years of a century already badly begun with more and more frequent aggressions, perpetrated more frequently by the powerful against the weak, a century which teeters on the verge of world domination where anything at all would be allowed to the absolute master, without there being the slightest recourse against him, neither force nor rights, it seems important to precisely define three factors:

- modern scientific methods, in particular in the realms of biochemistry and miniaturization, are such that the powerful are not assured of remaining powerful indefinitely, nor the weak, weak;
- these scientific methods are systematically placed in the service of political causes presented as the only "good", the annihilation of the adversary is from then on considered to be desirable, certain and moral (unlike in past centuries where potentates desired the submission and not the destruction of their adversaries);
- some techniques of media coverage are exactly to this point; allowing dissemination to one and all that force and right are necessarily on the same side.

Before treating an illness, supposing that this is possible, it is necessary to make the diagnosis. Thanks to the authors for bringing their diagnosis to our attention, however disturbing it is…

Vladimir Volkoff
International Peace Prize, 1989

Appendix: Questions and answers

Patrick Barriot

Question 1: You have mentioned the constraints placed on resuscitation with oxygen on site in the event of a chemical disaster. What types of equipment can reduce these constraints?

In the decontamination zone, the provision of oxygen is limited by the number of bottles which can be transported by the responders. The size D bottles used by the majority of the emergency services contain 340 liters of compressed oxygen. Steel bottles can be replaced with lighter aluminum or Kevlar bottles, which allow one to increase the oxygen pressure. The fire services are equipped with size J bottles. In the cold zone, oxygen can be stocked in liquid or solid form. Certain ventilators can be powered by compressed oxygen, but also by filtered ambient air. The 'CompPac' respirator functions with filtered air which is compressed by a battery-powered compressor. It is possible to ventilate a patient with air enriched with oxygen (FiO_2 50 per cent). The stand-alone capabilities of this type of ventilator varies according to the FiO_2 looked for, but it is much greater than that of portable ventilators functioning by means of a compressed oxygen bottle.

Question 2: Which antidote should be stockpiled for mass casualty poisoning with cyanide?

We have seen that two principal antidotes exist: dicobalt EDTA (Kelocyanor® from SERB Laboratories) and hydroxocabalamin (Cyanokit® from Lipha Santé Laboratories). Dicobalt EDTA exposes patients to the risk of adverse effects and there is no pediatric form, but its price is moderate, which is a good thing when it comes to making up stockpiles that may never be used. Hydroxocabalamin has no adverse effects, but its higher cost cannot be ignored. It therefore seems reasonable to stockpile these two antidotes in order to find the best cost/efficacy compromise.

Question 3: A recent publication mentioned the necessity of increasing the dosing schedule of the antiviral Tamiflu® when it is prescribed for curative treatment. Some other publications have reported the appearance of viral resistances and disturbing adverse effects. What does all of this mean?

The use of Tamiflu as a curative treatment has reduced the mortality of patients infected by the H5N1 avian influenza virus by 30 per cent. However, a recent study

Treating Victims of Mass Destsuction   Edited by Patrick Barriot and Chantal Bismuth
© 2008 John Wiley & Sons, Ltd

from the consultation committee on human influenza of the WHO, published in the *New England Journal of Medicine*, suggested that the doses of the antiviral necessary for treating the severe influenzal syndromes caused by this virus should be multiplied by two. In this manner, it should not be 150 mg of Tamiflu per day to treat an adult but rather 300 mg. If one believes this study, the stockpiles should thus be reviewed and increased. It must be understood that a daily dosing schedule of 300 mg does not correspond to the recommendations of the French Marketing Authority for Tamiflu. The prescription of a high dose of Tamiflu requires temporary authorization for utilization.

Regarding resistance to antiviral medications, the work of Richard Bright's group from the Centers for Disease Control and Prevention (CDC) in Atlanta has shown an increase in resistant viruses over the last 10 years. The mutations of the viral genome, above all, appear to be resistant to an older family of antivirals, such as amantadine and ranitidine, with more than 10 per cent of viruses resistant. The case of resistance to medications belonging to the recent family of 'neuraminidase inhibitors' (Tamiflu and Relenza) remains limited because viral neuraminidase does not readily undergo genetic mutations. It would be in the order of 0.4 per cent in adults and from four to 18 per cent in children. Resistance has been mainly detected in Japan. It is necessary to understand that Japan is the largest consumer of Tamiflu, with 20 million doses prescribed in 2004. The prescription of the medication from dozens to hundreds of millions of persons inevitably sets in motion an important increase in resistance. Some cases of resistance to Tamiflu have been observed in a virus that is still sensitive to Relenza. For this reason, it seems prudent to simultaneously stockpile these two antivirals.

Concerning the adverse effects imputed to Tamiflu, particularly behavioral alterations and hallucinations, one should be extremely careful. Some fatal accidents have been reported in Japan in adolescents being treated with Tamiflu. Two adolescents presented 'abnormal behavior': a 17-year-old high-school student threw himself under a truck and a boy fell from the ninth floor of his apartment building. However, as of today, investigation has not allowed the establishment of a cause-and-effect relationship between taking Tamiflu and fatal accidents in a country where 20 million doses of this antiviral medication were prescribed in 2004.

Question 4: Do we have an idea of the funds allocated to the antiterrorist effort, in particular for CBRN materials, and the manner in which they are allocated?

It is difficult to respond to this question as concerns France. In the United States, the Independent Congressional Investigation Commission on the September 11, 2001 attacks released its last report on the response of the government to recommendations made 16 months earlier on December 5, 2005. The President of the Commission, considering that the United States was always vulnerable to an attack stated: "More than 4 years after September 11, we are not as secure as we should be. This is unacceptable. Many things essential to preventing a new September 11 have simply not been done, neither by the President nor by the Congress." The Vice-President of the Commission, on his part, predicted that a new attack could occur, considering that "the nation is not well prepared. " This report denounces, amongst other things, a poor utilization of funds intended for the antiterrorist battle. In this fashion, one city used these funds to install air conditioners in garbage collection trucks, another to buy bullet-proof vests for its police dogs! Strong statements of recommendations by the competent authorities are frequently disregarded. We have a duty to take the example of the United States and demand an independent commission to evaluate the relationship between the recommendation of the health authorities and the use of public funds for each sector of the antiterrorist struggle, in particular that which concerns the CBRN threat.

Question 5: Are ethical problems taken into account in a general fashion in response plans and more particularly in the management of stockpiles?

It is a crucial question because the stability of institutions and social cohesion depend on it. A group of Canadian researchers at the Center for Bioethics at the University of Toronto has pointed out the national plans for the fight against a future influenza pandemic should imperatively integrate an ethical dimension, which currently is sorely lacking. During the SARS epidemic in 2003, an ethical problem was raised in France regarding the mandatory hospitalization for contagious illnesses. The Minister of Health, Jean-François Mattei, announced on April 22, 2003, the publication of a decree permitting the mandatory hospitalization of patients afflicted with contagious disease, on order of the Prefect and in perfectly defined exceptional emergency situations. Professor Didier Sicärd, President of the National Consultative Committee for Ethics, stated in the daily newspaper *Le Monde* on May 16, 2003: 'The circumstances of the transmission of the coronavirus are, however, well identified; physicians have died from contact with patients afflicted with acute pulmonary infection; rigorous isolation measures must be taken, even by constraint, in anticipation of a suspected case.' Placing in preventive quarantine, by the Armed Forces, of 'populations at risk' of many thousands of persons, poses a very serious problem.

Another ethical problem concerns the management of stockpiles in the event of a pandemic, more precisely the distribution of expensive antivirals stockpiled in Western countries. Who are the priority beneficiaries of the distribution of Tamiflu and Relenza? Persons who have already contracted the infection or, as a preventive measure, government workers useful for the effective functioning of the group? It is a matter of one question among many others. The Canadian researchers from the Center for Bioethics at the University of Toronto considered that measures which appeared to be 'fair and equitable' should be publicly discussed and clearly disseminated.

Question 6: The exclusivity of the patent on Tamiflu: can it oppose the importation of a generic medication to poorer countries?

The agreement on the aspects of the intellectual property rights regarding commerce (TRIPS) signed on April 15, 1994, and which came into force at the beginning of 2005, prohibits the production of generic copies of recently developes medications. In the event of a health emergency, it is theoretically possible to depart from the rules of the

TRIPS agreement and to suspend the patent exclusivity in order to manufacture generic medications (paying royalties of five per cent). An accord signed in 2003 with the WHO should allow the importation of generic medications into poor countries which do not have pharmaceutical industrial capacity. In reality, this accord has never been truly applied and each year 11 million persons die of infectious diseases because of the lack of access to essential medications. We note that in October 2001, after the bioterrorist episode with letters contaminated with anthrax spores, the American government evoked this suspension of patent of the German laboratory Bayer for ciprofloxacin, an efficacious antibiotic, judged to be too expensive by Washington.

Question 7: You have not mentioned the problems of potable water supplies and decontamination of water in the event of a chemical disaster such as that, for example, which occurred recently in China.

An accidental explosion in a petrochemical complex in the north of China, on November 13, 2005, spilled tens of thousands of tons of benzene into the Songhua River. This river, which flows into the Amur River, supplies potable water to millions of persons downstream, from the Chinese city of Harbin to the Russian city of Khabarovsk. The layer of benzene which came from China affected Siberia and polluted the waters of the Amur River. In eastern Siberia alone, one million persons found themselves in the contaminated zone. A newspaper in Moscow described the situation in these terms: 'Since several days ago, the people have made do with stocks of bottled water, still or sparkling, fruit juice, milk, beer and other drinks. The inhabitants of apartment buildings grouped together to get tank trucks and buy water wholesale. The refugees took to assaulting the suburban buses in order to reach wells in the outlying villages where they stretched out in long queues. In deciding to limit access to water points and to guard the wells night and day by armed police, the responsible authorities provoked a groundswell of indignation. André Tchirkin, head of the representation of the Khabarovsk region to Moscow, explained that the water points had become strategic.' Certain persons even used water from heating circuits for drinking or cooking. The pollution probably lasted all winter and, in the spring, thawing resulted in release of toxicants trapped in the snow. To the drinking water contamination was added contamination of fish from streams and rivers. Faced with situations of this type, it is crucial to have available a number of filtration systems for toxicants in suspension as well as dissolved toxicants, in particular filtration devices based on the principle of reverse osmosis.

Index

Treating Victims of Mass Destruction   Edited by Patrick Barriot and Chantal Bismuth
© 2008 John Wiley & Sons, Ltd